Urologic Pathology: The Prostate

Urologic Pathology: The Prostate

MYRON TANNENBAUM, M.D., Ph.D.

Departments of Pathology and Urology
Columbia-Presbyterian Medical Center
New York, New York

Lea & Febiger • 1977 • Philadelphia

616.994
U 78

Library of Congress Cataloging in Publication Data

Main entry under title:

Urologic pathology.

   Includes index.
   1.   Prostate gland—Cancer.   I. Tannenbaum, Myron.
[DNLM: 1.   Prostatic neoplasms.   WJ752 U73]
RC280.P7U76   616.9′94′63   76-5466
ISBN 0-8121-0546-X

Printed in Great Britain by Henry Kimpton Publishers, London

PRINTED IN THE UNITED STATES OF AMERICA

Print number: 3   2   1

To my wife Sheila Carol

PREFACE

I would like to quote portions of a letter that I received from one of my colleagues, a surgical pathologist at Rochester General Hospital: "A lot of times, or at least it seems to me that way, when we have seen borderline lesions in the prostate, we usually pass the slides around to all of our pathologists before we come up with an answer that reassures us all. I don't know whether it is the lack of fine morphology or just the inexperiences of picking up early lesions, but I certainly personally do not feel as confident about making a diagnosis in urologic pathology, especially with prostate, as I would about cervical, endometrial, or breast lesions." Not only has this idea been expressed by many other pathologists throughout the country but I have especially encountered it during my last ten years of teaching.

Urologic Pathology: The Prostate was conceived with the expectation of bridging the communication gap that currently exists between the general practitioner of urology and the surgical pathologist. It is also hoped that those in various disciplines such as biochemistry, radiology, and other basic sciences interested in diseases of the genitourinary system, especially the prostate, will find some illuminating and rewarding information in at least one of the chapters. Perusal of the table of contents demonstrates that the authors—experts in their respective fields—have addressed themselves to numerous themes that are pertinent to prostatic diseases. Special emphasis has been placed on issues that are of utmost importance to both the basic researcher and the clinician in order that the disease problems relating to tumor and infection may be better understood. Although this approach may inevitably be accompanied by some overlapping, the chapters were chosen because they would be of practical help to the urologist whether he is in the operating room or reviewing the slides together with the pathologist. Consequently, this text not only provides information regarding the history and epidemiology of prostatic disease but also presents diagrams that will show the pathologist in what manner the urologist approaches the surgery of the prostate gland.

My interpretation of the problems of prostatic disease, as well as the editorializing in this book, is based on a 15-year personal experience and the accumulative teaching from my mentors in surgical pathology. They include the late Dr. Arthur Purdy Stout, Dr. Raffaele Lattes, and Dr. Meyer M. Melicow. Even though I am the editor, *Urologic Pathology: The Prostate* represents the cooperative efforts of numerous other people. They not only have contributed to what I know will bring new understanding and insight to the readers but also have made many suggestions about the format of the chapters. I also want to thank my many other colleagues from various parts of the country whose loyal and enthusiastic support have made this effort possible. In addition, my gratitude is due to those people who have supported the contributing authors and especially to my secretary, Mrs. Edith Crespi. To Dr. John K. Lattimer, I wish to express my indebtedness for liberally supplying both space and clinical material from which numerous photomicrographs were taken. His contribution is represented by the atlas at the end of this volume. Likewise I wish to express my appreciation to my wife, Sheila, to whom I am greatly indebted, not only for her practical help with the chapters, but for her deep understanding which has sustained me during the writing and editing of this book. To my publishers, Lea & Febiger, I wish to impart my gratefulness for their encouragement, cooperation, and persistence in guiding me through this effort.

New York

Myron Tannenbaum

CONTRIBUTORS

Richard J. Ablin, Ph.D.
Associate Professor
Department of Microbiology
University of Health Sciences
The Chicago Medical School
Chicago, Illinois

John G. Batsakis, M.D.
Professor of Pathology
Department of Pathology
The University of Michigan Medical School
Ann Arbor, Michigan

David Brandes, M.D.
Associate Chief, Pathology
Baltimore City Hospitals
The Johns Hopkins School of Medicine
Baltimore, Maryland

Irving M. Bush, M.D.
Professor and Chairman
Divisions and Departments of Urology
The Chicago Medical School and
Cook County Institutions
Chicago, Illinois

Ronnie Beth Bush, Ph.D.
Department of History and Philosophy of Medicine
The Chicago Medical School and
Cook County Institutions
Chicago, Illinois

David P. Byar, M.D.
Head, Clinical and Diagnostic
Trials Section, Biometry Branch
National Cancer Institute
Bethesda, Maryland

John G. Connolly, M.D.
Chief, Division of Urology
Women's College Hospital
Toronto, Ontario, Canada

George W. Drach, M.D.
Associate Professor of Urology
University of Arizona Medical Center
Tucson, Arizona

L. M. Franks, M.D.
Head, Department of Cellular Pathology
Imperial Cancer Research Fund Laboratories
Lincoln's Inn Fields
London, WC2A PX, England

Donald F. Gleason, M.D., Ph.D.
Chief, Anatomic Pathology
Veterans Administration Hospital
Associate Professor
Department of Laboratory Medicine and Pathology
University of Minnesota
Minneapolis, Minnesota

Erol O. Gursel, M.D.
Department of Urology
Columbia-Presbyterian Medical Center
New York, New York

Clarence V. Hodges, M.D.
Professor of Surgery/Urology
Head, Division of Urology
University of Oregon Health Sciences Center
Portland, Oregon

Dieter Kirchheim, M.D.
Department of Urology
University of Washington Medical School
Seattle, Washington

Paul W. Kohnen, M.D.
Section of Urology
Department of Surgery and
Department of Pathology
University of Arizona Medical Center
Tucson, Arizona

Ilse Lasnitzki, M.D., Ph.D., Sc.D.
Sir Halley Stewart Fellow
Fellow of Lucy Cavendish College
Cambridge University
Cambridge, CB1 4RN, England

Maguid R. Megalli, M.D.
Department of Urology
Columbia-Presbyterian Medical Center
New York, New York

C. W. Moncure, M.D.
University of Virginia Medical School
Richmond, Virginia

Gerald P. Murphy, M.D., D.Sc.
Institute Director
Roswell Park Memorial Institute
New York State Department of Health
State University of New York at Buffalo
Buffalo, New York

George R. Prout, Jr., M.D.
Chief of the Urological Service
Massachusetts General Hospital
Professor of Surgery
Harvard Medical School
Boston, Massachusetts

W. D. Rider, M.B.
Director, Radiation Oncology
The Princess Margaret Hospital
Toronto, Ontario, Canada

Myron S. Roberts, M.D.
Associate Clinical Professor of Urology
Department of Urology
Columbia-Presbyterian Medical Center
New York, New York

Thomas M. Sodeman, M.D.
Professor of Pathology and Microbiology
Director of Clinical Laboratory
West Virginia Medical School
Morgantown, West Virginia

Myron Tannenbaum, M.D., Ph.D.
Associate Professor of Pathology
Division of Surgical Pathology,
Department of Pathology and
Department of Urology
Columbia-Presbyterian Medical Center
New York, New York

Ralph V. Veenema, M.D.
Professor of Clinical Urology
Department of Urology
Columbia-Presbyterian Medical Center
New York, New York

CONTENTS

PART III MANAGEMENT OF PROSTATIC DISEASE

PART IV SURGICAL PATHOLOGY OF THE PROSTATE

Part I

Introduction

Chapter 1

Prostatic Cancer

CLARENCE V. HODGES

Prostatic cancer continues to be the malignant disease seen most frequently by urologists. Approximately 17,000 men die of prostatic cancer every year, but perhaps 10 times this number would show prostatic cancer histologically at any given time, Many of the statistical peculiarities related to prostatic cancer may be alluded to in the following chapters, such as its greater incidence among Negroes, its lesser incidence among Orientals when they live in their native countries but rising to equal that of Caucasians when they live in a Caucasian environment, the poorly validated suggestion that prostatic cancer occurs more in males who begin sexual activity early and practice it more often than the usual pattern, and the fascinating hints that a viral cause may link it with cervical cancer.

An early 20th century clinician said "Whatever you do for prostatic cancer is bound to be wrong." Except for increased urologic skills in removing or bypassing tumor-caused obstruction, this situation remained true until 1941 when Huggins and his group at the University of Chicago culminated a long series of animal experiments and a study of hormonally treated human patients with the announcement that prostatic cancer, being a growth of adult epithelial cells, behaved similarly in the dog prostate and could be *inhibited* by castration or administration of estrogens or *stimulated* by androgens such as testosterone.

To someone as privileged as I was to watch a succession of seeming miracles in hitherto incurable patients, it seemed that the millennium had indeed come! Patients were eased of their bone-racking pain, regained their appetites and reentered the human race. Paraplegics walked again, decubiti were healed, solid muscles replaced atrophic ones, and tumor-laden bone marrows became normal. It heralded not only the birth of hormonal therapy for prostatic and, subsequently, breast and uterine cancer, but chemotherapy of all tumors as well. One might well have waxed poetic over man's conquest of cancer.

It soon became apparent, however, that the conquest was only a temporary cease-fire, or at best an armistice. About 80% of the patients responded initially to hormonal therapy by either orchiectomy or estrogen administration but, within a year, about 80% of them showed exacerbation of their disease, which was no longer

3

amenable to the previously effective measures. Sadly, there has been no *fundamental* improvement in the control of prostatic cancer since that time. Cooperative groups have labored mightily but ultimately have only redocumented this statement. "Cadres" and "Task Forces" have made sorties and forays against outcroppings and pockets of enemy tumor, elimination or temporary suppression of which will then be recounted with an impressive display of statistics, but when the dust has settled, no one can claim real progress. Whether we explain this failure to control tumor by either the loss of androgen dependence by tumor cells or the persistence of clones of cells that never were dependent on androgen stimulation or to varying hormonal levels or ratios between hormone levels, 34 years have demonstrated that the old enemy is still there, implacable and irresistible. The rare patient who survives for 10 to 15 years after responding to administration of hormonal therapy only points up the extent of our frustration; for an answer is surely there if we could find it. Basic scientists and clinicians will, in the succeeding chapters, attempt to document pertinent problem areas and suggested solutions.

One of the main thrusts of this monograph is to bridge the gaps that lie between the clinician and the pathologist. As one who has always believed that the study of all clinical disease must rest on pathology, that every good urologist personally evaluates his patient's pathologic tissues whenever possible, and who has for years maintained in his training program a four-month rotation of the urology resident through pathology, it is a welcome task to introduce the hope that finer communications can be made to prevail between the disciplines of basic science and clinical medicine.

PROBLEMS OF MUTUAL CONCERN

What problems are there that share the common interest of the two disciplines?

Perhaps the most basic is that of determining whether malignancy exists. Fortunate is the urologic surgeon who has absolute trust and confidence in his pathologist, so that when the answer is "yes" or "no" on the basis of frozen section biopsy, the dichotomy is securely resolved. The answer of "maybe," or the reversal of position after further examination or consultation, or both shakes the urologist and is absolutely heartrending to patient and family. It is particularly important for the urologist to review with his pathologist all slides accompanying the patient from an "outside" source.

One would hope most sincerely that pathologists, as time goes on, will gain more expertise in evaluating the biologic potential of malignant cells. As already stated, only about one in 10 histologic cancers become clinical cancers, but which ones are they? We have become accustomed to thinking that stage A (or I) carcinoma does not represent a clinical threat and we are currently advised by statisticians that such patients need no treatment. However, it is sobering to recognize that all carcinomas must have been at this stage at some interval and it is frightening to find that an occasional patient who certainly fell in this category initially has suddenly joined the clinically significant and perhaps already incurable group.

We should be most appreciative if pathologists could tell us from their study of the cells in the biopsy specimen whether the tumor is likely to have already metastasized. Urologists employ many imperfect clinical studies such as digital rectal palpation of the primary lesion, cystoscopy, serum and bone marrow acid phosphatase, bone surveys and scans, lymphangiography, and surgical staging; could pathologists, by more sophisticated grading of tumors, improve and shorten the staging procedure?

We should like the pathologist to tell us after his examination of the tumor cell whether—and which type of—hormonal therapy would influence tumor growth and spread and whether radiation therapy might be reasonably considered.

We should particularly like them to study the occasional patient whose metastases disappear with either short- or long-term hormonal therapy and who lives for years in apparently perfect symbiosis with his tumor, for he embodies the goal toward which we strive.

Our hope in 1977 is that by the year 2000, or even perhaps by the next decade, communication between urologists and pathologists will lead to another great leap forward similar to the one that occurred in 1941.

Chapter 2

Early Developments in the History of Prostatic Disorders

RONNIE BETH BUSH and IRVING M. BUSH

The history of prostatic diseases is a fascinating story in the development of medical thought and knowledge. Spanning three thousand years, it highlights man's search to cure himself of the ills bestowed upon him by nature (old age, e.g.,) and by other human beings (venereal disease).

Early investigators did not have a clear concept of the prostate's anatomy and function. It is easy to understand their difficulties. In man the prostate is not readily visualized on peritoneal examination. In mammals its configuration and structure vary, but the afflictions in which the prostate is involved appear ageless. The agony that they have caused over the centuries could not be ignored and as a result, "physicians" from the beginning of written history have been involved in the analysis and treatment of many of the clinical entities that we see and treat today.

There have been several good general reviews of the history of prostatic disease to which the reader is referred.[1-6] In this chapter we should like to highlight some aspects of the story that are not well known or that seem to deserve emphasis.

MAGICAL AND DEVOUT MEDICINE

In the Mesopotamian society that inhabited the "fertile crescent" between 3400 and 1200 B.C., there were two groups charged with medical care: the *asu* (physicians) and the *asipu* (magical experts). In the oft-broken tablets that record their medical prescriptions, many references to venereal disease and several references to possible prostatic disorders have been identified:

"[. . .] day and night he cannot sleep [. . .] (. . .) this man has choking of the bladder [. . .]."

(asutu)

"If a man stands up to urinate too often, in wine or beer he shall drink (. . .) (drugs)."

(asutu)

"If his urine is repeatedly blocked off, he dies."

(asiputu)

"If a man (is) urinating water and it is very little but he stands up (to urinate) too often, his bladder is contracted."

(asutu)

"If a man: in his sleep (?) (or) in his walking has seminal discharge and he does not know that he went to his wife and his penis and his 'cloth' are full of seminal fluid, (. . .) he will recover."

(asutu)

"When he walks his semen flows out without his knowing it as if he had gone into a woman (. . .)."

(asutu)[7]

In the Bible there are several references to diseases of the genitourinary system (fertility, venereal-like disease, bladder stone, penile trauma, cryptorchidism) but not to any disorders related specifically to the prostate. In the Midrash (commentaries on the old testament written after 400 B.C.), there may be a reference to urinary obstruction owing to prostatic enlargement. It states that "old men have to strain to pass their water and . . . occasionally [need to] defaecate before they can urinate."[8] This may also reflect an awareness of the association between urinary obstruction and constipation. In any event the Midrash indicates that there was a great fear of urinary retention, and the "people were advised to urinate at the first urge since any delay might lead to retention and swelling of the abdomen."[8]

CLASSICAL WISDOM

Although human anatomical studies were not being practiced in the Asklepieion of Cos, Hippocrates or the writers of the Hippocratic tracts knew of the symptom complexes caused by narrowing of the bladder neck:

"Those whose bowels are loose and healthy, whose bladder is not feverish, and the mouth of whose bladder is not over narrow, pass water easily, and no solid matter forms in their bladder. But feverishness of the bowels must be accompanied by feverishness of the bladder. For when it is abnormally heated its mouth is inflamed. In this condition it does not expel the urine, but concocts and heats it within itself. The finest part is separated off, and the clearest passes out as urine, while the thickest and muddiest part forms solid matter, which, though at first small, grows in course of time. For as it rolls about in the urine it coalesces with whatever solid matter forms, and so it grows and hardens."[9]

He also observed that older men suffered from difficult urination and stranguria:

"Old men suffer from difficulty of breathing, catarrh accompanied by coughing, strangury, difficult micturition, pains at the joints, kidney disease. . . ."[10]

Hippocrates described several conditions associated with strangury which may have had a prostatic etiology:

"When the urine is thick, full of clots, and scanty, fever being present, a copious discharge of (comparatively) thin urine coming afterwards gives relief. This usually happens in the case of those whose urine contains a sediment from the onset or shortly after it."[10]

"When there are swelling and rumbling in the hypochondria, should pain in the loins supervene, the bowels become watery, unless there be breaking of wind or a copious discharge of urine. These symptoms occur in fevers."[10]

"If there be blood and clots in the urine, and strangury be present, should pain attack the hypogastrium and the perineum, the parts about the bladder are affected."[10]

"When tumours form in the urethra, should these suppurate and burst, there is relief."[10]

"Those who, after strangury, are attacked by ileus, die in seven days, unless fever supervenes and there is an abundant flow of urine."[10]

"When a patient passes in the urine blood and clots, suffers strangury and is seized with pain in the perineum and pubes, it indicates disease in the region of the bladder."[10]

Hippocrates discerned a difference in patient's suffering from dysuria owing to stone and those who suffered from a tumor about the bladder (prostate?). In the former the patient might adopt a position in which the stone would not obstruct the urethra "while the latter patient would suffer no matter what attitude be assumed."[12]

Aulus Cornelius Celsus was born about the year 25 B.C. Very little is known about his life except that he was acquainted with the poems of Ovid and that he was probably the editor of a general encyclopedia which, besides *De Medicina*, included treatises on agriculture, military arts, rhetoric, philosophy, and jurisprudence.[13] Although Celsus was probably not a physician, the author(s) or translator(s) of *De Medicina* must have been a skilled physician or surgeon, or both. He seems to have had knowledge of his Greek predecessors, and in many passages he expressed personal opinions and used first-hand examples of patient experiences. He was well versed in urology, which is demonstrated by his treatment of kidney disorders and urine abnormalities:

"As regards the kidneys, these when they have become affected, continue diseased for a long while. It is worse if bilious vomiting is added. The patient should rest, sleep on a soft bed, keep the bowels loose ... even using a clyster when they do not act otherwise; he should sit frequently in a hot bath; take neither food nor drink cold, abstain from everything salted, acid, acrid, and from orchard fruit; drink freely; add whether to the food or to the drink pepper, leeks, fennel, white poppy; which are the most active in causing a discharge of urine ..."[13]

"But when the urine exceeds in quantity the fluid taken, even if it is passed without pain, it gives rise to wasting and danger of consumption; if it is thin, there is need for exercise and rubbing, particularly in the sun and before a fire. The bath should be taken but seldom, and the patient should not stay in it for long; the food should be astringent, the wine dry and undiluted, cold in summer, lukewarm in winter, and in quantity the minimum required to allay thirst. The bowels also are to be moved by a clyster or by taking milk. If the urine is thick, exercise and rubbing should be more thorough, and the patient should stay longer in the bath; food and wine should be of the lighter kind. In both affections, everything that promotes urine should be avoided."[13]

His description of lithotomy was used almost unchanged to the early 1800s. Celsus also described the condition of spermatorrhea:

"There is also a complaint about the genitals, an excessive outflow of semen; which is produced without coition, without nocturnal apparitions, so that in course of time the man is consumed by wasting. Salutary remedies in this affection are: vigorous rubbings, affusions, and swimming in quite cold water; no food and drink taken unless cold."[13]

and may have known about prostatic obstruction and the need for longer, curved catheters in these patients:

"Sometimes we are compelled to draw off the urine by hand when it is not passed naturally; either because in an old man the passage has collapsed, or because a stone, or a blood-clot of some sort has formed an obstruction within it; but even a slight inflammation often prevents natural evacuation; and this treatment is needed not only for men but sometimes also for women. For this purpose bronze tubes are made, and the surgeon must have three ready for males and two for females, in order that they may be suitable for every body, large and small; those for males should be the longest, fifteen fingerbreadths in length, the medium twelve, the shortest nine; for females, the longer nine, the shorter six. They ought to be a little curved, but more so for men, and they should be very smooth and neither too large nor too small. Then the man must be placed on his back, in the way described for anal treatment, on a low seat or couch; while the practitioner stands on his right side, and taking the penis of the male patient in his left hand, with his right hand passes the pipe into the urethra; and when it has reached the neck of the bladder, the pipe together with the penis is inclined and pushed on right into the bladder; and when the urine has been evacuated, it is taken out again. The woman's urethra is both shorter and straighter, like a nipple placed between the inner labia over the vagina, and this requires assistance no less often though it is attended by somewhat less difficulty."[13]

Hippocrates, Galen, and Celsus laid the foundation of medical and surgical care for 1500 years.

TWILIGHT OF THE ANCIENT WORLD

Rufus of Ephesus (98–117 A.D.) lived in Alexandria during the reign of Trajan. Alexandria had been a medical center for

300 years. Herophilus had in the fourth century B.C. conducted his anatomical studies and may have used human cadavers for some of his observations. Among his many discoveries he described the cerebrum and the cerebellum, the meninges, the retina, the pulmonary artery (arterial vein), the duodenum, and the ovary and may have been the first observer to discuss the seminal vesicles or the prostate, or both.[14] Erasistratus (ca. 310–250 B.C.) considered by some researchers to be the first experimental physiologist, had studied digestion, respiration, and blood circulation and had coined the terms *pneuma* and *plethora*. He treated urethral strictures with an "S"-shaped catheter of his own design.

Rufus, who noted that the pulse, heartbeat, and systole are synchronous, used apes for anatomical studies. He was considered to be a competent surgeon and seems to have been the first investigator to describe the prostate as a gland, which he referred to as the *parastates glanduleux*, and delineated the anatomical relationships of the vas deferens. Several fragments of his work have been preserved in a 1554 text (Paris). They include a *Treatise of the Diseases of the Kidney and the Bladder*, which was translated into French by Daremberg and Ruelle in 1879. Two extracts, one on inflammation of the bladder (possibly owing to prostatic hypertrophy) and the other on prostatic abscess (tumors of the bladder) were translated into English by Bitchai and Brodny in 1956:

On Inflammation of the Bladder

Of all the disturbances of the bladder, the most dangerous and most fatal is inflammation; the patients are taken with a violent fever, insomnia, and delirium and vomit pure bile; they cannot urinate; the hypogastric region becomes hard; sharp pain invades the pubis; the hands and feet cannot be warmed; pain is especially felt at the level of the pubis and a little lower; death comes quickly, if a great quantity of thick and purulent urine

is not passed, if the inflammation is not carried outside in part, or if the pain does not stop.[15]

Swellings of the Bladder

As for tumors of the bladder, it is necessary to bring them to maturity. The best method is to try to dissolve them right from the beginning, before they arrive at suppuration; but if they cannot be dissolved, we must bring them promptly to maturity by the methods I have mentioned concerning the kidneys. It is not difficult to recognize all types of these tumors by the pain, the weight, by percussion, and by palpation; in fact, those destined to suppurate became at once hard, tumefied, and hotter than other tumors. The secretions are directed toward the center and necrotize in the center; those which turn toward the exterior, point at the exterior, some by the rectum, others at a point toward which they have extended. These cases are generally fatal; internal ruptures are the most fatal ... The patients suffer constantly, especially when they start to urinate and when they finish, and the urine passes undiluted; they cannot stand straight nor lie down. ...[15]

THE GLORY OF SPAIN

Francisco Diaz, author of the first text devoted completely to urology, was born between 1510 and 1515, at the dawn of the golden age of Spain. The disparate strands of Spanish culture draped in gold and silver from the new world somehow blended to create a glorious renaissance. This was true in medicine as well as in the arts and literature.

Diaz received his bachelor of medicine degree in Alcala de Henares in 1551 and his doctorate in 1558. After graduation he attempted to secure a hospital position. When he was unsuccessful, he went into private practice in Burgos.[16] Later in his life he compared hospital and medical private practice and concluded that only in private practice could the best physician-patient relationship be achieved. Private physicians have the necessary time. The hospital physician was always in a hurry and lacked the time needed to establish rapport with his patients.

Diaz was an unusually capable physician, and because of his growing reputation, he was awarded the degree of Surgeon to His Majesty, King Philip II, a post that he continued to hold from 1570 to 1588. Diaz wrote three works: a *Compendium of Surgery*, an anatomy text, and a three-volume work on urology. Only the *Compendium of Surgery* and the urology text have survived.

The urology text was written in the vernacular, following renaissance tradition, in the hope that it would reach the largest possible audience (Figure 2–1). The first volume dealt with conditions of the kidney, and the second with diseases of the bladder including stones, inflammation, and ulcers. In the third volume he described strictures of the urethra and prostatic obstruction, which he called "carnosities and calluses." He attributed them to inflammation, passing of stones, sexual abuse, and humoral alterations. The symptoms included a weak stream, stranguria, burning on urination, retention, the sensation of incomplete emptying of the bladder, and infertility. Diaz thought a carnosity of the prostate was due to an increase in the flesh of the bladder neck, so much so that "it occludes the canal and causes the suppression of the urine which occasionally terminates somewhat miserably."[17] Treatment was to be threefold: careful diligent dilatation, local application of caustics, and his "instrumento cisorio," which he devised to punch through the prostate · into the bladder (Figure 2–2).[17]

There has been much confusion about the concept of carnosities of the bladder neck, because of which historians until recently have tended to discount the whole concept. The problem has been one of what the early authors called the bladder neck. The neck of the bladder in the 1500s is the prostatic urethra of today. Therefore the instrument that Diaz used to tunnel through the prostate and the instrument of Ambrose Paré, which was used to chip out the carnosities at multiple sittings — just as the latter punch instruments would be used — were in reality the first instruments for transurethral resection of the prostate. Guthrie, who in 1834 established a differential between hypertrophy of the glandular tissue of the median lobe and the bar at the neck of the bladder, devised an instrument to cut the median bar and/or punch his way through the prostate into the bladder.[18] It bears a strong resemblance to the instrument devised 250 years earlier by Diaz.

Diaz was concerned that patients with carnosities should not be neglected or fall

TRATADO
NVEVAMENTE
IMPRESSO, DE TODAS
LAS ENFERMEDADES DELOS
Kiñones, Vexiga, y Carnofidades dela verga, y Vrina, diuidido en tres libros. Compueſto por Franciſco Diaz Dotor en Medicina, y maeſtro en Filoſofia, por la inſigne vniuerſidad de Alcala de Henares, y Cirujano del Rey nueſtro Señor.

DIRIGIDO AL DOTOR VALLE
Protomedico del Rey nueſtro Señor, y Medico de ſu Camara, &c.

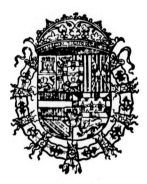

CON PRIVILEGIO.

Impreſſo en Madrid por Franciſco Sanchez.

Año. 1 5 8 8.

Figure 2–1. Title page of the first textbook of urology. De Todas Las Enfermedades De Los Riñones, Vexiga, y Carnosidades de la verga, y Urina, written by Francisco Diaz (Madrid, 1588).

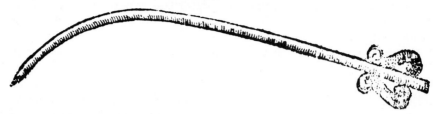

Figure 2-2. "Instrumento cisorio" of Francisco Diaz, used to treat urethral obstructions including carnosities and calluses of the bladder neck.

into the hands of unskilled physicians or artisans. He warned that if treatment was delayed the patient would "lose his life" or when he would later "want to remedy it, the occasion of the cure [would have] passed, because a carnosity hardens forming in this manner a hard uncurable callus."[19]

THE BEGINNING OF UROLOGIC PATHOLOGY

One of the 18th century's greatest teachers was Giovanni Battista Morgagni (1682–1771). He is referred to by some medical historians as the "Father of Pathologic Anatomy" because of his ability to correlate the patient's medical history and symptomatology with the pathologic findings found at autopsy and with previous case reports. He played a significant role in many of the medical advances of the late 18th and early 19th centuries.[20] When his classic pathology text was published in 1761, "there were no professional pathologists in the modern sense, no men who devoted themselves entirely to the study of 'morbid anatomy.' "[21]

Morgagni's *Seats and Causes of Diseases Investigated by Anatomy* was written as a series of letters. In it, he described a multitude of urinary tract problems. Prominent among these were those associated with the prostate. In letter 41 he presented the case of:

"... [a] man, of seventy years of age, having labour'd under a long difficulty of making water; so that he discharg'd no urine but by the help of the catheter; finding his disorders increase every day, was oblig'd to come into the hospital of St. Mary de Vita at Bologna. There, while the lithotomist was endeavouring to procure an exit for the urine, by means of the catheter, without effect, he died with a laborious respiration and a stertor.

The fibres of the urinary bladder had so increas'd, as to resemble the strong bundles of fibres in the heart; and that both in figure and magnitude. An excrescence of the prostate gland, in the form of a pear, and scarcely leaving any passage, had been affected with an inflammation in the lower part; from the continual impetus of the catheter."[22]

Morgagni distinguished between (1) excrescences (caruncles) of the prostate gland; (2) tubercles which form "sometimes in the bladder, or at its neck" which may "easily be changed into pus and leave the passage free and open"; and (3) "scirrhus [sic] tumours, or tumours verging to the hardness of a scirrhus such as are often found in the prostate gland, or frequently grow out therefrom:

"A physician, who was his kinsman, took great pains to administer relief by clysters, baths, and bloodletting from the haemorrhoidal veins; and even by such remedies as increas'd the intestinal discharges, which were at the same time diminish'd: but to no purpose. He therefore, at length, order'd the catheter to be introduc'd: which was done without great difficulty, both then, and afterwards. And at each time of introducing it, almost seven pints of urine were drawn off, on the first days from the time it began first to be introduc'd; notwithstanding he had but little given him to drink.

On the intermediate days, for he liv'd, in all, about fifteen, the quantity was somewhat less: and on the last days the quantity again amounted to seven pints. When, therefore, we came to inquire into the cause of this suppression, it appear'd to be at the lower part of the bladder. That is to say, the prostate gland was universally swollen out in a preternatural manner, and had attain'd to such a state of hardness, as to seem to those who cut into it, to consist of the substance of cartilage and ligament mix'd together as it were. This tumefied gland was of a white colour; except that, in some places, but particularly on both surfaces, it was blackish, from blood stagnating in the vessels; and that most on the right side, where the scrotum was, in part, distended with a large enterocele."[22]

Morgagni was also aware of differences in the types of prostatic growth:

"But the whole prostate gland is not always tumid. For frequently, only the superior circumference of it either grows out on every side, or on a particular part; and swells to such a degree, as to prevent the exclusion of the urine. I think I can point out examples from the Sepulchretum, of its being so tumid as to have this effect: and I have many observations of its beginning to grow out: and these, that you may know what are the small beginnings of great disorders, I will take the trouble to subjoin here, in order, after the former."[22]

and emphasized the isolated occurrence of hypertrophy of the middle lobe of the prostate (so-called Morgagni tubercle):

"And when the anterior paries of the bladder was cut asunder longitudinally; in that part of the opposite paries, which is nearest to the orifice, and in the very middle of this part, a roundish protuberance appear'd: being of the bigness of a small grape, cover'd over with the internal coat of the bladder. What this protuberance was I readily suppos'd; and by forcing the knife into it, I cut through this and the contiguous prostate gland, at the

same time, lengthways, and show'd that it was of the same nature with that gland: that it was very evidently continued from it; and that there was no doubt, but, if it had grown out to a greater degree, it must have been a very considerable impediment to the discharge of the urine."[22]

One of the more interesting letters that Morgagni wrote detailed the public demonstration of the body of a 54-year-old man who was found to have a smaller than usual urinary bladder. In this "first" report of prostatic corpora amylacea he stated: "In the urethra was nothing particular observed except granules of tobacco as it were at the orifices of the prostate gland . . .[22] The seminal caruncle had, at the side of it, granules of the kind I am speaking of; from some of which, that were dissolv'd, as I suppose, by the moisture of the place, not only the other parts, which lay near, but even the orifices of the seminal ducts, were yellow."[22]

Morgagni's unusual ability to perceive the gross pathologic verification of genitourinary disease led to many of the subsequent advances in urologic knowledge.

EARLY AMERICAN INTEREST

The first American publication exclusively devoted to the prostate seems to be one written by Robert M. Sullivan as a dissertation for the degree of doctor of physic from the College of Physicians and Surgeons in the University of the State of New York (May, 1816). Sullivan was a pupil of Wright Post (1766–1828), the professor of anatomy and surgery at the college and surgeon to New York Hospital, and Valentine Mott (1785–1865), who was then professor of surgery at the College of Physicians and Surgeons. In *The Sclerocele of the Prostate Gland with an Inquiry into the cause of This Disease and also why this affection Occurs more particularly in old and sedentary men* he reviewed "current" theory and the philosophical problems involved in understanding prostatic enlargements and obstructions. Under the influence of Ramsden (on testicular tumors) and Tissot, he postulated that sclerocele of the prostate ("hard growth") was due to rectal irritation, venereal disease, bladder calculi, strictures, onanism or other mechanical violence, and old age. He distinguished sclerocele from "schirrus" in the following manner:

> "The term schirrus has been applied for the same reason; the disease being an indurated gland. One author describes a *Schirrus* of the prostate in the following words: 'it is often found of a cartilaginous texture; but more frequently of the *appearance of hog's skin*, and appears filled with a kind of inspissated lymph.
>
> Sometimes it is increased to double, sometimes triple its natural size. Sometimes we find the whole gland affected with schirrus, and at others we find it only partially affected with this kind of induration.
>
> The hardness of the gland can sometimes be discovered by the introduction of the finger into the rectum, which is attended with little pain.
>
> The definition given by writers of schirrus, is nearly as follows: a hard tumour, with craggedness of surface, with a red or livid appearance, attended with severe lancinating pain, and derangement of general health."[23]

Quoting mainly from Morgagni, Home, Dessault, and Mott, Sullivan described prostatic calculi, bladder stone owing to prostatic growth, and varicose swellings at the bladder neck. He also pointed out that middle lobe enlargements were an uncommon form of growth. Although he favored "treatment 'by the urethra' with the bougie,"[23] he does not indicate that he personally treated any patients with prostatic disease. Sullivan also presented the case of Dr. John Fothergill, who was reported by Everard Home to have had a fungus of the middle lobe of the prostate (Figures 2–3 and 2–4). His opinions disagreed in part with those expressed later in a report by his teacher Valentine Mott.[24]

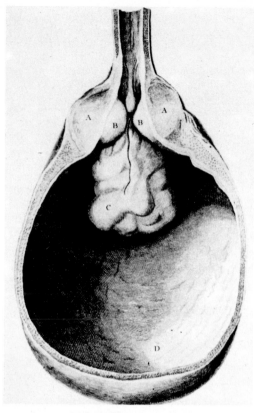

Figure 2–3. "The valvular part of the bladder so increased as to form a considerable tumour, projecting into the cavity of the bladder. The prostate is also enlarged. This tumour had been the occasion of several severe suppressions of urine, and had often been the cause of a failure in drawing off the water with the catheter, by that instrument most probably passing into its substance so deep as to hinder the urine entering its opening. The dark line passing along the tumour from the urethra was probably made by this means, but now collapsed." (Plate 7 from Hunter, J.: A Treatise on The Venereal Disease. Edited by Everard Home (3d ed.). London, 1810.)

PROSTATIC CANCER DEFINED

Little is generally known about George Langstaff (1780–1846), English morbid anatomist and surgeon. He practiced in the era of Astley Cooper and John, Charles, and Benjamin Bell, when surgeons did not think they were adequate unless they followed their patients to the postmortem table. In 1817, Langstaff described several cases of malignant growths, including what may be the first

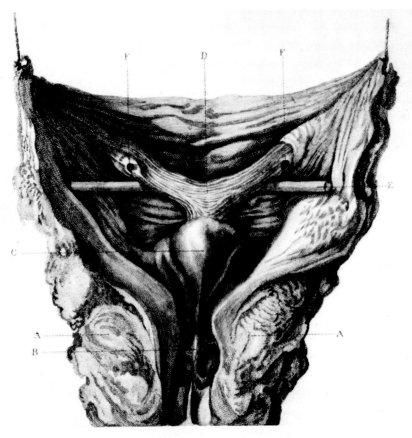

Figure 2–4. ". . . the diseased prostate gland and part of the bladder. The third lobe of the prostate is enlarged, and the connection of the muscles of the ureters with it is very distinct." (Plate 6 from Bell; C.: Account of the muscles of the ureters and their effects in the irritable states of the bladder. Medico-Chirurgical Transactions 3:171, 1812.)

clear description of a case of prostatic cancer with possible metastasis to the liver and lungs (Figure 2–5). He used the term *fungus haematodes,* proposed initially by Hey, to describe (1) tumors that bleed, slough, and cause absorption of the surrounding integuments; (2) pulpy or medullary tumors; (3) combinations of the above; and (4) carcinomas:

> Case of Fungus Haematodes in the Urinary Bladder, Liver, and Lungs.
>
> I. B. a pauper, sixty-eight years of age, had laboured under an affection of the bladder upwards of five years, and had been under the care of several surgeons without experiencing any essential relief. During the last six months of his life, he had suffered the most excruciating pain in

the region of the kidnies [sic] and bladder, attended with almost constant desire to void urine, which was effected with the greatest difficulty, either by drops, or in a very small stream, and generally coloured with blood. He also felt much pain in the rectum, which was greatly aggravated by costiveness, and was teased with a frequent dry cough, accompanied with dyspnoea.

> An examination per rectum, proved that there existed an enlarged state of the prostate gland, and slight pressure occasioned great pain. . . .
>
> The symptoms daily increased, . . . He became feverish; . . . [and] [i]n this miserable state he lived four days.
>
> Dissection
>
> The first thing on opening the abdomen, which attracted particular notice, was a

CASES

OF

FUNGUS HÆMATODES,

WITH

OBSERVATIONS;

By GEORGE LANGSTAFF, Esq.

AND

AN APPENDIX

CONTAINING

TWO CASES OF ANALOGOUS AFFECTIONS.

By WILLIAM LAWRENCE, Esq. F.R.S.

PROFESSOR OF ANATOMY AND SURGERY TO THE ROYAL COLLEGE OF
SURGEONS, &c. &c.

Read May 27, 1817.

HAVING devoted a considerable portion of my time during the last fourteen years, to the prosecution of the study of morbid anatomy, and having with considerable labour and attention obtained specimens illustrating most of the diseases to which the human body is liable, I am induced to offer the following cases to the Society; and shall feel much gratified, should they be considered as throwing any light upon the hitherto incurable disease, they are intended to describe.

Figure 2–5. Initial page of George Langstaff's 1817 presentation of "Fungus Haematodes." In this report published in the Medico-Chirurgical Transactions 8:1820, he presented a case of prostatic cancer.

bloody effusion beneath the peritoneum, on the right side of the body, extending from the seat of the kidney as far as the pelvis. The fluid proved to be offensive smelling urine mixed with blood, and measuring altogether three pints in quantity.

My great desire now was, to ascertain the course of this unnatural escape of urine. The kidney was large, very pale coloured, but healthy in structure; its pelvis had been dilated to a considerable extent, as was the whole course of the ureter; the latter from over distension had sloughed and burst about midway between the kidney and where it enters the bladder.

The bladder and urethra were next examined. The former felt like a solid substance: on laying it open, it was found to contain a tumor as big as a large orange, the surface of which was covered with recently coagulated arterial looking blood, which being removed, exhibited layers of concentrated coagulated blood, similar to what is seen in aneurisms. After minutely examining the tumor, it was discovered to derive its origin from the prostate gland, chiefly from the middle, or third lobe. A perpendicular section was made into the tumor, which was composed principally of loose coagulated blood mixed with a white pulpy substance; but its base on the posterior part of the bladder, was of a dense, hardish consistence, and had produced a firm union and considerable thickening of that part of the muscular coat.

The fungus extended laterally, and had completely plugged up both ureters; on the right side half an inch beyond where it penetrates the muscular coat of the bladder. The prostatic urethra was nearly closed with the same growth, the remaining part of the tube being quite healthy.

In the liver there were several tubera near its surface, some as large as a gooseberry. They were vascular, of a reddish colour, pulpy consistence, and when squeezed, exactly like the soft part of the tumor of the bladder. There were several of those tubera in the lungs, but they did not possess capsules.[25]

Appended to Langstaff's work was a report of William Lawrence (1783–1867), professor of anatomy and surgery to the Royal College of Surgeons, of two analogous afflictions and what seems to be a lymphoma and a tumor of the testicle.

FIRST AMERICAN UROLOGIC TEXT

A second American contribution to development of the understanding of prostatic disease appears in the first American urologic text, which was written by Dr. Joseph Parrish (1779–1840) as part II of his *Practical Observations on Strangulated Hernia, and Some of the Diseases of the Urinary Organs* (1836). He was a pupil of Caspar Wistar (one of early America's leading surgeon/anatomists) and colleague of Philip Syng Physick (first professor of surgery at the University of Pennsylvania). Parrish was a noted lecturer on chemistry and materia medica in addition to surgery. In 1811 he edited an American edition of William Lawrence's work on hernia.

In his introduction to his urologic text he stated that:

"On diseases of the urinary organs, I would simply observe, that an accurate anatomical knowledge of the parts, both in a natural and morbid condition, is of the highest importance. Without this, a practitioner would fail in his efforts to relieve a patient from great suffering and danger, at a moment when his services were imperiously demanded. With it, he may prove the instrument of speedy relief from one of the most painful conditions to which the human frame can be subjected."[26]

A careful physician, Parrish made postmortem examination a part of his clinical teaching. As one of the most successful private medical lecturers, he was influential in the speed of scientific medicine and urologic knowledge. In his discussion of the prostate gland he stated:

"Among the diseases peculiar to advanced life, is an enlarged condition of the prostate gland. This gland is situated at the neck of the urinary bladder, and is called into action in every effort to evacuate its contents.

The morbid condition of this structure which we are about to notice, first manifests itself by a frequent desire to void urine, obliging the patient to rise several times in the course of the night. This disposition slowly increases, until the calls become very frequent, accompanied with severe pain and straining. As the disease advances, retention of urine to a greater or less extent, not unfrequently takes place, requiring the use of the catheter (Figure 2–6).

A post mortem examination reveals the cause of the symptoms just described. The prostate gland, which in a natural state does not exceed the size of a horse-chestnut, may be found equal in bulk to a large pear. Sometimes the enlargement is most conspicuous in the lateral lobes, while in other instances the third lobe seems to have been principally affected. The latter form is the more serious, from the fact of this lobe forming, in a natural state, a small projection towards the

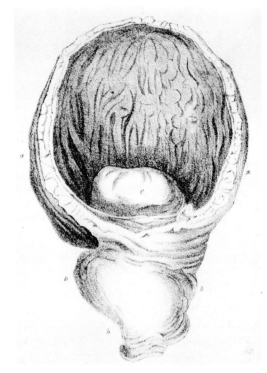

Figure 2–6. "Interior view of the bladder, with enormous development of the third lobe of the prostate gland." (Plate 2 from Parrish, J.: Practical Observations on Strangulated Hernia and Some of the Diseases of the Urinary Organs. Philadelphia, 1836.)

urethra, which, when increased by disease, constitutes a large triangular body, overhanging the opening of the urethra into the bladder. This lobe acts the part of a valve, which, under certain morbid conditions, may completely close the opening from the bladder into the urethra; offering a most serious mechanical impediment to the introduction of the catheter."[26]

Parrish discussed the suggestion of Guthrie and Blizzard to drain prostatic abscesses by perineal incision. He also gave a lively discussion of the relationship between bladder calculi with prostatic enlargement:

"Although my own experience does not furnish a case of stone complicated with enlarged prostate, in which an operation was performed, yet a striking instance has lately occurred in this city, in the person of the late Chief Justice Marshall. This highly distinguished and excellent man, was subjected to the operation of lithotomy by Dr. Physick, and a large number of calculi were removed from the bladder. The prostate gland was considerably enlarged at the time of the operation, and the third lobe was distinctly felt projecting into the bladder.

The venerable patient recovered most happily, resumed his official duties, and enjoyed a considerable share of health for several years. He died with a disease unconnected with the urinary organs. A post mortem examination was made, and the prostate particularly examined. Dr. Physick, (whose opinion on this point was requested,) explicitly states, that the size of the gland was not diminished by the operation. The preparation is now in his possession.''[26]

He particularly emphasized the hypertrophy of bladder musculature due to prostatic obstruction and the use of indwelling suprapubic tubes in the patients with enlarged prostates (Figure 2–7):

"I am now willing to suggest the result of my own reflections on this subject, after premising that they are predicated on a case related to me by my beloved and departed preceptor, Dr. Wistar. He tapped the distended bladder of an elderly gentleman above the pubis, in consequence of

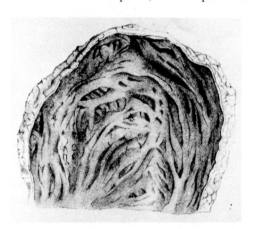

Figure 2–7. Section and interior view of fundus of bladder taken from subject with enlarged prostate gland, showing columns of mucous coat, caused by long continued dysuria and resembling the muscular columns of the heart. (Plate 3 from Parrish, J.: Practical Observations on Strangulated Hernia and Some of the Diseases of the Urinary Organs. Philadelphia, 1836.)

his inability to introduce a catheter; the difficulty being caused by an enlargement of the prostate gland. In this instance the patient wore a gold tube, in the opening made by the operation, through which the urine was discharged without difficulty. From having been the subject of great suffering for years, he was by this means enabled to enjoy comparative comfort; his health improved, and was so far restored that he was in the practice of riding out to his country seat, several miles from the city, not only in his carriage, but sometimes on horseback. Nearly two years elapsed under this favourable change. In the interim the diseased prostate had so far recovered, that the patient could pass water through the urethra freely and without pain. Thinking that the disease was cured, he removed the tube, and relied entirely upon the natural passage. The consequence was, a renewal of the disease in the prostate, of which he finally died. A small fistulous opening continued above the pubis, but the bladder never rose sufficiently high to admit of a repetition of the tapping, and the tube could not be replaced.''[26]

A MODERN UROLOGIST

Sir Benjamin Collins Brodie, born June 8, 1783, came to London in 1801 at the age of 18 to study medicine under Wilson and Abernethy. John Abernethy, at the time, was drawing large audiences to his lectures at St. Bartholomew's Hospital and at his home in "Bartholomew Close."[27] After two years, Brodie entered St. George's Hospital to learn from Sir Everard Home, brother-in-law of the great John Hunter. Here, he was successively: pupil (1803); house-surgeon (1804); assistant-surgeon (1808); and full surgeon (1822). From this position his gifts as a surgeon reached their fullest development and were recognized by his peers. "Brodie reigned supreme in the world of surgery for a quarter of a century,"[28] holding all the major offices the surgical world had to offer including: President of the Royal Medical and Chirurgical Society (1839); the Royal College of Surgeons (1844); and the Royal Society (1858–1861). In 1832, on the death of Sir Everard Home, he was made sergeant-surgeon to William IV, a position he continued to hold under Queen Victoria.

He believed diseases of the urinary organs required special attention and acted upon that belief throughout his career.[28] His notes from his student days at St. George's are still extant and show his concern with urologic problems. They are filled with detailed observations and careful notes on unusual cases (Figure 2–8):

Case of Enlarged Prostate Gland

Bernelli, an Italian, status 68, has had a difficulty in voiding his urine for some time. As far as he recollects, he first experienced it about the end of November, 1805. . . . He has through the progress of the complaint had considerable irritation

L E C T U R E S

ON

THE DISEASES

OF

THE URINARY ORGANS.

BY

SIR BENJAMIN C. BRODIE, Bart. F.R.S.
SERJEANT-SURGEON TO THE QUEEN.

Third Edition,

WITH ALTERATIONS AND ADDITIONS.

LONDON:
PRINTED FOR
LONGMAN, BROWN, GREEN, AND LONGMANS,
PATERNOSTER ROW.
1842.

Figure 2–8. Title page of Benjamin Brodie's text on The Diseases of The Urinary Organs initially published in London in 1836.

about the neck of the bladder: — the attempts to empty that viscus have been attended with great pain and distress: — the urine has been very frequently bloody and has always had floating in it a white ropy mucus resembling white of egg.. . .[29]

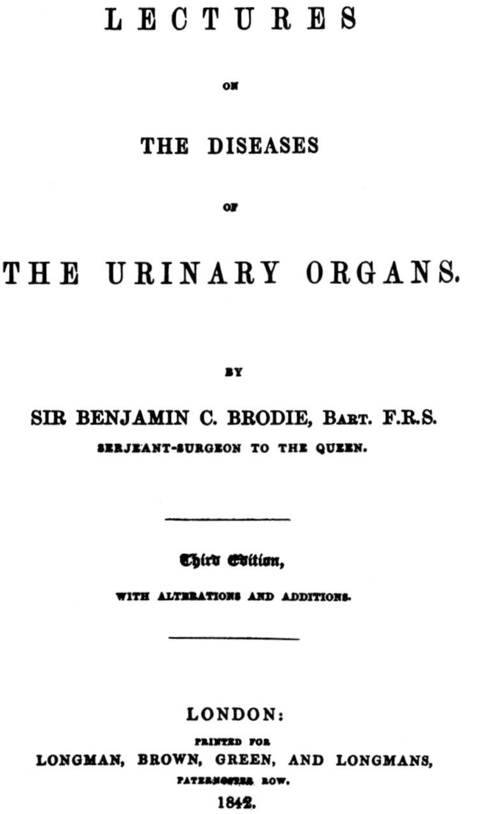

Brodie was a careful observer trained in the autopsy verification of his clinical findings. Regarding prostatic disease, he was instrumental in clearly delineating the etiology, symptoms, and treatment of patients with prostatic abscesses and the effect of all prostatic enlargements on the gross structure and function of the upper urinary system. Pertaining to this, he presented in his *Lectures on the Diseases of the Urinary Organs* (1832) several cases which highlighted his argument that urethral obstruction not only caused renal damage but also obstructions to the ureters "which principally baffles our skill and renders vain all our efforts for the patient's relief."[30] In a case perhaps similar to Langstaff's he stated:

"At last, however, we satisfied ourselves that the catheter drew off no urine, because there was none in the bladder. The patient died, and Mr. Stanley examined the body. He found a growth of medullary fungus immediately behind the internal orifice of the urethra, projecting into the bladder, and extending to the orifices of the ureters. It seemed that this disease, at the termination of the ureters, had impeded the flow of urine into the bladder from the kidneys, both ureters being much enlarged, and distended with urine through their whole extent. The kidneys were very soft and vascular, but contained no large accumulation of urine."[30]

He felt that malignant diseases of the prostate were rare and that the term "scirrhus" should not be used to describe what he called, "chronic enlargement of the prostate gland."[30] He felt that chronic enlargement of the prostate was similar to chronic enlargement of the thyroid:

"Malignant diseases of the prostate are of very rare occurrence, and it is certainly a great mistake to apply the term scirrhus to the cases which are now under our consideration. The chronic enlargement of the prostate may be said to be a disease of a peculiar kind, having no exact resemblance to what we meet with in any other organ. It may, however, in some respects, be compared to the chronic enlargement of the thyroid gland, known by the name of bronchocele. Like the latter, it is generally slow in its progress; and frequently, after having reached a certain point, if proper treatment be employed, it remains almost stationary for many years. It is on the whole a rare occurrence for it to terminate in ulceration or abscess; and the symptoms, to which it gives rise, are, with a few exceptions, to be referred to the influence which the disease exercises over the functions of the parts in the neighbourhood."[30]

Brodie reported two cases of patients with urinary difficulties and stony hard prostates. In one patient the prostate was "not very much enlarged" and had no retention but had a large lymph node in the groin. In the other, Brodie reported urinary retention and possible metastasis to the spine causing lower limb paralysis:

"A gentleman, about sixty years of age, who had been long in India, consulted me a few years ago, respecting what appeared to be a chronic enlargement of the prostate gland. There was nothing unusual in his symptoms, and I merely recommended to him the regular use of the catheter. From this treatment he derived much benefit, and he persevered in it ever afterwards.

It was not less than five or six years after this period that I was requested to see him again, in consultation . . . He now could void no urine without the assistance of the catheter. There was a constant and most severe pain, referred to the neck of the bladder, which was not relieved on the urine being drawn off. The prostate gland, examined by the rectum, was found to be much enlarged, and of a stony hardness. From these circumstances we were led to suspect that the prostate had become affected with a true scirrhous disease; and, in confirmation of this opinion, we found the patient complaining of excruciating pains in various parts of the body, sometimes in one part, sometimes in another, which could be compared to nothing except the pains under which persons

afflicted with carcinoma occasionally labour. Altogether, I may say, that I have never seen a human being whose sufferings were more intense; and they were scarcely mitigated by the exhibition of very large doses of opium. I continued to visit him occasionally, in consultation, for nearly a year, at the end of which time he suddenly lost the use of the muscles of his lower limbs, and died in a fortnight afterwards. Permission was not obtained to examine the body; but it is worthy of notice, that a lady, whose case is related in the eighth chapter of the last edition of my work on Diseases of the Joints, and who had long laboured under carcinoma of the breast, died after a similar attack of paralysis of the lower limbs, and that in her it was ascertained by dissection, that the cause of the paralysis was a conversion of the bones of the spine into the scirrhous structure."[30]

In regard to chronic enlargement of the prostate gland Brodie contended that at different periods in human life changes take place in the body's organs which demonstrate "that the individual has entered on that downward course, which is to end in his dissolution."[30]

"When the hair becomes grey and scanty, when specks of earthy matter begin to be deposited in the tunics of the arteries, and when a white zone is formed at the margin of the cornea, at this same period the prostate gland usually, I might perhaps say invariably, becomes increased in size. This change in the condition of the prostate takes place slowly, and at first imperceptibly, and the term *chronic* enlargement is not improperly employed to distinguish it from the inflammatory attacks to which the prostate is liable in earlier life."[30]

Brodie emphasized the occurrence of bladder diverticula (bladder cysts) in patients with prostatic obstruction and postulated the reason for overflow incontinence. Although he favored conservative therapy with the intermittent use of a gum catheter, he proposed and used forcible entry into the bladder through the prostate with sharp hollow instruments initially proposed by Diaz and again demonstrated in England by Mr. Hunter and Mr. Home.[30]

In conclusion, we may say that by the 1850s knowledge of the gross pathology of the prostate and its physiologic consequences were well known. The introduction of the microscope into pathologic examination, anesthesia, roentgenography, operative surgical extirpation of the prostatic adenoma or carcinoma, endoscopic diagnosis and surgery, hormonal manipulation, and antibiotics would, in the subsequent one hundred years, revolutionize the prognosis of patients with prostatic disease. Yet the approach of the physician to diseases of the prostate has not materially changed from the beginning of recorded history.

ACKNOWLEDGMENT

We would like to thank Dr. John Blake, Mrs. Dorothy Hanks, and Mr. Patrick Dore of the History of Medicine Division of the National Library of Medicine for making the collection accessible to us and for answering our requests with knowledge and dispatch. We would also like to thank Miss Georgia Price, Mr. Anton Olson, and Miss Joan Davis for their help.

Ms. Brenda Shore, Mrs. Mary Bochek and Mrs. Muriel Moore deserve our recognition. Mrs. Barbara Sanders and Mrs. Marge Blazier made this chapter a reality.

References

1. Desnos, M. E.: Dysurie, strangurie, ischurie vessie et prostate. In Histoire de L'Urologie, in Encyclopédie Française D'Urologie. Paris, Octave Doin, 1914, pp. 123–134.
2. Herman, J. R.: The prostate: Surgical Approaches. and TUR: The Development of Instruments. In Urology: A View Through the Retrospectroscope. Hagerstown, Harper & Row, 1973, pp. 111–129.
3. Hunt, V. C.: Prostatism and prostatic surgery. In History of Urology. Edited by Ballenger et al. Baltimore, Williams & Wilkins, 1933, pp. 91–136.
4. Murphy, L. J. T.: The prostate. In The History of Urology. Springfield, Ill. C. C Thomas, 1972, pp. 378–453.
5. Shelley, H. S.: The enlarged prostate; a brief history of its treatment. J. History Med. Allied Sci. 24:452, 1969.
6. Wershub, L. P.: Surgery of the prostate and further advances in bladder surgery. In Urology from Antiquity to the 20th Century. St. Louis, W. Green, 1970, pp. 252–264.
7. Bush, R. B., and Bush, I. M.: Urology in the "Fertile Crescent". Chicago: Privately printed, 1969.
8. Sussman, M.: Diseases in the Bible and the Talmud. In Diseases in Antiquity. Edited by D. Brothwell and A. T. Sandison. Springfield, Ill., C. C Thomas, 1967, p. 215.
9. Jones, W. H. S., (trans.), and Page, T. E. (ed.): Air Waters Places, IX. In Hippocrates, Vol. 1. Cambridge, Harvard University Press, 1962, pp. 95, 97
10. Jones, W. H. S. (trans.), and Page, T. E. (ed.): Aphorisms. In Hippocrates, Vol. 4. Cambridge, Harvard University Press, 1962, pp. 135, 137; 153; 155; 157; 189; 201.
12. Desnos, E.: L'histoire de L'urologie. In The History of Urology. Translated and edited by L. J. T. Murphy. Springfield, Ill., C. C Thomas, 1972, p. 21.
13. Spencer, W. G. (trans.), and Page, T. E. (ed.): Introduction. In Celsus De Medicina, Vol. 1. Cambridge, Harvard University Press, 1960, pp. vii; Book IV, 419, 451; Book VII, vol. 3, 425, 427.
14. Garrison, F. H.: An Introduction to the History of Medicine, 4th ed. rev. Philadelphia, W. B. Saunders, 1929, p. 103.
15. Bitschai, J. and Brodny, M. L.: A History of Urology in Egypt. New York, Riverside Press, 1956, pp. 18; 19–20.
16. Casas Motra, D. A.: Algunos datas bibliograficas de Francisco Diaz, trabajos de la catedra de historia critica de la medicina 6:231, 1934.
17. Diaz, Francisco: Tratado Nuevamente Impresso, De Todas Las Enfermedades De Los Riñones, Vexiga, y Carnosidades de la verga, y Urina. Madrid, 1588, pp. 323; 352.
18. Guthrie, G. J.: On the Anatomy and Diseases of the Neck of the Bladder and of the Urethra. London, 1834, p. 275.
19. Diaz, Francisco: Tratado Nuevamente Impresso, de Todas Las Enfermedades de los Rinones, Vexiga, y Carnosidades de la verga, y Urina. Madrid, 1588, p. 324.
20. Klemperer, P.: Introduction. In The Seats and Causes of Disease Investigated by Anatomy. Edited by J. B. Morgagni and translated by B. Alexander, Vol. 1 (1769). Reprinted edition in New York, Hafner, 1960.
21. King, L., ed.: A History of Medicine, Selected Readings Harmondsworth, Penguin Books, 1971, p. 167.
22. Morgagni, J. B.: The Seats and Causes of Disease Investigated by Anatomy. Translated by B. Alexander, Vol. 2 (1769). Reprinted edition New York, Hafner, 1960, pp. 454; 461–462; 467; 468; 611; 611–612.
23. Sullivan, R. M.: A Dissertation on the Sclerocele of the Prostate Gland, with an Inquiry into the Cause of This Disease, and also, Why This Affection Occurs More Particularly in Old and Sedentary Men. New York, Forbes, 1816, pp. 28; 51.

24. Mott, V.: Disease of the prostate gland. South. Medical Surg. J. n.s. 15:28, 1859.

25. Langstaff, G.: Cases of fungus haematodes with Observations. *In* Medico-Chirurgical Transactions (2d ed.), Vol. 8. London, 1820, pp. 279–282.

26. Parrish, J.: Practical Observations on Strangulated Hernia, and Some of the Diseases of the Urinary Organs. Philadelphia, Key & Biddle, 1836, pp. 4; 250–251; 256; 259–260.

27. Smith, G.: The Concise Dictionary of National Biography. London, Oxford University Press, 1939, p. 3.

28. Riches, E.: A Manuscript of Benjamin Collins Brodie's Surgical Lecture, 1822; with Some Notes on the History of Stricture and Stone. Proceedings of the Royal Society of Medicine 51 Sectional 27, 1049, 1958.

29. Cases 1805–1807 by Benjamin Brodie, St. George's Hospital Medical School Library, London.

30. Brodie, B. C.: Lectures on the Diseases of the Urinary Organs (3rd rev. ed.) London, 1842, pp. 151–152; 154; 164; 167; 182; 194–195.

Note: Reference 11 deleted.

Chapter 3

Etiology and Epidemiology of Human Prostatic Disorders

L. M. FRANKS

As with most other forms of cancer, little is known about the cause of prostatic carcinoma. The dramatic effects produced by hormones in some patients with prostatic cancer has focused attention on the endocrine system, but epidemiologic and clinical studies suggest that there are other factors involved, particularly age and race, both of which seem to influence the development of the disease. A major obstacle to experimental investigations is the absence of a suitable model system, since cancer of the prostate occurs in few species other than man.

DEFINITION OF TERMS

There is also confusion about the terms used to describe the disease. Under the microscope and to the naked eye, all cases of prostatic cancer are similar but biologically, i.e., in the patient, three types can be distinguished, including: *Clinical.* Any case in which a firm clinical diagnosis of prostatic cancer is made and confirmed by histology should be described as a clinical cancer. *Latent.* These tumors by definition exist but do not become manifest, i.e., they produce no

clinical evidence of disease. They are found *incidentally. Occult.* These tumors manifest themselves by their metastases. The primary tumor remains hidden (occult).

These definitions have no direct relationship to size, growth rate, histological structure, local invasion, or distant metastases. They are concerned *only* with the method of presentation. It seems likely that all types have the same etiology and differ only in the degree of biologic malignancy. This may be a result of changes in the tumor cells or in the host response.

INCIDENCE

The incidence of prostatic cancer is influenced by age and race. It is predominantly a disease of the elderly, and both latent and clinical cancers are rarely found before the age of 50 years. The incidence of both types of cancer then increases rapidly. There are many reported series showing an increased incidence of latent cancers with age.[1,2] The figures range from 14 to 46% of all autopsies on men over 50 years old, the

Table 3–1

Increasing incidence of prostatic carcinoma with age (postmortem studies)

| Age Group (yrs) | Cases studied | | No. in which carcinomas were found | | | |
| | Gaynor | Present series | Number | | Percentage | |
			Gaynor	Present series	Gaynor	Present series
20–29	15	4	0	0	0.0	0.0
30–39	25	8	1	0	0.4	0.0
40–49	122	18	6	0	4.9	0.0
50–59	241	38	25	11	10.4	28.9
60–69	312	53	54	16	17.3	30.2
70–79	237	70	67	28	28.3	40.0
80–89	93	17	36	12	38.7	70.6
90+	5	2	2	2	40.0	100.0
Totals	1050	210	191	69	18.2	32.9

exact figure being largely determined by the number of sections of the gland examined. Table 3–1 gives the age distribution from 2 series[1,3] of European patients. In the yellow races the figures are similar.[2,4,5]

In clinical cases the pattern is similar. Doll[6] has summarized figures of rate of increase in 11 different areas and discussed figures for selected areas in Great Britain in more detail. The pattern seems to be similar in all areas for which satisfactory statistics are available. Little,[7] using figures from Connecticut and New York, calculated a serial rate of increase which illustrates the pattern very well. In age groups between 20–29 and 30–39 years the rate increased 9.5 times. Between 40–49 and 50–59 years the increase was 18-fold. Between 50–59 and 60–69 the increase was six-fold, i.e., 2052 times the rate of the 20–29 year group. Between 60–69 and 70–79 there was a further increase of 3.3 times, and over 80 years an increase of 1.9 times. The slowing of the rate in patients over 80 years may be of significance even though the figures are small, since some evidence suggests that the disease may be "less malignant" in these patients, i.e., metastases are less frequent and death occurs less often from cancer.[8]

RACE AND TUMOR INCIDENCE

The difficulties involved in any comparative study on cancer incidence in different countries are well known. Even in a country like Denmark, which has a fairly homogeneous population, is small, and has a well-established system of medical care, both in general practice and in hospitals, there are wide variations in tumor incidence at different sites, as reported to a central cancer registry.[9] Differences between rural areas, small towns, and large towns may be owing to differences in diagnostic facilities, the availability of histologic and autopsy services, and so on. Fashions in diagnosis, particularly histologic, may produce an apparent but spurious increase in incidence of a given tumor. The prostate of course is a good example of this. Prostate glands from men over 50 years are commonly found to have "latent" cancers on histologic examination. Thus, increasingly effective histologic studies will increase the incidence of prostatic cancers diagnosed. These must find their way into the total incidence figures, since histologically there is no way of distinguishing them from any other cancer.

Similarly, there appears to be an increased incidence of cases of prostatic cancer in patients with bladder tumors. It is possible that this only reflects the increased likelihood of a prostatic examination in patients being routinely examined for another genitourinary cancer.[10] Even assuming that all cases are diagnosed correctly and reported to a central registry, they must be related to the total population so that accurate census figures are also required. Given that the conditions in Denmark are likely to be the best that can be obtained in an imperfect world, there are still variations in incidence in cancers of various sites which follow a Poisson distribution,[9] so that figures for a sufficiently long period must be collected.

In less well-developed societies these problems are even more marked. An obvious problem in the investigation of a disease of the elderly in such a society is that only a small proportion survives to old age. Although this may be corrected statistically, it cannot allow for an element of selection. A less obvious problem is concerned with the social acceptance of illness. This is well illustrated in a series of cases reported from Indonesia by Tan.[11] He showed that prostatic hyperplasia and cancer were present quite frequently in an Indonesian population, although clinical prostatic disease was said to be very rare. In biopsies from 337 patients over 40 years of age, prostatic cancers were found in 28, and 55 of 208 patients were found to have benign nodular hyperplasia. Further questioning of these Indonesian patients showed that they did indeed have complaints but that they had grown accustomed to their symptoms and had accepted them as a natural thing. Any interpretation of statistics on the incidence of prostatic disease must therefore be treated with caution, and it must take into account factors of this sort in addition to the more obvious causes of underdiagnosis in less prosperous societies.

Even taking these possible sources of error into account, there seem to be some remarkable racial and geographical differences in incidence. The racial incidence of prostatic cancer was discussed by Steiner,[12] who reviewed the earlier work on this subject. It has been recognized for over 40 years that the clinical entity was very rare in the yellow races. Nagayo (quoted by Steiner) reported that in over 12,000 autopsies in Tokyo only 5 prostatic cancers were found (0.45% of all cancers in males). In China too the incidence was low: no case in 106 autopsies or in 303 surgical specimens,[13] and only one case in 821 histologically diagnosed carcinomas.[14]

Steiner also reported that the disease was rare in Filipinos and Mexicans. More recent work has amplified and extended these findings. Mortality and morbidity data are similar. The only consistent finding is the low incidence in yellow races, but there is a remarkable variation in incidence in other races. The highest rate (age adjusted morbidity rate) is that for Negroes in one particular area of the United States (Alameda County) of 65.3, whereas the whites in the same area have a rate of 38.0. This compares with a rate for 10 cities in the United States of 49.9 for non-whites and 34.8 for whites. The regional variations are even more striking, varying from 17.1 for non-Latin Texans to 37.8 for urban inhabitants of Iowa. The extremes in Canada range from 17.0 in Newfoundland to 39 in Saskatchewan. In South and Central America, Chile has a rate of 11.3 and Colombia, 23.3.

Other continents show a similar variation. In Africa the rate varies from 4.4 in Uganda to 29.1 in Rhodesia. There are apparently inexplicable variations such as a rate of 19.2 for Bantu in Cape Province compared with 9.4 for Bantu in Johannesburg. The rate in Indians (6.5 in Bombay, 9.4 in Natal) is low, as is that in eastern

Europe (e.g., Poland, 4.6–12.8) and Israel (3.1 for non-Jews to 10.8–13.2 for Jews). New Zealand has a consistently high rate — 40.0 for Europeans and 40.3 for Maoris. The Japanese in Japan have a consistently low rate (3.2–4.3). There are no comparable figures for China, but the rate for Chinese in Singapore is 0.9.

SIGNIFICANT DIFFERENCES IN RACIAL DISTRIBUTION

It is difficult to place any reliance on minor differences, but the incidence in yellow races is so greatly and consistently lower than it is in other groups that it can be confidently accepted, even though more critical studies may introduce minor variations in detail. It seems likely too that the high incidence in some groups of American blacks and in New Zealand can probably be accepted. The significance of lesser differences, e.g., between eastern and western Europe is less certain. If the differences are owing to environment, they should be affected by migration. Unfortunately, available results at present are confusing. Haenszel and Kurihara[15] made an exhaustive comparison of the incidence of cancer and other diseases in Japanese in Japan, Japanese immigrants to the United States (Issei), and their United States-born offspring (Nissei and Sansei). The pattern of change in incidence was not consistent. The stomach cancer incidence remained about the same, but colon cancer incidence increased. Breast cancer in women remained low. Prostate cancer incidence rose but to nowhere near the incidence in Caucasians. The figures given by Haenszel and Kurihara[15] are:

	(age specific mortality rates)	
	65–74 yrs	75 yrs and over
Japan	11.6	28
Issei	40.2	130.0
U.S. whites	92.6	307.5

There are no figures as yet for descendants of Japanese migrants. The original paper should be consulted for details and for a discussion of the influence of an "imported environment."

Other migrants from low incidence areas, particularly from eastern Europe, also show a rise in incidence.[16] This American experience with migrants and the high incidence in two dissimilar racial groups in New Zealand suggest that possible environmental factors may be concerned. Yet other figures, e.g., from Hawaii where significant environmental factors appear to vary little between the races, give widely varying incidence between the races, but the figures for Japanese are higher than for native Japanese: Caucasians (43.4), Hawaiians (30.0), Filipinos (17.6), Japanese (13.9), and Chinese (9.8).

A final but important point is that the incidence of latent cancers is much higher than that of clinical cancers in all races. Even in the yellow races it is not uncommon, as has already been noted. Akazaki and Stemmermann[2] also report that the proliferative type of latent carcinoma is commoner in Hawaiian Japanese and suggest that growth factors may be environmental in origin.

AGE AND RACIAL INCIDENCE

Ashley made a mathematical study of age-associated incidence rates of latent and clinical prostatic cancers.[17] When the data for latent tumors were plotted on a double logarithmic scale, there was a straight-line relationship between frequency and age, frequency varying with the third power of the age. When a similar plot was made for clinical cancers, a similar relationship was found but the slope was steeper, corresponding to the seventh power of the age. According to the "multiple hit" theory of carcinogenesis originally proposed by Armitage and Doll,[18] Ashley suggests that this supports the idea that latent cancer is the result of smaller number of hits than clinical cancer.

Doll[6] discusses the mathematical basis for the multiple hit theory and concludes that:

1. A rapid and progressive increase in incidence of cancer with age suggests that the tissue is regularly exposed to a carcinogenic agent over a long period.
2. For those cancers that increase rapidly in incidence with age, the relationship between incidence and age can be described by the equation:

$$I = b(t - w)^k$$

where I is the incidence, t is the age, w is the sum of the preexposure period and the time between the beginning of the tumor and clinical recognition, b is proportional to the mean daily dose of the agents, and k is approximately 4. $(t - w)$ can also be defined as the duration of effective exposure and b as the mean dose per mitotic cycle.
3. An unusually rapid increase in incidence with age may be owing to a long preexposure period, a prolonged development time, or a reduction in the exposure of successive cohorts to environmental carcinogens.

Latent cancers even in low incidence groups suggest that in accepting the multistage hypothesis of carcinogenesis, the initiation stage may commonly occur. As Doll[6] suggests, the increasing frequency with age may be due to the increased exposure to a hypothetical carcinogen or it may be a direct or indirect consequence of the process of aging. The further development of the neoplastic process may then depend on promoting factors which may be environmental or genetic. The fact that other hormone-related cancers such as breast, ovary and endometrium are also low in Japan,[16] does not suggest that there may be a possible common endocrine basis. This again may be owing to differences in the endocrine environment, i.e., hormone secretion pattern, or to differences in cellular responsiveness. Both are well-known phenomena in different strains of experimental animals. Although differences in endocrine pattern have been reported in Japanese, there is little information about other low incidence groups.

HORMONES AND PROSTATIC CANCER

Since the hormones were first shown to have an effect on the prostate, they have usually been considered to play a primary role in prostatic carcinogenesis, although the evidence for this is slight. Much is known about the endocrine control of prostatic growth and function in animals,[19,20] but little of this information is directly applicable to changes in man because of the wide variation in species response to different hormones. Studies in man have been less extensive and most concerned with the measurement of steroid hormone levels in blood or urine. These have shown that there seems to be no direct relationship between steroid hormone levels — estrogens, androgens, or adrenal steroids — in the blood or urine and the development of prostatic cancer.[21-23] Pituitary hormones, which may possibly be involved, have not been intensively studied mainly because suitable methods have only recently become available.[24]

An added drawback to endocrine studies is that most of them have been carried out after the disease has been diagnosed and it is probable that if there is an endocrine basis, the critical changes may have taken place many years before clinical symptoms appear. All of these endocrine studies are based on the assumption that changes occur in the humoral environment, but we must also consider the possibility that there may be a primary cellular change in responsiveness to hormones. A detailed study using modern methods[25] of changes in steroid metabolism by prostatic cells during aging may give useful information.

Sommers[26] and Harbitz and Haugen in a large series of cases (see reference 27 for review and references) approached the problem in a different way by a morphometric analysis of the prostate and a series of endocrine organs.

They studied the interrelations between certain morphologic characteristics of the pituitary gland, the adrenal glands, and the testes in men with benign hyperplasia, carcinoma, atypical glandular proliferation, and normal histology of the prostate in an autopsy series and analyzed the findings by the use of multiple regression. As estimated from the quantitative morphology of the testes and the adrenal glands, small pituitary adenomas, which were frequent in patients with carcinoma of the prostate, were apparently not related to an insufficiency in these organs. In the analyses of the relationships between several endocrine parameters, only few significant correlations emerged. In men with benign hyperplasia, carcinoma plus benign hyperplasia and atypical glandular proliferation plus benign hyperplasia, a strong, positive relationship between the seminiferous tubule weight and the number of Sertoli cells was observed. It is suggested that hormones produced by the Sertoli cells are of major importance for the maintenance of the germinative epithelium and may also be involved in the pathogenesis of hyperplastic and neoplastic growth of the prostate.

From their comprehensive study, it is concluded that both benign hyperplasia and carcinoma are associated with a progressive involution of the gonads, which most likely originates in the testis itself. Their findings indicated that the stimulus to benign hyperplasia could come from nonandrogenic hormones (estrogens?), either alone or together with pituitary trophic hormones. The marked decline of the Leydig cell mass with age, observed in individuals with carcinoma, suggests that prostatic carcinoma develops against a background of progressive androgen deprivation.

Since prostatic cancer and benign enlargement do not occur in eunuchs or true eunuchoids,[28] some androgenic stimulation seems to be necessary. It is reasonable to assume that the main part played by the hormones is to stimulate the development and maintenance of the prostatic epithelium so that a sufficient number of cells is present in which malignant change can occur. The hormones may play no part in the actual process of carcinogenesis. Once a tumor has developed, the neoplastic cells may remain responsive to the factors that control normal growth, provided the cells still retain these particular normal differentiated characters.[29]

LOCAL AND OTHER INFLUENCES ON INCIDENCE

Many other factors have been considered, including socioeconomic status, marital status, fertility, social and sexual habits, previous diseases, height, weight, hair distribution, religion, place of birth, family history, diet, blood group, and others (summarized by King et al.[30] and by Wynder et al.[16]). No significant relationship has been found.

So far all the factors herein discussed have been general factors which influence all cells in the gland. But since cancer is a focal disturbance, we must also consider cellular factors that influence the development of a tumor in one localized area, although admittedly in cells that may have been altered by general factors. Again, we have no real knowledge of possible localizing factors, but there is a suggestion[31,32] that a type of atrophy associated with focal fibrosis may be followed by a precancerous hyperplasia. There is little evidence to incriminate other localizing factors, although many have been suggested.

A further unexplained fact is the finding that prostatic cancer almost invariably begins in the outer zone of the gland — the prostate proper[1] — although there is still some confusion over the terminology used to describe the various prostatic lobes.[33] Since benign prostatic enlargement begins in the inner glands, there seems to be a local cellular predisposition to malignant change in the outer glands.

References

1. Franks, L. M.: Latent carcinoma of the prostate. J. Pathol. Bacteriol. 68:603, 1954.
2. Akazaki, K., and Stemmermann, G. N.: Comparative study of latent carcinoma of the prostate among Japanese in Japan and Hawaii. J. Natl. Cancer Inst. 50:1137, 1973.
3. Gaynor, E. P.: Zur Frage des Prostatakrebses. Virchows Arch. Pathol. Anat. 301:602, 1938.
4. Misa, Y.: A histopathological study on latent carcinoma of the prostate among the Japanese. Jap. J. Cancer Clin. 7:304, 1961.
5. Tazaki, H.: Pathological studies on the prostate glands of Japanese, with special reference to latent malignancy. Keio J. Med. 11:253, 1962.
6. Doll, R.: The age distribution of cancer in man. In Thule International Symposia — Cancer and Aging. Stockholm, Nordiska Bokhandelns Förlag, 1968. p. 15.
7. Little, C. C.: The relation of age to the incidence of cancer of certain sites. Proc. Natl. Acad. Sci. 52:865, 1964.
8. Franks, L. M.: The spread of prostatic cancer. J. Pathol. Bacteriol. 72:603, 1956.
9. Clemmesen, J.: Statistical studies in the aetiology of malignant neoplasms. Acta Pathol. Microbiol. Scand. Suppl. 174, I & II, 1965.
10. Clemmesen, J. and Nielsen, A.: Cancer incidence in Denmark 1943 to 1953. Dan. Med. Bull. 3:33, 1956.
11. Tan, R. E.: Prostatic disease in Indonesia. J. Urol. 86:428, 1961.
12. Steiner, P. E.: Cancer: Race and Geography. Baltimore, Williams and Wilkins, 1954.
13. Heine, J.: Über Geschwülste bei Chinesen. Z. Krebsforsch. 33:529, 1931.
14. Hu, C. H., and Ch'in, K. Y.: A statistical study of 2,179 tumors occurring in the Chinese. Chin. Med. J. 50:43, 1936.
15. Haenszel, W., and Kurihara, M.: Studies of Japanese migrants. 1. Mortality from cancer and other diseases among Japanese in the United States. J. Natl. Cancer Inst. 40:43, 1968.
16. Wynder, E. L., Mabuchi, K. and Whitmore, W. F. Jr.: Epidemiology of cancer of the prostate. Cancer 28:344, 1971.
17. Ashley, D. J. B.: On the incidence of carcinoma of the prostate. J. Pathol. Bacteriol. 90:217, 1965.
18. Armitage, P., and Doll, R.: A two-stage theory of carcinogenesis in relation to the age distribution of human cancer. Br. J. Cancer 11:161, 1957.
19. Ofner, P.: Effects and metabolism of hormones in normal and neoplastic prostate tissue. Vitam. Horm. 26:237, 1968.
20. Farnsworth, W. E.: The normal prostate and its endocrine control. In Some Aspects of the Aetiology and Biochemistry of Prostatic Cancer. 3rd Tenovus Workshop. Edited by K. Griffiths, and C. G. Pierrepoint. Cardiff, Tenovus Workshop Publications, 1970. p. 3–15.
21. Bulbrook, R. D., Franks, L. M., and Greenwood, F. C.: Hormone excretion in prostatic cancer: The early and late effects of endocrine treatment on urinary oestrogens, 17-ketosteroids and 17-ketogenic steroids. Acta Endocrinol. (Kbh) 31:481, 1959.
22. Marmorston, J., Lombardo, L. J. Jr., Myers, S. M., et al.: Urinary excretion of neutral 17-ketosteroids and pregnanediol by patients with prostatic cancer and benign prostatic hypertrophy. J. Urol. 93:276, 1965.
23. Robinson, M. R. G., and Thomas, B. S.: Effect of hormonal therapy on plasma testosterone levels in prostatic carcinoma. Br. Med. J. 4:391, 1971.
24. Reynoso, G., and Murphy, G. P.: Adrenalectomy and hypophysectomy in advanced prostatic carcinoma. Cancer 29:941, 1972.
25. Ruokonen, A., Laatikainen, T., Laitinen, E. A., et al.: Free and sulfate-conjugated neutral steroids in human testis tissue. Biochem. 11:1411, 1972.
26. Sommers, S. C.: Endocrine changes with prostatic carcinoma. Cancer 10:345, 1957.
27. Harbitz, T. B., and Haugen, O. A.: Endocrine disturbances in men with benign hyperplasia and carcinoma of the prostate. In Endocrine Aspects of Benign Hyperplasia and Carcinoma of the Human Prostate. Oslo, 1974.
28. Moore, R. A. In Endocrinology of Neoplastic Disease, New York, Oxford University Press, 1947. p. 194.
29. Franks, L. M.: Some comments on the long-term results of endocrine treatment of prostatic cancer. Br. J. Urol. 30:383, 1958.
30. King, H., Diamond, E., and Lilienfeld, A. M.: Some epidemiological aspects of cancer of the prostate. J. Chron. Dis. 16:117, 1963.
31. Moore, R. A.: The evolution and involution of the prostate gland. Amer. J. Pathol. 12:599, 1935.
32. Franks, L. M.: Atrophy and hyperplasia in the prostate proper. J. Pathol. Bacteriol. 68:617, 1954.
33. McNeal, J. E.: Origin and development of carcinoma in the prostate. Cancer 23:24, 1969.

Part II

Evaluation of Prostatic Disease

Chapter 4

Immunobiology of the Prostate

RICHARD J. ABLIN

Clinical and experimental investigations, notably from studies of leukemic,[1] melanotic,[2] and sarcomatous[3] tissue, have brought forth a substantial body of evidence suggesting that factors of host resistance, mediated to a large extent by parameters of specific, as well as nonspecific immunologic responsiveness, are involved in the development and modulation of malignancy. The concept that host resistance and immunobiologic factors might be associated with malignancy was considered as early as 1900 by Ehrlich.[4] Since the initial demonstration of tumor-specific antigens in animal-induced neoplasms by Foley[5] and by Prehn and Main,[6] the association of malignancy and immunology has led to a better understanding of some of the intricacies of the tumor-host relationship. The identification of tumor-specific and tumor-associated antigens (TAA) and the ability of the host to develop an immunologic response to these antigens forms in part the basis of Burnet's theory[7] of immunologic surveillance, i.e., tumor cells arising on a continuing basis in the host are eliminated because of their foreignness. However, when these tumor cells evade the host's immunologic surveillance system or when the system becomes impaired, whether as a result of genetic defect, infection, or immunosuppression, they may proliferate and lead to overt malignancy.

The immunologic surveillance system, as we know it now, may functionally be manifested into two components: cell-mediated and humoral immunity. This dichotomy into a cellular and a humoral response traces its origin to a common precursor stem cell found in liver and spleen prior to birth and in the adult bone marrow. As a consequence of the influence of different microenvironmental factors on this stem cell population, two separate lines of cell populations are suggested to have arisen.

Lymphocytes concerned with cell-mediated responses appear to come under the influence of the thymus and are thus referred to as *thymic-dependent*. Thymic-dependent lymphocytes (T-cells) may react directly with antigens on foreign cells and initiate a cytotoxic reaction leading to their destruction. T-cells are associated with the familiar delayed-type hypersensitivity reaction to tuberculin and homograft rejection and also may function as "helper" cells in the humoral antibody response to certain antigens.

The second component, humoral immunity, is characterized by specific immunoglobulins (Ig), e.g., IgG, IgA, and IgM, in the blood and tissue fluids synthesized by plasma cells. Those cells concerned with the formation of immunoglobulins and serum antibodies appear to come under the influence of the bursal-dependent system (in birds) commonly referred to as *thymic-independent*. When stimulated, thymic-independent lymphocytes (B-cells) differentiate into plasma cells. Circulating antibodies may then combine with antigens, facilitating their elimination.

To be effective, both components of specific immunologic responsiveness depend on polymorphonuclear leukocytes and macrophages, which may also participate nonspecifically. In general, the response of the host to bacterial infections appears to be largely dependent on humoral mechanisms. The response to viruses and perhaps, as suggested from recent studies, to tumor cells also depends predominantly on cellular mechanisms. The potential role of cytotoxic antibodies in tumor destruction or antitumor antibody as a means by which antitumor agents may be transported to the tumor surface should not be discounted.

These brief introductory comments with regard to some of the fundamental considerations of the immune response, while obviously far from complete, shall hopefully serve as a background. For more details the reader may refer to a recent synopsis of basic immunologic definitions and concepts employed in the majority of the studies to be presented[8] or to other more comprehensive treatises on the subject.[9-11]

RATIONALE

Investigative efforts of genitourinary tumors, notably of the bladder and prostate, have received increasing attention within the past few years. In this regard it would appear that: (1.) attention to the diverse behavior of the natural history of prostate adenocarcinoma in man suggested that host responses may play a significant role in the pathogenesis of this disease;[12] (2.) the advent and successful application of cryosurgery for the treatment of many, otherwise inoperable cases of benign and malignant diseases of the prostate[13-32] prompted questions about the possible immunologic effect of cryogenic destruction of prostatic tissue;[33-37] and (3.) observations of localized eradication of prostatic malignancy and of metastatic tumor cell destruction in patients following cryotherapy of their primary prostatic tumor[22,24,25,27] suggested that some form of augmented host resistance, possibly of an immunologic nature, existed as a plausible explanation for cellular destruction occurring beyond the freeze site.[22,24,25] These and other factors recently reviewed[8,38] have prompted clinical and experimental investigations suggestive of the participation of immunobiologic factors in prostatic diseases.

Ethical considerations, as well as the lack of readily accessible or adaptable animal models, have limited initial investigations of the immunologic properties of prostatic tissue and other associated sexual glands to various animal species. Nevertheless, invaluable information has been obtained. These data, although not completely applicable to man, have contributed much to the development of methodologies suitable not only for investigating immunobiologic factors in the pathogenesis of the human prostate, but also for implementing improved methods of diagnosis, prognosis, and therapies.

Two recent reviews have dealt with much of the early experimental developments leading to our present state of knowledge of the immunologic properties of prostatic tissue of various laboratory animal species.[8,38] To avoid being repetitious I will consider in the "Experimental" section only those investigations which have not, for the most part, previously been considered and which would appear to contribute to our understanding of similar, but as yet unresolved, problems in man. As concerns consideration of data which I believe to fall under the broad heading of "Clinical," I will again attempt to focus primarily on salient findings heretofore not considered. However, for the sake of completeness, and thus by necessity, there will be some repetition.

Admittedly, while the investigations presented are those with which the author is most familiar, it is hoped that they may be regarded as reasonably comprehensive. In this regard I believe it appropriate at this juncture to state frankly that, as the body of knowledge in this field is growing so rapidly, complete coverage of the present subject is rapidly approaching book proportions.

EXPERIMENTAL CONSIDERATIONS

The study of prostatic cancer in man, despite the successful application of various disciplines, has been restricted in part due to ethical considerations but perhaps more so because there is no suitable experimental animal model of human prostatic cancer. Therefore as I visualize it two divergent experimental approaches to this dilemma have been pursued.

In the first approach, there have been continued efforts on the part of numerous investigators to pursue studies of comparative biochemistry, histology, and morphology of the prostate and to induce a model prostatic tumor in animals that would resemble its human counterpart in terms of acid phosphatase production, chromosomal composition, hormonal responsiveness, and pathology.

In the second instance (perhaps an indirect approach), the natural history of prostatic cancer in man suggested that host responses, possibly of an immunologic nature, may play a significant part in the pathogenesis of the prostate.[12] This observation, together with other factors previously enumerated, has led several investigators to consider evaluation of the immunologic properties of prostatic tissue, as well as the participation of various parameters of cellular and humorally mediated immunologic responsiveness. In this regard, investigation of the autoimmune response obtained following parenteral hetero-, iso-, and autostimulation with preparations of prostatic tissues and secretions or cryo (freezing in situ) stimulation in laboratory animals seems to have been of value.

Induction of Prostatic Cancer

Except for recent reports, prostatic induced cancer in laboratory animals has not been evaluated immunologically.[39–41b]

In one report, tumor specific transplantation immunity to an acid phosphatase-secreting tumor of hamster prostatic tissue transformed in vitro with simian virus 40 [SV40 (an oncogenic DNA virus)] model introduced by Paulson et al.[42] has been evaluated following in situ cryosurgical tumor destruction and surgical excision.[39] As such, discussion of this model is deferred to the subsequent consideration of the effect of cryosurgery on prostatic induced tumors (page 43).

Abdalla and Oliver[39a] have reported on the induction and transplantation of a 3-methylcholanthrene-transformed human prostatic tumor from benign human prostatic tissue in Syrian golden hamsters possessing characteristics of its human counterpart. Studies directed toward demonstrating tumor-specific antibodies were negative.[39a] Experience with this model in our laboratory resulted in development of an anaplastic cell sarcoma rather than a carcinoma.[39b]

MA160 cells derived in tissue culture from a benign prostatic adenoma have been successfully transplanted into nonimmunosuppressed hamsters.[40]

Chromosomal studies of these tumors showed that their make-up was similar to that of man, and immunologic tests failed to implicate any of the common DNA or RNA hamster tumor viruses. Sera from tumor-bearing hamsters did not react by immunofluorescence or complement-fixation with the T or neoantigen of SV40 viruses. In addition, no complement-fixation reaction was observed between sera from tumor-bearing animals and extracts of tumors induced with Moloney sarcoma virus.

Of particular interest was the observation that progressive tumor growth of this transplanted tumor was dependent on a globulin antibody present in the serum of tumor-bearing animals. This was observed, by immunofluorescence, to bind to the membrane of viable tumor cells. The intensity of the immunofluorescence staining appeared to be related to the size of the tumor. By contrast, in those animals in which tumor had regressed, reaction between their sera and viable tumor cells was negative. In view of the absence of demonstrable complement-dependent or independent cytotoxicity of the sera against MA160 tumor-derived tissue culture cells, the possible tumor "enhancing" nature of this globulin may be of particular significance as related to circulating antibodies observed in patients with prostatic cancer reactive with the cytoplasmic membrane of prostatic secretory epithelial cells (Figure 4–5 [148,149a]).

Irradiated male adult hamsters previously immunized with cell suspensions from 10-day-old Syrian golden hamster fetuses, were challenged with SV40 transformed hamster prostatic tissue.[41] The development of tumors in control animals (not previously immunized) and of animals immunized with normal kidney and liver cells, in contrast to failure of animals immunized with fetal tissue to develop tumors, suggested to these investigators the presence of cross-reactivity between TAA present in SV40 transformed prostatic tissue and fetal antigens.[41]

Results of a recent study[41a] of the antigenic characteristics of methylcholanthrene-induced prostatic tumors in the rat disclosed the presence of species-specific antigens. However, as in a previous study of methylcholanthrene-induced prostatic tumors,[39a] tumor-specific antigens were not identifiable.[41a]

Absence of tumor-specific antigens in methylcholanthrene-induced prostatic tumors, the inability of such tumors to engender a specific immune response, and the earlier comments by Bishop[41b] of the failure of prostatic (accessory gland tissues) implants to be rejected, may provide some explanation for the failure of patients with prostatic cancer to reject their tumors, as perhaps best exemplified in patients with occult carcinomas. These observations, together with our present understanding of the nature of the immune response following experimental cryosurgery,[38] essentially form the basis in part for the recent hypothesis[267] of the prostate as an immunologically privileged site. Interestingly, the rather early and astute observations of Bishop[41b] have not been cited in this regard.

Parenteral and Cryostimulation

By parenteral or cryostimulation an immunologic response to prostatic, other accessory gland tissues, and secretions of reproduction of various laboratory animals was developed. The evaluation of this response by parameters of cellular and humoral-mediated immunity has provided a most suitable means for investigating their antigenic properties and the immunopathogenic effects of prostatic and other accessory gland antibodies.[8] Studies have been directed toward the: (1.) Elucidation of in situ autosensitization following cryostimulation of the prostate. (It should be noted that the portion of the prostate subjected to in situ freezing in the male rabbit was the anterior prostate, more commonly referred to as the coagulating gland.) This involves identification and mechanism of release of the autoantigen. Does its antigenicity depend upon in situ freeze-thaw induced molecular alteration and its subsequent encounter with immunologically competent cells (T- and/or B-cells)? (2.) Androgenic and ontogenic dependence of the antigenicity of accessory gland tissues and secretions; (3.) Immunopathogenic effect of accessory gland antibodies; and (4.) Effects of cryosurgery on experimentally induced prostatic and nonprostatic tumors.

The Immune Response Following Cryostimulation

Immunologic studies of rabbit accessory gland tissues and secretions[43-46] have led to the identification of a secretory product of the coagulating and prostate glands which has been termed "coagulo-prostatic fluid" (CPF).[47] Coaguloprostatic fluid possesses the major soluble autoantigenic components of the coagulating and prostate glands. Whether CPF may be synonymous with or related to the heat-labile enzyme termed "vesiculase" secreted by the coagulating gland of the rat and guinea pig[48] or to the kallikrein-like enzyme "cobayin" present in the coagulating, prostate, and seminal vesicles of the guinea pig[49] remains to be determined. Evaluation and comparison of hetero- and isoimmune sera to CPF with sera obtained following cryostimulation demonstrate a common specificity for these antibodies.[46] This initial observation led Ablin et al.[34] to suggest that the development of antibodies following in situ freezing may be attributed to the liberation of this normally sequestered secretory product from prostatic epithelial cells after freezing damage. Additional evidence in support of this hypothesis comes from studies in which the intensity of the immune response following cryostimulation was shown to be dependent upon the concentration of androgenically and ontogenically dependent autoantigens present in the target organ at freezing time,[50,50a,52a,54] and of the

response of rabbits to endogenous secretions introduced into the abdominal cavity through cannulation of the coagulating gland.[53a]

Fractionation studies of CPF identifying an antigen-rich fraction sensitive to freeze-thaw treatment led Bronson et al.[51] to suggest that the immune response following cryostimulation may alternately be attributed to denaturative changes as the result of in situ freeze-thaw alterations rendering "self" into "non-self."

Further elucidation of the mechanisms operative in the development of an immune response following cryostimulation has evolved from attempts to characterize some of the physicochemical properties of CPF.

Gel diffusion precipitation and immunoelectrophoretic studies employing monospecific antisera to rabbit immunoglobulin G (IgG) and whole rabbit serum, initially suggested the presence of IgG in CPF.[44] It was confirmed by immunofluorescence that the in vivo rabbit IgG is bound to focal accumulations of secretory granules lying within the lumina of coagulating and prostatic tissue acini (Figure 4–1A) and also to secretory granules in preparations of CPF smears (Figure 4–1B).[45]

Collation of these findings, i.e., (1.) the identification of the common specificity of parenterally[46] and cannulated[53a] induced antibodies to CPF and to antibodies developed following cryostimulation[34] and (2.) the presence of IgG in CPF,[44,45] together with histologic studies[52] (Figure 4–2), suggests that both hypotheses of the mechanism(s) operative in the development of an immune response following in situ freezing may be applicable. CPF, normally a potent sequestered antigen, may upon release owe a portion of its antigenicity to its autologous IgG content, which as a result of freezing damage may undergo structural modification from its native state in the circulation.

Cryosurgical procedures designed to

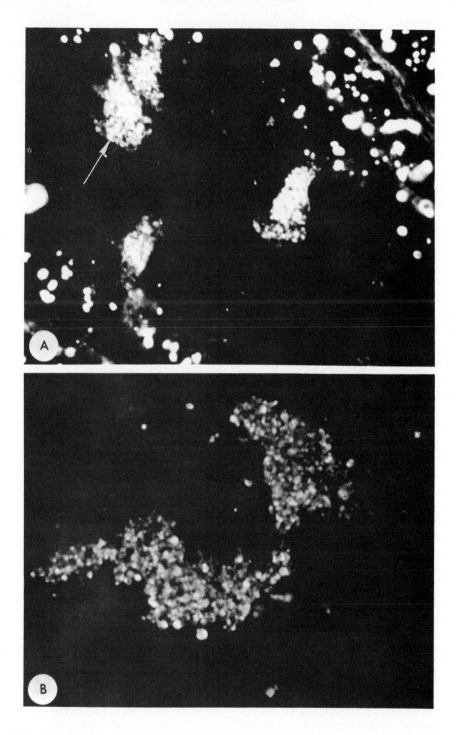

Figure 4–1. Photomicrographs of direct immunofluorescent staining reactions demonstrating in vivo binding of rabbit immunoglobulin G to *(A)* accumulations of secretory granules (arrow) in the lumina of the acini of the rabbit coagulating gland (× 600 with oil); and to *(B)* secretory granules present in preparations of smear of coaguloprostatic fluid (× 400 with oil). (From Ablin.[45])

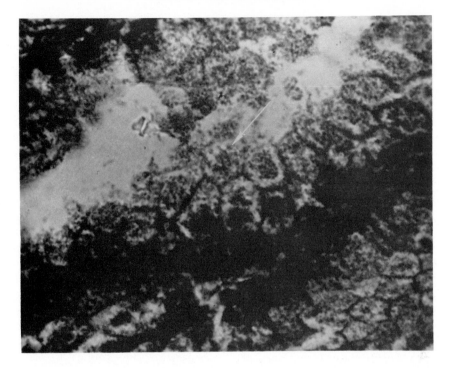

Figure 4–2. Photomicrograph of cross-section of hematoxylin and eosin preparation of rabbit prostate illustrating liberation of secretory granules (arrow) following in situ freezing (× 400 with oil).

evaluate the effects of multiple in situ freezing of the canine and subhuman primate prostate (the latter of which is considered further under Androgenic and Ontogenic Dependence of Antigenicity) have been carried out. Although both species appeared to develop antibodies, notably more so in the monkey, following in situ freezing of their prostate glands, these antibodies were not of the intensity or specificity of those previously described in the rabbit following comparable treatment.

Androgenic and Ontogenic Dependence of Antigenicity

Studies to determine the mechanism(s) of in situ autosensitization following cryostimulation have suggested that the development of antibodies may be attributed to the liberation of the naturally occurring but yet sequestered secretory product of prostatic epithelial cells termed CPF.[47,52] Until recently, however, factors determining observations of the variance in the incidence and magnitude of the antibody response following cryostimulation were not fully resolved. Earlier observations suggesting a correlation between the intensity of the immune response and differences in the size, i.e., fullness of glandular secretions (observed at the time of surgery[33,34]), and physiologic activity of the prostate,[53] together with knowledge of the source of the autoantigen and of the androgenic dependence of the prostate, suggested that factors altering its synthesis would affect its antigenicity, and thus the incidence and magnitude of the immune response elicited. This suggested androgenic and ontogenic dependency has been evaluated by comparison of the development of the immune response as determined by tanned cell hemagglutination of cryostimulated and subsequently parenterally stimulated normal, androgen- (testosterone), and estrogen-treated orchidectomized and nonhormonally-treated orchidectomized and androgen-treated immature (prepuberal) and nonandrogen-treated immature and mature rabbits.[50,50a,52a,54]

Androgen-treated orchidectomized animals yielded consistently high titers of antibody following cryostimulation and secondary (anamnestic) responses following subsequent parenteral stimulation. In contrast, cryostimulation of estrogen-treated orchidectomized and normal animals yielded low, variable primary antibody titers followed by a secondary antibody response to parenteral stimulation which was of the magnitude and immunoglobulin class (as characterized by its sensitivity to 2-mercaptoethanol) of a primary response.

Higher titers of antibody, although of a greater variation in magnitude, were observed in mature than in immature animals following cryostimulation. However, following receipt of androgen supplementation for 4 weeks, beginning at 4 weeks of age, immature animals not responding (e.g., at 8 weeks of age) did respond equally well or better than normal mature animals. Similar observations employing parenteral stimulation alone have recently been reported.[54a]

Observations of these recent studies point to the presence of androgenically and ontogenically dependent autoantigens of the prostate, presumably present in CPF. The presence of analogs of such antigens in man and their relationship to the development and magnitude of the immune response elicited following cryostimulation may be significant in the consideration of the patient with prostatic cancer for cryosurgery, if he has previously received estrogenic and/or surgically ablative hormonal therapy. As such, these factors have been considered to be contributory to what has been termed the "cryosensitivity"[34,54,54b] of the host.

Further documentation of the significance of cryosensitivity at the experimental level may be gleaned from recent studies of humoral immunologic responsiveness in the monkey following cryostimulation of the prostate.[57]

Immunologic studies demonstrating cross-reactivity of human and monkey prostatic tissue-specific antigens[56] and antibodies to human prostatic fluid[50] and in prostatic cancer patients[148-149a] reactive with monkey prostatic tissue suggested the monkey as a potential experimental model for the induction of prostatic cancer and the subsequent evaluation of the treatment of prostatic malignancy by cryotherapy. In an initial inquiry of this possibility, a representative proportion of monkeys developed circulating antibodies to prostatic tissue following multiple in situ freezing of their prostate.[57] The intensity of the humoral response was considerably modest, however, when compared to that obtained in rabbits following similar treatment.[33,34,36] Furthermore, this response did not appear to increase to any significant degree following multiple freezing.[33a,34,37] By way of explanation, the possible relationship of the modest humoral response to the cryosensitivity of the target organ and of the animals evaluated—i.e., the concentration of glandular secretions (autoantigens), androgenic and ontogenic dependence, and immunocompetence—has been considered in view of their age and secretory activity.[57]

Other factors not evaluated but previously discussed[33a,34,35] may contribute to a variation in the intensity of the immune response following cryostimulation. This could include time-temperature profile (freeze-thaw velocities), genetic variation of a given animal responding to a given antigenic stimulus, and the inherent variance in antigenic preparations from one pool to another, or their adherence to coated erythrocytes, or both.

Nonetheless, it is important to reiterate that these empiric observations in the rabbit and monkey appear to be of particular significance in considering cryotherapy for treatment of the elderly human adult male with prostatic cancer or for that matter by other therapeutic modalities suggestive of being immunopotentiating. As such the concept of "cryosensitivity" shall be given further consideration in the subsequent discussion of the "prospective" approaches to immunotherapy of prostatic cancer.

Immunopathogenicity of Prostatic and Accessory Gland Antibodies

Although the immunologic properties of prostatic and other associated accessory gland tissues and secretions of various species have been studied extensively through the production of antibodies via parenteral or cryostimulation, few reports suggest the immunopathogenic effects of accessory gland antibodies in the "antibody producer." Antibody producer is specified in order to distinguish between histologic alterations observed following inoculation with antisera, e.g., in prostatic tissue, following isoimmunization with antisera possessing antibodies to prostatic tissue,[58,59] and prostatic fluid,[60] as considered in a recent review,[8] from alterations in the antibody producer.

Reports of histologic alterations in the antibody producer following immunization with components of accessory gland tissues or secretions: the production of autoimmune orchitis in the rabbit following autoimmunization with seminal plasma;[61] and infiltration and atrophy of the tubules of the guinea pig seminal vesicles following isoimmunization with guinea pig vesicular fluid, did not reveal any pathologic changes in the prostate.[62] Of interest, but apparently not associated with histologic alterations in the prostate, is the recent report of reproduction impairment in female rabbits following inoculation with CPF.[63] These observations, as well as those of Rosenmann et al.,[64] raise speculation about the existence of a hypersensitive state due to the possible presence of cross-reactivity of seminal plasma and prostatic fluid antigens in patients with diseases of the prostate, and the possible relationship of such a state to infertility as suggested initially by Flocks and co-workers.[65]

The initial report of the pathologic effect following immunization — isoimmunization in this case — with prostatic tissue and implicating the possible participation of cell-mediated immunologic responses was that of Nagakubo,[66] who observed atrophy and an eosinophilic staining of prostatic epithelial cells suggesting diminished secretory activity.

In a recent report, Yantorno et al.[67] observed a delayed type of hypersensitivity response with mononuclear infiltration and flattening and desquamation of prostatic epithelial cells in the rabbit following immunization with extracts of rabbit male accessory glands. However, similar histologic alterations were observed in other rabbits included in this study who received autologous native and chemically modified seminal plasma. The question arises of the relationship between the observed histologic alterations and their specificity, i.e., were these changes, as observed in the prostate, due to specific prostatic tissue antigens or to those of other accessory gland tissues and secretions included in the inoculum? Had these investigators immunized with specific tissue or secretory components or even evaluated their antisera and skin hypersensitivity assays with extracts of specific tissue or secretory components, the observed histologic alterations might have been more meaningful, at least in terms of specificity.

Immunopathogenic effects of antibodies implicated with the development of contralateral aspermatogenic orchitis[67a,67b] and epididymo-orchitis[67c] following cryosurgery of the rabbit testis and epididymis have been observed. Interestingly, the immunologic response in these

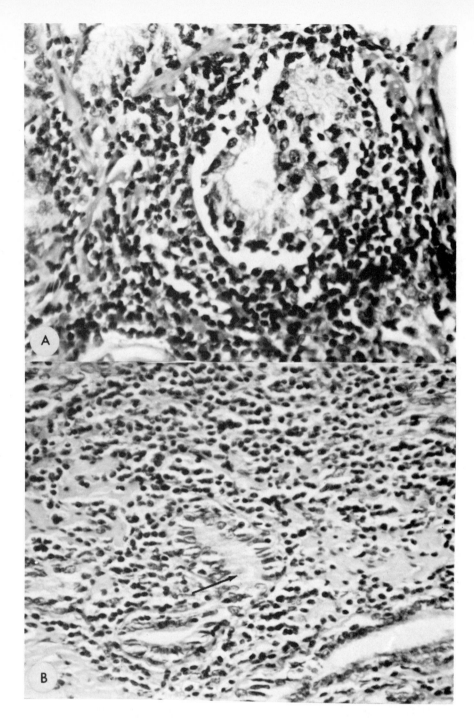

Figure 4–3. Photomicrographs of hematoxylin and eosin preparations of monkey prostatic tissue obtained at autopsy following multiple in situ freezing of the prostate. *A,* Section of caudal lobe containing large foci of cellular infiltrates composed predominantly of lymphocytes concentrically arranged around prostatic acinus as seen 41 days following the third of three independent freezes of the prostate. Separation of the basal lamina and destruction of acinar epithelial cells by lymphocytic infiltrates may also be seen (× 160). *B,* Caudal lobe in another animal as seen 49 days following the third of three independent freezes of the prostate, illustrating similar, but extensive and generalized, lymphocytic infiltration compared with that shown in *A.* Neutrophilic exudates (arrow) were observed in the lumina (possibly proteinaceous material admixed with neutrophils, the former observed in the section of rabbit prostate shown in Figure 4–1A) of some prostatic acini as yet not completely destroyed (× 160). (From Ablin and Reddy.[57a])

animals occurred predominantly at the cellular, rather than at the humoral, level.

Observations of the development of a modest response following cryostimulation of the monkey prostate[57] suggested, in light of the responses of the testis and epididymis, the possible occurrence and predominance of an immunologic response at the cellular rather than at the humoral level and of the ensuing immunopathologic effects of this response on the prostate. Investigation of this possibility disclosed a reduction in the size of the monkey prostate and histologic alterations characterized by what appeared to be specific periacinar foci of lymphocytic infiltrates.[57a] These lymphocytes were observed, as shown in Figure 4–3A, to infiltrate onto acinar epithelial cells, resulting in their subsequent separation from the basal lamina and epithelial cell destruction. This cellular response, though reasonably consistent in the animals evaluated, was, as shown from Figure 4–3B, illustrating similar but more extensive damage by surrounding lymphocytes, variable to some degree from one animal to another.

In consonance with observations of the prostate following cryosurgery,[13,27,67d] histologic alterations in the prostate of the animals evaluated were further characterized by stromal fibrosis, periodic presence of inflammatory cells, and proliferation of regenerating glands. Although present in the cranial and caudal lobes of the prostate, alterations were more frequently observed in the latter. Circulating prostatic antibodies were present in only one of the animals at the time at which histologic alterations were made.

It has been suggested[57a] that the cellular response observed in the monkey prostate was immunologically mediated through the reaction of lymphocytes that had become sensitized to prostatic epithelial cell antigens following freezing. These observations may be of potential significance toward further elucidating observations of the eradication of human prostatic carcinomas following cryosurgery.[24,25,27–28a,30–30b]

Cryosurgery on Prostatic and Nonprostatic-Induced Tumors

The effects of cryosurgery on in situ tumor destruction have been evaluated in animals with experimentally induced prostatic tumors[39] and nonprostatic induced tumors.[68–69c]

Following the initial report by Myers et al.,[68] demonstrating that tumor-specific transplantation immunity of methylcholanthrene-adenocarcinomas in syngeneic mice was greater following in situ freezing than surgical excision, Blackwood and Cooper[69] have confirmed these observations in rats possessing myosarcoma MT449A and carcinosarcoma Walker 256 transplanted tumors. They also demonstrated complement fixing antibodies in the sera of animals with complete tumor regression following cryosurgery. When tumors developed in animals possessing complement fixing antibodies induced by parenteral immunization with tumor antigen and transplanted with viable tumor cells, the complement fixing antibodies were not solely responsible for the observed tumor regression or inhibition of tumor growth when cryosurgically treated animals were challenged with viable tumor. Nevertheless, the presence of complement fixing antibodies in association with tumor regression following cryosurgery offers support to the earlier suggested implication of the participation of complement-mediated cytotoxic antibodies in patients with prostatic cancer as an explanation for observations of destruction of metastatic lesions following cryotherapy of their prostatic tumor.[24,25]

Of further interest were observations that suggested a threshold of antigenic stimulation, i.e., when tumors were grown at two loci and cryosurgery of one site induced regression in the second, the rate of tumor regression was inversely proportional to the amount of necrotic tissue remaining. Such findings are suggestive of the participation of antigen excess leading to the adsorption of antibody in vivo, thereby removing it from the circulation, and are consistent with the reported elution of cell-bound antibodies following cryosurgery.[150]

The effects and comparison of tumor-specific transplantation immunity following in situ freezing and surgical excision of hamster SV40 transformed prostatic tumors have been evaluated.[39] This tumor resembles human prostatic cancer in histology and by its production of elevated levels of serum acid phosphatase. Interestingly the levels of acid phosphatase and tartrate-inhibitable acid phosphatase were observed to return to normal in hamsters in which cryosurgery or surgical excision resulted in a cure. However, in contrast to the observation of greater tumor-specific transplantation immunity in syngeneic mice possessing nonprostatic chemical- and virus-induced tumors following cryosurgery, no differential immunity was observed when compared with that obtained following surgical excision of SV40 transformed hamster prostatic tumors.[69–69c] As an explanation for this difference, it is suggested that absence of differential immunity in the hamster model may be attributed to a functionally larger antigen dose per tumor cell in the SV40 tumors.[39]

CLINICAL CONSIDERATIONS

Based on the identification of a cellular and humoral basis of immunologic responsiveness, evaluation of parameters of these two broad categories has been applied toward investigating the possible participation of immunobiologic factors in the pathogenesis of human prostatic diseases. In the course of such investigations, some of these parameters — although limited at present — have shown promise not only of serving as adjunctive

aids to existing methods of diagnosis and prognosis, but also of providing a basis for implementing new and improved modes of therapy for treating patients with prostatic cancer.

Humoral Aspects

Serum and Urinary Proteins

Albumin, α_1-, α_2-, β- and γ-globulin. Observations of alteration of serum protein levels in a variety of diseases have been the subject of innumerable reports.[70,71] Electrophoretic separation and quantitation of five serum proteins (albumin, α_1-,α_2-, β- and γ-globulin) have been evaluated in patients with benign prostatic hypertrophy[72] and carcinoma of the prostate (Levy, Nora and Sandor, unpublished observations cited by Sandor[71] and other investigators.[71–73]). Patients with benign prostatic hypertrophy were observed to possess decreased levels of albumin and increased levels of α_1- and α_2-globulin, with elevated levels of α_2- and β-globulin being noted in patients with prostatic cancer. No significant alteration in the level of γ-globulin was noted in either group.

Systematic evaluation of serum protein levels in patients with prostatic cancer as related to the stage[74] of their malignancy[73] showed associated increased levels of α_2-globulin, and to a lesser extent of β-globulin. Increased levels of β-globulin may have been reflective of elevated levels of IgA and C'3 [β_{1A} (which migrate in the β-globulin area)] observed in these patients.[94–94b,98] Patients exhibited an elevation of these proteins with the progression of their malignancy.

Elevations, in particular of α_2- and β-globulin, may be considered one of the more common alterations of protein metabolism in malignant neoplasms, and are not pathognomonic for prostatic cancer.[70,71] However, the striking association of their progressive increase, notably of α_2-globulin, with progression of malignancy and the occasional mention of paraproteinemia in patients with epithelial rather than reticuloendothelial neoplasms suggested that further investigation of alterations of these proteins with regard to their usefulness was warranted.[75]

In this regard preliminary observations of the association of a reduction in the level of α_2-globulin and evidence of remission of metastatic lesions in four patients following cryotherapy of their primary prostatic tumor[76-78] directed our attention to the α_2-globulin level and its: 1.) immunoregulatory function and interference with mechanisms of host resistance, i.e., immunologic surveillance[76-84] and 2.) prognostic value following cryotherapy.[85]

The possible role of α_2-globulin in interfering with mechanisms of host resistance has been evaluated by parameters of cell-mediated immunologic responsiveness. This particular aspect of its suggested significance will be dealt with in the discussion of "Cellular Aspects."

With regard to the possible prognostic value of α_2-globulin, we have observed[85] a decrease in the level of this protein in 14 (78%) of 18 patients with prostatic cancer following cryotherapy (Table 4–1). Of these 14 patients, 11 (79%) showed a "favorable" clinical response. Of the other three patients showing a reduction, one showed no change from his preoperative status and two had a "poor" response. In contrast, of the four (22%) patients in whom α_2-globulin increased following cryotherapy, one showed a "favorable" response, two showed "none," and one a "poor" response. Thus it appears that patients in whom the level of α_2-globulin declined following cryotherapy have a more "favorable" clinical response. However, this interpretation may have been skewed by the fewer patients in whom the level of α_2-globulin increased postoperatively and who were, thereby, available for comparison of their postoperative alteration in α_2-globulin and clinical response to cryotherapy.

In support of the suggested correlation between increased levels of α_2-globulin and its association with a progression of malignancy and prognostic potential are the earlier studies of Juret and Frayssinet,[86] and those of patients with breast,[87,87a] gastric,[87b] ovarian,[87c] and renal cell[87d] carcinomas. In addition, but difficult to extrapolate to man, are studies of experimentally induced tumors demonstrating a correlation between an increase of protein components with an

Table 4–1

Correlation between alteration in level of α_2-globulin and clinical response following cryotherapy[a]

Pre- to postoperative level of α_2-globulin	Number of patients	Clinical response[b]		
		Favorable	None	Poor
Increased	4(22%)	1(25%)	2(50%)	1(25%)
Decreased	14(78%)	11(79%)	1(7%)	2(14%)
Overall	18	12(67%)	3(17%)	3(17%)

[a] Adapted from Ablin et al.[85]
[b] Evaluation of clinical response indicated was made following completion of the patient's total course of cryotherapy, i.e., in a patient receiving two freezing treatments, clinical response indicated was that obtained following second freeze and judged as: *Favorable*, by either—Symptomatic improvement (feeling of well-being and palliation of pain as expressed by patient); Diminution in size of patient's initial primary tumor or regression of metastases. *None*, No change in patient's disease from preoperative status. *Poor*, Progression of patient's disease from preoperative status.

electrophoretic mobility of α_2-globulin on metastatic development and a reduction in these components on regression or extirpation of the tumor.[88-90]

Individual levels of α_2-globulin, as well as other serum proteins, which in general were characterized by a reduction in albumin and β-globulin and an increase in α_1- and γ-globulin from their preoperative levels following cryotherapy, and the effect of the number of freezing treatments and relationship of these alterations to the stage of prostatic malignancy treated have been delineated elsewhere.[85,91,92] With regard to these alterations following cryotherapy, it is of interest to note that in contrast to the general trend in serum proteins observed following surgical trauma, where one observes a transient decrease in albumin, an increase in the α_1- and α_2-globulin fractions with β- and γ-globulin remaining essentially unchanged, our observation of the striking *reduction rather than increase* and the moderate-to-high alterations in α_2- and γ-globulin, respectively, following cryotherapy, suggests further the possible clinical significance of these changes.

With regard to other studies reporting alterations in serum proteins following cryoprostatectomy, there is, with exception of our preliminary report[91] and the formal communication of this report,[92] the study of Drylie and co-workers.[93] They reported the levels of three serum proteins [albumin, ceruloplasmin, and γ-globulin (IgG, IgA, and IgM)] in pre- and postoperative serum specimens of patients with benign prostatic hypertrophy and carcinoma of the prostate treated by cryoprostatectomy. However, any meaningful comparison of this with other studies is most difficult as: (1) no distinction was made between patients with benign and malignant disease and (2) no quantitative measurement of the serum proteins was made other than an indication of the "percent of change" from pre- to postoperative level. It may be stated

that they observed a decrease in albumin and an increase of α-globulin (which they measured by ceruloplasmin).

Immunoglobulins and Complement. In addition to the general evaluation of the serum protein levels in patients with prostatic cancer, the level of the three major classes of immunoglobulins, i.e., IgG, IgA, and IgM in the serum[94-96] and urine[97] and of the third component of complement $-C'3$ (β_{1A}-globulin) in the serum,[94a,98] the latter also in patients with benign prostatic hypertrophy,[98] have been evaluated by radial immunodiffusion. A recent report has included evaluation of IgG, IgA, and IgM, as well as that of IgE, the latter by radioimmunoassay.[98a]

The greater proportionate elevation of serum immunoglobulins in these patients was observed in the IgA fraction, with 22% (five of 23) of the patients studied, having levels ranging from 365 to 550 mg/100 ml. Levels of serum IgG and IgM, although slightly decreased, were within the normal expected range for age-related healthy adults.[94]

On the whole, there were no statistically significant differences in the levels of immunoglobulins within each of the stages of carcinoma evaluated.[94a,98a] However, there were variations in each of the immunoglobulins which deviated from the normal age-related values and when taken on an individual basis may, with support from other corroborative studies, be suggestive of aberrations of immunologic responsiveness. The initial expressed[94] possible significance and pathologic manifestations of the observed elevation of serum IgA has been somewhat lessened by the recent survey[99] of immunoglobulins in healthy older individuals (aged 40 years and older), indicating that approximately two-thirds of the subjects studied exhibited an elevation in serum IgA.

In another survey of serum immunoglobulins in prostatic cancer,[95] higher levels of IgG were observed in patients with locally invasive cancer (Stage III) than in patients with advanced disease (Stage IV). Decreased levels of IgM in Stage IV vs Stage III suggested to these investigators that less debilitated patients are in a state of antigenic stimulation and/or that they may possess a more competent immunologic system, or both. Levels of IgA, while elevated in a small percentage of patients in this study, were generally within the normal range.[95]

After increases in γ-globulin in four patients showing remission of metastatic lesions following cryotherapy, the levels of specific immunoglobulins were quantitated.[76–78,91,94b] Evaluation of immunoglobulins in these patients disclosed somewhat moderate increases in the level of IgG. Three of the four patients showed increases in IgM ranging from 72%, i.e., from 145 to 250 mg/100 ml, to 384%, i.e., from 62 to 300 mg/100 ml over their preoperative levels. The fourth patient showed an 18% reduction of IgM from his preoperative level of 146 mg/100 ml to 120 mg/100 ml.[94b] It is of interest that the observed increases of IgM in these patients, with the one exception, in whom remission of metastatic lesions following cryotherapy was observed, is in agreement with recent observations by Gursel et al.[96] They stated that there were increased levels of IgM in patients with prostatic cancer following cryotherapy in whom disappearance or decrease of bone pain was associated. This increased concentration in γ-globulin observed following cryotherapy could represent an active immunologic response by the host against tumor either in the form of 'blocking' factor(s)[173a] or possibly cytotoxic antibody.

In an earlier study, Drylie et al.[93] observed initial decreases in IgG and IgM 7 days following cryosurgery followed by a rise toward their preoperative levels. IgA showed a trend suggesting an elevation. Further comment or meaningful comparison of this report to others is most

difficult, because in their evaluation of serum proteins[93] no level or distinction between patients with benign vs. malignant disease was made.

In a recently completed study of urinary immunoglobulins in patients with prostatic cancer,[97] exceptionally high levels of all three major immunoglobulin classes were observed as compared to the levels of urinary immunoglobulins in age-related healthy adult males. Of particular interest was the finding that patients with prostatic cancer with levels of CEA-like antigen in their urine $\geq$ 20 ng/ml, also had elevated levels of urinary immunoglobulins. Subsequent correlation of the amount and type of immunoglobulin excreted in the urine with the stage and grade of prostatic cancer and the presence and relationship of urinary CEA-like antigens in the absence of infection may be of diagnostic value.

Immunochemical assay of the level of C'3, i.e., measurement of biologically inactive antigenic components, e.g., β_{1A}-globulin, in patients with prostatic cancer disclosed elevated levels, $\geq$ 195 mg/100 ml (normal mean of 134 mg/100 ml plus 2 SD) in 27% (six of 22) of the patients.[98] The mean level of C'3 for all patients of 181 mg/100 ml was statistically significant ($p < 0.05$) compared to the level of 135 mg/100 ml in patients with benign prostatic hypertrophy and of 134 mg/100 ml in a control population of healthy adults. As in evaluation of immunoglobulins, differences observed in the mean levels of C'3 for each stage of prostatic cancer were not statistically significant. However, a noticeable trend from a significantly mean elevated level of 230 mg/100 ml in Stage I, toward mean levels within the range of normal with a progression of malignancy was observed.[94a]

While elevated levels of β_{1A}-globulin may be evidence against the possible presence of antigen-antibody complexes as a contributing factor to the as yet unknown etiology of prostatic cancer, other components of C', both biologically active and inactive, must be evaluated before any definitive conclusions may be made. In this regard, we may note that McKenzie et al.,[99a] in evaluating the biologic reactivity of C', observed significantly elevated levels of the hemolytic reactivity of C' in four patients with prostatic cancer. Possible explanations of elevated levels of C' in malignancy have been considered.[94a,98]

In contrast to observations of C' in prostatic cancer, reduced levels of C'3, i.e., <72 mg/100 ml (normal mean of 134 mg/100 ml less 2 SD), in some patients with benign prostatic hypertrophy[98] may be a reflection of the possible in situ adsorption (deposition) of C' in prostatic tissue analogous to the fixation of C'3 seen in various nephritic syndromes. Observations by Tannenbaum and Lattimer[116–118] of the in vivo binding of C'1q and C'3 (the latter also observed in the author's laboratory) in the secretions and luminal borders of benign prostatic tissue are in keeping with this suggestion.

"Oncofetal Associated Antigens." Considerable interest has been directed toward the identification of specific antigens, or perhaps more accurately termed TAA, elaborated by tumors into the serum and tissue fluids of patients with malignancy, e.g., alpha-fetoprotein (α-FP) and carcinoembryonic antigen (CEA), whose appearance seems to be the result, not the cause, of neoplastic transformation. However, their presence, as in the case of α-FP in hepatoma or embryonal testicular tumor[100] and CEA in colonic cancer,[101] may provide a means for early diagnosis. In addition, measurement of subsequent alterations of these TAA has also been shown to bear some relationship to prognosis and serve as an adjunctive aid in the assessment of the efficacy of treatment.[102] Other TAA include: alpha H ferroprotein; fetal sulfoglycoproteins; Regan isoenzyme and T globulin. The association of these TAA with a suggested loss of suppressor genes, the regression of the cell to a more embryonic state, and the finding of these macromolecules in embryonic and tumor tissue have led to a suggestion that they might be more appropriately referred to as "oncofetal associated antigens."[103]

Of those oncofetal associated antigens which have been evaluated for their diagnostic and prognostic ability in patients with urologic tumors, it was initially thought that CEA was the most promising. In addition to CEA, brief mention will also be made of α-FP and T globulin.

Carcinoembryonic Antigen. First described in 1965 by Gold and Freedman,[104] elevated levels, i.e., ≥2.5 ng/ml, of CEA have been observed by several investigators in the plasma of patients with prostatic cancer.[105–107] These studies have, in the main, employed a modification by LoGerfo et al.[105] of the original assay for CEA (employing the Farr technique[104]) using zirconyl phosphate gel, more commonly referred to as the "Hansen assay." The result was the detection of a CEA molecule possessing somewhat different physicochemical properties from that of the Gold assay. I believe it more appropriate to refer to CEA reported in such studies as CEA-like antigen.

In studies attempting to correlate levels of CEA-like antigen with the stage and grade of prostatic malignancy,[108,109] it has been found that patients with higher stage tumors were more often positive than those possessing lower stage tumors. However, the accuracy of CEA-like antigen in diagnosing prostatic tumors has been less than promising, ranging in various studies from 25[108] to 59%,[109] with poor accuracy for low-stage tumors. No correlation has as yet been noted between grade and CEA-like antigen.[108,109]

In view of the fact that the findings already mentioned may have been a reflection of the limitations of retrospective analysis rather than of a prospective study, 200 consecutively admitted male urogenital patients (studied in two separate series of 100 patients each[110,111]) were evaluated for acid phosphatase and plasma CEA-like antigen. In these studies, CEA-like antigen and acid phosphatase detected less than 50% of the histologically diagnosed carcinomas of the prostate, with both detecting only high stage tumors. It is known that acid phosphatase is less accurate in detecting early prostatic malignancy, and from the results of these two recent studies it appears that such is the same for CEA-like antigen.

The possible effects of hormonal therapy on levels of CEA-like antigen have been suggested;[109] however, these results are somewhat borderline and shall require further confirmation.

Observations of elevated levels of CEA-like antigen[109,110] and α_2-globulin[72,73] in the serum of patients with prostatic cancer and the recent report by Hsu and LoGerfo[112] pointing to a suggested correlation of increased levels of CEA-like antigen and α_2-globulin in patients with colonic cancer, prompted a retrospective study of the possible occurrence and significance of this relationship in prostatic cancer. Preliminary studies thus far of 21 patients with various stages of histologically confirmed prostatic cancer have disclosed 10 (48%) and six (29%) patients with an elevated level of CEA-like antigen and α_2-globulin, respectively. Only two (10%) patients possessed a concurrent elevation of both.[113]

Elevated levels of CEA-like antigen have also been observed in the urine of patients with prostatic cancer,[114,115] particularly in association with elevated levels of urinary immunoglobulins.[97] However, the possibility as to whether such elevations may be related to concurrent infection has to be clarified.

In a rather interesting approach, CEA has been localized histologically in malignant prostatic tissue by immunoperoxidase staining.[116-118]

At present the initial promise of the CEA test as a screening procedure for the early detection of prostatic malignancy has been lessened somewhat by the incidence of 'false positives.' Also by the finding that it is usually only positive in patients with clinically advanced malignancy in whom the diagnosis is obvious by other means. There is also the recent result that detection of CEA-like antigen is less, or at least no more, accurate than acid phosphatase in detecting carcinoma of the prostate.[110,111] It is reasonable to state that perhaps the present limitations and usefulness of the identification of CEA-like antigen in prostatic cancer lies in the question of specificity, and the fact that the test antisera employed have been developed against CEA isolated from colon carcinoma. The recent immunohistologic studies of Tannenbaum and co-workers[116-118] demonstrate binding of an anticolonic CEA serum to prostatic tissue and may mean that CEA released from different tumors is indistinguishable as far as tissue-specificity is concerned.

Not to leave this particular discussion from a totally pessimistic point of view, a favorable prognostic indication of the detection of CEA-like antigen in patients with prostatic cancer may be found in the recent findings of Wechsler and co-workers.[119] In their study the failure of TAA (their choice of terminology for what I have referred to as CEA-like antigen) to disappear from the serum of patients in whom it had been present prior to therapy, correlated closely with either incomplete surgical extirpation of tumor or its incomplete destruction by radiotherapy. They have suggested that TAA "may prove useful as a test for incompleteness of tumor death or removal or of recurrence."[119] However, in this regard I wonder if this persistence is not simply related to the normal process of tissue regeneration. In addition Gursel et al.[30] have recently reported a correlation between the preoperative level of circulating TAA (again here they prefer this term to CEA, and this is the same I believe to what I have referred to as CEA-like antigen) and the clinical response of patients with prostatic cancer following sequential cryotherapy of their primary prostatic tumor, i.e., an "excellent" response was noted in patients with normal preoperative levels of TAA (<2.5 ng/ml) which decreased postoperatively. In contrast those patients giving a "moderate" or "poor" response possessed above-normal preoperative levels of TAA, which in the majority of patients became further elevated following cryotherapy.

Alpha-Fetoprotein and T Globulin. Initially alpha-fetoprotein was studied in hepatoma.[120] With the exception of a single case report of the presence of α-FP in a patient with gastric and prostatic carcinomas,[121] recent studies by Guinan et al.[121a] have disclosed no evidence of α-FP in 18 patients with carcinoma of the prostate. However, the recent report of the immunohistologic localization of α-FP in prostatic tissue,[118] suggests that certainly further studies are warranted.

A serum globulin designated as T globulin found in association with a variety of malignancies has been observed in five cases of prostatic cancer evaluated.[122]

Tissue Proteins

In vivo-Bound Immunoglobulins and Complement. Immunohistochemical studies[116–118,123,124] have demonstrated in vivo-bound immunoglobulins and complement in normal, benign, and malignant human prostatic tissue by immuno-fluorescent[118,123,124] and immunoperoxidase[116,117] staining. These studies have disclosed the presence of: (1) IgG and IgA in focal accumulation of secretory granules within the ductal lumen of prostatic acini;[123] (2) IgG in the cytoplasm of basal secretory epithelium;[123] (3) IgA in plasma cells in the fibromuscular stroma;[123] (4) IgM in the cytoplasmic membrane of

basal epithelial cells in benign[124] and in hyperplastic tissue adjacent to areas of malignant tissue;[116–118] and (5) C'1q and C'3 in the secretions and luminal borders.[116–118]

The possible significance of the localization of these immunoglobulins, particularly that of IgA, regarding their possible origin and antibacterial function in acute and chronic diseases of the prostate has been considered.[124] Immunoglobulins in the prostate and its secretions suggest the existence of a local immunologic system, perhaps similar to the gastrointestinal tract, parotid glands, lactating breast, and respiratory tract. The possible relationship of IgG in secretory granules in man[123,124] as related to the mechanism of the development of an immune response after in situ freezing of the prostate has recently been discussed.[38]

Isoantigens A, B, and O (H). Initially,[125] and more recently, through utilization of what has been termed the specific red-cell adherence test,[126] loss of blood-group isoantigens A, B, and O (H) has been interpreted as evidence of immunologic and physiologic dedifferentiation, analogous to the morphologic dedifferentiation of anaplasia. The specific red-cell adherence test has been most valuable in borderline cases wherein a question may exist as to the morphologic interpretation of the benign or malignant nature of a primary tumor and also in diagnosis, prognosis, and assessment of potential tumor growth. Studies of numerous tissues, e.g., cervix, lung, and pancreas, suggest that absence of specific adherence favors the diagnosis of malignancy and suggests the increased probability of metastases.

Recently[127] the specific red-cell adherence test has been applied to evaluate changes in normal and pathologic prostatic tissue. In these studies it was observed that isoantigens in the normal prostate exhibit a considerable increase with the onset of benign prostatic hypertrophy. Whereas in contrast to cases of primary and metastatic cancer, it was observed that A, B, and O (H) isoantigens were not detectable. Whether the absence of A, B, and O (H) isoantigens in malignant prostatic tissue may be related to the inability of malignant cells to synthesize or maintain their normal level of A, B, and O (H) antigens, or whether the process of malignancy itself may alter or destroy these antigens requires further study.

Prostate-Specific Antigens. Studies suggesting the existence of tissue-specific antigens of the prostate gland and its characteristic secretory product–prostatic fluid in man and in experimental animals have been the subject of recent reviews.[8,50,128]

Of particular interest are studies demonstrating that saline extracts of normal human prostatic tissue possess prostate-specific antigens.[56,129] Two antigens were found to be specific for prostatic tissue, whereas a third occurred in both prostatic tissue and prostatic fluid.[56,129] Utilization of the adjunct specificity of antigen-antibody interaction in gel-precipitation and enzymatic analysis permitted the identification (Figure 4–4) of one, and possibly two, of the prostatic tissue-specific antigens as acid phosphatase. As the phosphatase staining of this precipitation(s) was inhibited by L-tartaric acid, which is specific for prostatic acid phosphatase, but not for plasma or erythrocytic phosphatase; and as the line(s) of precipitation was removed by absorption with prostatic tissue, this antigen was initially identified as prostatic acid phosphatase.[56] However, recent studies[130] demonstrating that renal acid phosphatase is also subject to selective inhibition by L-tartaric acid, raise some question as to the enzymatic specificity of this antigen. However, as antisera used for these studies were absorbed with kidney which did not remove the line(s) of precipitation, the likelihood that this was a renal acid phosphatase is remote.

Specifically absorbed heteroimmune sera to saline extracts of pooled normal human prostatic tissue, and those derived from benign and malignant tumors, have been employed in an attempt to facilitate comparative studies of the antigenic composition of these tissues.[131] Here, as with studies of normal prostatic tissue, specific immunochemical staining applied to the gel-precipitation patterns obtained were utilized. Results of these

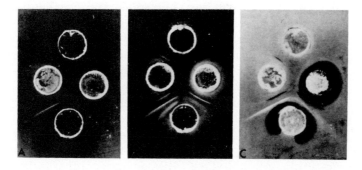

Figure 4–4. Photograph of gel diffusion precipitation reaction illustrating utilization of adjunct specificity of antigen-antibody interaction and enzymatic analysis for the identification and characterization of tissue-specific antigens of the prostate. Reactions identical in *A, B,* and *C.* Lower well, antiserum to normal human prostatic tissue absorbed with normal human serum, liver, and kidney: upper well, the same antiserum further absorbed with human prostatic fluid; left and right wells, extract of normal human prostatic tissue and human prostatic fluid, respectively. Precipitation reactions shown following: *A,* 48 hours at room temperature; *B,* incubation in buffer-substrate mixture, and *C,* staining for acid phosphatase. (From Ablin et al.[56])

preliminary studies suggest that benign and malignant prostatic tissues are antigenically deficient in comparison to normal prostatic tissue, i.e., normal prostatic tissue-specific antigens may be either present in reduced concentrations or absent in these pathologic tissues. The possible deficiency of normal prostate-specific antigens — particularly of prostatic tissue-specific acid phosphatase antigens following studies with preparations of malignant prostatic tissue — is particularly interesting in view of previous chemical and histochemical reports of diminished quantities of acid phosphatase in patients with advanced carcinoma of the prostate.[132-135]

The diagnostic and prognostic use of the detection of the antigenic deficiency of specific prostatic tissue-specific acid phosphatase antigens exists as a definite possibility, pending the determination as to whether there is an association between these antigens and various stages and grades of growth patterns of carcinoma of the prostate. Loss of tissue-specific antigens has also occurred in other experimental and human malignancies, and their absence has been suggested as possibly indicating absence of a particular growth-controlling factor from malignant cells.[136] If control of normal growth requires such a 'self-marker', its absence may indicate uncontrolled malignant growth.[136] In this regard, recent development of a radioimmunoassay for human prostatic acid phosphatase may be of assistance in facilitating such an analysis, which would possibly serve as a sensitive diagnostic tool.[137]

Somewhat similar studies on human prostatic tissue–acid phosphatase employing other methodologies have also been reported.[138-141] Of particular interest in these studies are the: 1.) identification of two molecular forms of aminopeptidase localized in the α_1- and α_2-globulins. (Based upon gel-precipitation studies,[140] the aminopeptidase localized in the α_1-globulin fraction was called the prostatic type, while aminopeptidase found in the α_2-globulin fraction was called the 'renal type'. Comparable studies of malignant prostatic tissue revealed that the activity of the prostatic type was greatly reduced.) And 2.) the suggested variable loss of normal prostatic acid phosphatase isoenzymes in extracts of primary and metastatic prostatic cancer tissue.[141]

In addition to the studies already mentioned, antigens resembling in their properties T transplantation antigens of experimentally viral-induced neoplasms, have recently been detected in malignant prostatic as well as in other malignant genitourinary tissues.[142] These antigens were observed to: (1) be typical for a given type of tumor; (2) be absent from tumors of a different histogenetic origin; (3) induce formation of humoral antibodies and cellular immunity; and (4) cross-react with antigens present in different tumors of the same histogenetic origin.[142]

Circulating and Cell-Bound Antibodies

Nuclei and Bile Canaliculi. In perhaps what may be the first serological screening of patients with prostatic cancer, circulating antibodies to various components of nuclei — e.g., nuclear membrane, nucleolus, and canaliculi of hepatic bile ducts — were observed by the fluorescent antibody method in 25% (six of 24) and 71% (17 of 24) of patients studied.[143]

An attractive hypothesis put forth by Burnham[144] and Zeromski et al.[145] is that an association may exist between malignancy and the presence of circulating antibodies to various components of nuclei in the absence of connective-tissue disease and/or other factors, or both, e.g., medication, such as hydralazine, associated with the induction of circulating antibodies to various components of nuclei and that "they may have possible diagnostic, prognostic and pathogenetic implications."[144] However, it is discouraging in this regard to note the presence of circulating antibodies to various components of nuclei also in patients with benign prostatic hypertrophy, in whom connective-tissue disease either has been excluded or was unconfirmed.[143] This finding is not meant to imply that circulating antibodies to various components of nuclei should be completely disregarded in patients with malignancy in the absence of connective-tissue disease. But, in view of their association with a wide variety of diseases, with the incidence approaching as high as 10% of the general populace, they may be representative, i.e., "markers," of nonspecific indicators of other immunologic aberrations in these patients.

Regarding antibodies to bile canaliculi, it was initially suggested that, as none of the evaluated 17 patients with prostatic cancer who possessed these antibodies were known to have any hepatic abnor-

mality, their relatively high incidence might be of some pathologic significance.[143] However, upon further consideration, it has been suggested[146] that antibodies to bile canaliculi may be pathologically related to the normal processes of aging rather than to a specific disease entity, e.g., lupoid hepatitis. With the decline of cellular and humoral-mediated immunologic responsiveness with age,[147] does the host gradually lose the ability to differentiate "self" from "nonself"? Therefore, in the instance of antibodies to bile canaliculi, are these antibodies developed in response to what the host no longer recognizes as "self" products of catabolism due to the occurrence of age-related immunogenetic changes in the somatic cells of the host?[146]

Cell Surface and Cytoplasm. Circulating antibodies reactive with the cytoplasmic membrane or intercellular areas

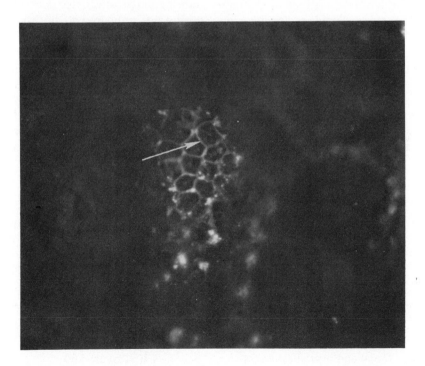

Figure 4–5. Indirect immunofluorescent staining reaction illustrating binding of antibodies from patient with prostatic cancer to cytoplasmic membrane or intercellular areas (arrow) of monkey prostatic secretory epithelial cells. Granules of various sizes fluorescing, are lipofuscin granules (× 400 with oil). (From Ablin.[149a])

of secretory epithelial cells of subhuman primate (monkey) prostatic tissue have been identified by immunofluorescence as shown in Figure 4–5, in the serum of slightly over half of 24 patients with various stages of prostatic malignancy (Table 4–2).[148] In contrast, only 11 (10%) of 106 patients with other than prostatic cancer possessed prostatic antibodies.[149a] This included eight (73%) patients with a genitourinary disease (5 with benign prostatic hypertrophy and 3 with carcinoma of the bladder). While not possessing sufficient specificity for diagnosis, the high incidence of prostatic antibodies, 92% positive in patients with advanced disease (Stage III), suggests it may be useful as a prognostic index of patients with metastatic disease. Whether a relationship exists between the higher incidence of prostatic antibodies in advanced disease and the presumably greater tumor mass or surface area and proportionate increase in tumor-specific antigens or TAA shed remains to be determined.

Immunofluorescent studies of sera from two patients with metastatic carcinoma of the prostate included in this series were shown to possess antibodies which reacted with their own (autologous) prostatic tissue.[148–149a] This finding, while limited to the study of only two patients, is suggestive of the role, in part, of autoimmune processes in the pathogenesis of carcinoma of the prostate. Subsequent immunofluorescent studies of sequential serum specimens obtained following cryotherapy of the primary prostatic tumor in one of these patients disclosed, among other changes, a gradual reduction in the immunofluorescent staining titer of antiprostatic epithelial antibodies.[150] This gradual reduction in the titer of circulating antibodies to prostatic tissue following cryotherapy prompted us to examine the possibility that they might have, due to the liberation of prostatic tissue (tumor?)-specific or TAA following in situ freezing of the primary prostatic tumor, become cell-bound in the presence of antigen excess. In this regard an acid eluate prepared from the patient's prostatic tissue obtained at autopsy disclosed by immunofluorescence, antibodies reactive with autologous prostatic tissue.[150] These eluted antibodies appeared to be immunohistologically indistinguishable from those observed prior to operation, and as long as 10 days after the first of two independent cryosurgical treatments of the patient's prostatic tumor (Figure 4–5). Electrophoretic analysis of this eluate disclosed a single line of precipitation in the IgG region of the electrophoretic field.[25]

Table 4–2

Summary of indirect immunofluorescent staining titers of antibodies in patients with prostatic cancer reactive with cytoplasmic membrane or intercellular areas of primate prostatic secretory epithelial cells as related to stage of malignancy[a]

Stage of carcinoma[b]	No. of patients	No. (%) positive/range in immunofluorescent titer
I	5	1(20%)/20[c]
II	7	1(14%)/20
III	12	11(92%)/10–160
Total and overall range	24	13(54%)/10–160

[a] Adapted from Ablin et al.[148]
[b] According to classification of Flocks.[74]
[c] e.g., 1(20%)/20 means that one patient or 20% had an indirect immunofluorescent staining titer of 1:20.

The demonstration of the elution of cell-bound antibodies from malignant prostatic tissue following cryotherapy that are reactive with autologous tissue provides evidence of a preliminary nature that, in man as in the rabbit[34,46] prostatic tissue (tumor?)-specific or TAA is liberated into the circulation following freezing damage. It would be of interest to determine the possible role of these antibodies in carcinoma of the prostate. Are they of a cytotoxic nature as previously hypothesized,[25] or do they possibly interfere with complement-mediated cytotoxicity and function in the capacity of "blocking" factors,[151] recently observed in patients with prostatic cancer?[173a] Furthermore, their relevance to recently observed 'unbound' antibodies in patients with benign and malignant diseases of the prostate reactive with other sources of epithelium remains to be elucidated.

The observation of antibody activity for prostatic epithelial cells suggested the possibility of similar reactivity with other epithelial tissues. A preliminary survey[152] of serum from patients with carcinoma of the prostate, employing frozen sections of esophagus as a source of epithelial tissue, disclosed immunofluorescent staining of the intercellular areas of stratified squamous epithelium as initially described in patients with pemphigus.[153] In addition, a granular type of immunofluorescent staining of the intercellular areas of stratified squamous epithelium accompanied by a somewhat linear staining of the border of the basal cell layer or the membrane of basal cells, or both, recently described as a "nodular pseudoepidermal intercellular immunofluorescence"[154] was observed. Recent studies of previously unscreened sera from patients with carcinoma of the prostate have also revealed immunofluorescent staining of granular deposits (keratohyalin granules?) lying in the granular layer of epithelium of mouse esophagus.[155]

Intercellular antibodies were also observed in the serum of patients with benign prostatic hypertrophy;[155,156] however, they were of a much lower intensity and were not observed at titers greater than 1:40.

These studies were initiated to examine the possible tissue-specificity of antibodies reactive with primate prostatic secretory epithelial cells and have permitted the identification of antibodies reactive with four histologically identifiable components of stratified squamous epithelium: (1) basement-membrane zone (dermal-epidermal junction); (2) cytoplasmic membrane or intercellular areas (spaces); (3) keratohyalin granules; and (4) nuclear membrane.[155] Representative photomicrographs of each of these four types of immunofluorescent staining patterns are illustrated in Figure 4–6. The frequency and range in immunofluorescent titers of antibodies reactive with each of these epithelial components are presented in Table 4–3. The immunofluorescent staining reactions obtained with sera from some of the patients yielded a peripheral type of immunofluorescence, in contrast to the polygonal type characteristic of true intercellular immunofluorescence. This was shown by evaluating sera with this pattern on sections of liver, to be attributable to peripheral or membranous circulating antibodies to various components of nuclei masquerading as intercellular on squamous epithelium. These antibodies, as mentioned previously, have been referred to as "pseudo" intercellular.[152,154,155]

The significance of antibodies directed against components of epithelial tissue and their increased incidence in individuals with malignant neoplasms was also recently observed by Bystryn et al.[157] This appears to be particularly relevant in light of previous studies[158,159] pointing to the possible relationship between bullous dermatoses and malignant neoplasms, as first suggested by Bogrow in 1909.[160] The case presentations of Jordan et al.,[161] the

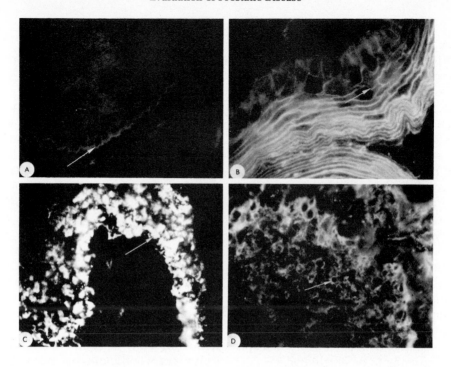

Figure 4–6. Representative photomicrographs illustrating four types of immunofluorescent staining reactions, as indicated by the arrows, obtained on sections of mouse esophagus with sera from patients with benign prostatic hypertrophy and carcinoma of the prostate: *A,* basement-membrane zone; *B,* intercellular; *C,* keratohyalin granules; and *D,* nuclear membrane (× 200 with oil). (From Ablin.[155])

recent reports of Saikia[162] and of Saikia and co-workers,[163] and the review of Cormia and Domonkus[164] suggest cutaneous reactions to be an indicator of internal malignant neoplasm and may, in many instances, antedate the actual identification of a malignant neoplasm. Further studies of antiepithelial antibodies, which might lead to the earlier diagnosis and initiation of therapy in select cases, are most certainly worthy of pursuit.[165]

Employing immunofluorescence and mixed hemadsorption, Dmochowski et al.[165a] have recently observed the presence of antibodies in sera from patients with prostatic cancer, benign prostatic hypertrophy, and carcinoma of the bladder reactive with autologous and allogeneic cells derived from these tumors. The relationship of these antibodies, possibly of a viral etiology,[165a] to those described

earlier to be reactive with prostatic and other epithelial tissues[148–149a] remains to be determined.

Cytotoxic. Lymphocytotoxic and leukoagglutinating antibodies to allogeneic cells have been observed in a very small proportion of patients (two of 22) studied with prostatic cancer.[166,167] However, this finding is of particular interest in view of the fact that comparable lymphocytotoxic activity for allogeneic cells was not demonstrable in serum from 28 patients with benign prostatic hyperplasia, from 18 patients with carcinoma other than prostate, or from 50 healthy adults included in these studies.

The finding of cytotoxic antibodies in the serum of patients with carcinoma of the prostate suggests that lymphocytotoxic antibodies may be one of many immunopathogenic manifestations of car-

Table 4-3

Immunohistologic localization, frequency, and range in immunofluorescent staining titers of antiepithelial antibodies[a]

Diagnosis	No. of Patients	No. (%) positive[b]/range in IF staining titer			
		Basement-membrane zone	Cytoplasmic membrane or intercellular	"Pseudo" intercellular	Keratohyalin granules
Benign prostatic hypertrophy	42	3(7%)/10–20[c]	11(26%)/10–40	2(5%)/10–20	0/<10
Carcinoma of prostate	24	0/<10	8(33%)/10–320	1(4%)/10	1(4%)/160
Carcinoma other than of prostate	18[d]	1(6%)/10	0/<10	1(6%)/20	0/<10
Healthy adults	25	0/<10	0/<10	0/<10	0/<10
Total and overall range	109	4(4%)/10–20	19(17%)/10–320	4(4%)/10–20	1(1%)/160

[a] From Ablin.[165] Copyright 1974, American Medical Association.

[b] If positive, i.e., Immunofluorescent titer ≥1:10, in blood group, A, B, or O individuals, serum was absorbed with blood group-specific substances A and B, or in case of AB individuals, sections were pretreated with anti-H prior to application of patient's serum and then reevaluated.

[c] E.g., 3(7%)/10/20 means that three patients or 7% had an indirect immunofluorescent staining in titers for the basement-membrane zone of stratified epithelium on mouse esophagus ranging from 1:10 to 1:20.

[d] Included six patients with carcinoma of bladder; two patients each with carcinoma of cervix, lung, and skin (melanoma); and one each with carcinoma of rectum, nasopharynx, brain, breast, colon, and endometrium.

cinoma of the prostate. In this regard it is of interest that, as antigens of lymphocytes are known to be present in or on other tissues, or both, the possibility exists that the occurrence of tissue damage observed in prostatic cancer — particularly metastatic carcinoma — may be a direct or indirect effect of cytotoxic antibodies. On the other hand, one might further speculate that cytotoxic antibodies are in fact the result of a defense mechanism of the host against self-destruction. These antibodies may act in a manner similar to the lymphotoxic factor recently observed in the sera of patients with multiple sclerosis.[168] If we assume that tissue (tumor?)-specific or TAA are present in the human prostate[56,129,131] or, on the basis of a recent report of the presence of IgG autoantibodies to prostatic tissue in the serum of patients with metastatic carcinoma of the prostate,[148–149a] then the destruction of lymphocytes that have presumably been stimulated by this antigen to produce autoantibodies would be a prophylactic response of the host in an attempt to prevent self-destruction.[166,167] As such, the presence of lymphocytotoxic antibodies are, as suggested by Yagoda,[169] a further indication of the possible potential role for immunotherapy in patients with prostatic malignancy.

Blocking Factor(s). Several studies demonstrate that serum from tumor-bearing animals can specifically vitiate the cytotoxic effect of sensitized lymphocytes on tumor cells in vitro and facilitate tumor growth when inoculated in vivo.[170,171] Serum from animals whose tumors have regressed or have been removed does not possess this blocking capacity. This has led to the identification of what has been termed the "blocking" factor. It is suggested that sera possessing blocking factor(s) mediate a form of immunologic enhancement in promoting or permitting tumor to grow in vivo.[172] Blocking factor(s) has been identified in patients with a variety of malignant con-

ditions, including bladder and kidney tumors and seminoma.[173]

Indirect evidence of blocking factor(s) in patients with prostatic cancer has been suggested by observations of: (1) inhibition of in vitro parameters of nonspecific cellular responsiveness by patients' serum[80–84,207,215] and (2) the concomitant abrogation or reduction of the inhibitory properties of their serum in association with a favorable clinical response following cryoprostatectomy.[250a,250b] However, only through demonstration of antitumor cell-mediated immunity in patients with prostatic cancer,[173a] and the interference (blocking) of this immunity by autologous serum,[173a] has direct evidence of blocking factor(s) in the vernacular initially described[173] been demonstrated in prostatic cancer. The blocking of cell-mediated immunity will be dealt with under "Cellular Aspects."

Potpourri. In addition, mention of other antibodies has been made in patients with diseases of the prostate. These have been placed under the heading "Potpourri."

Prostatitis-Arthritis. There is a paucity of evidence regarding the intriguing association of inflammatory disorders of the genitourinary tract, e.g., prostatitis, which have been observed to precede Reiter's syndrome. In this regard phenolic extracts of normal human prostatic tissue have been observed, as demonstrated by tanned cell hemagglutination, to react with sera from patients with prostatitis as well as with sera from patients with Reiter's syndrome, ankylosing spondylitis, and uveitis.[174] Grimble and Lessof have suggested that the presence of such antibodies in patients with arthritic disorders may represent an immunologic response to the release of a prostatic antigen that occurs with inflammation and may point to a possible underlying prostatitis.[174]

Anticoaguloprostatic Fluid. Precipitating antibodies to prostatic tissue or prostatic fluid in patients with prostatic cancer have, with exception of their reactivity with autologous malignant prostatic tissue in one of five patients studied,[149a] not been observed. However, gel diffusion precipitation reactions have been observed to occur between rabbit CPF and the sera of patients following cryoprostatectomy.[47] Staining of the precipitin bands employing a modification of the Gomori histochemical procedure reveals acid phosphatase activity.[56] Why sera from patients treated by cryoprostatectomy should precipitate with CPF is at present an enigma. It remains to be determined whether this type of cross-reactivity is similar to that observed in patients with acute rheumatic fever or those with glomerulonephritis following streptococcal infection, who possess antibodies reactive with streptococcal antigens.

Antiviral. Viruses have been implicated in the etiology of several tumors. Virus-like particles were initially observed in electron microscopic studies in benign prostatic cancer cells adjacent to malignant cells by Tannenbaum et al.[175] In continuing electron microscopic studies, these investigators have observed similar virus-like particles known to be associated with the Lucké tumor virus (which causes kidney tumors in experimental animals) in patients with carcinoma of the breast and prostate.[176] Although no mention of the possible presence of antibodies to these virus-like particles has been made, it is perhaps of interest to note that neutralizing antibodies to SV40 virus have been identified in two of 24 patients with prostatic cancer.[177]

With a view to investigating further the question of viruses in the etiology or its participation in prostatic cancer, Farnsworth[178] in evaluating extracts of benign and malignant prostatic tissue for RNA-viral activity by a reverse transcriptase assay, has observed potent RNA-dependent DNA polymerase activity in malignant tissue. When compared with the elution pattern of enzyme activity obtained with authentic virus, this extract possessed almost an identical pattern.

Employing a competitive radioimmunoassay with antiserum to interspecies antigens of the feline and murine leukemia viruses and saline extracts of benign prostatic tissue, protein components from the latter have been observed to compete with the interspecies viral antigens for binding sites on the antiviral globulins.[178a] Seal et al.[178a] suggested that these observations may indicate the presence of oncornavirus-like proteins in benign prostatic tissue.

Anti-Stilbestrol. Investigation of the participation of a humoral factor in the development of unresponsiveness to diethylstilbestrol observed in many prostatic cancer patients has been made.[178b] Prompted by the presence of anti-insulin antibodies in the development of insulin-resistant diabetes mellitus, Silk,[178b] employing paper electrophoresis with tritiated labeled diethylstilbestrol as a tracer, has observed the migration of diethylstilbestrol with γ-globulin in prostatic cancer patients who had previously received this hormone and has suggested this to indicate the presence of antibodies to diethylstilbestrol. Unfortunately, no correlation of the presence of these suggested "antibodies" and the clinical status of patients in whom they were observed was possible.

Anti-Gamma Globulin. Rheumatoid factor of the IgM class has been observed not only in patients with rheumatic disorders, but also in patients with other diseases including malignant disease.[179-181] Rheumatoid factor has also been observed in healthy adults in whom its incidence increases with age.[182]

In at least one case, high titered anti-gammaglobulin has been observed by latex agglutination following cryotherapy. Whether this may be related to age or to the release, as observed follow-

ing cryostimulation of the rabbit prostate,[38] of a sequestered antigen possessing
altered autologous gamma-globulin remains to be determined.

Cellular Aspects

Lymphocytosis and Lymphopenia

Evidence that the host maintains some
variable degree of control of tumor growth
does not, in itself, imply that this control
is of an immunologic nature. However,
some histologic observations indicate that
lymphoid or plasma cell infiltration of the
tumor affects prognosis. For example,
infiltration of mononuclear cells in and
around the tumor has previously been
reported to improve the prognosis of
patients with neuroblastoma, seminoma,
and other malignant tumors.[183-185] In two
recent studies of patients with carcinoma
of the bladder,[186,187] the presence of lymphocytes signified a greater chance of
survival and the absence of aggressive
tumor behavior, whereas lymphopenia
was found in association with poorer
survival and was most common during
the end stage of the disease.

Whether lymphocytosis is a consequence of mobilization by nonspecific
host defense mechanisms or is, in fact,
mediated by specific stimulation remains
to be determined. Nevertheless, the possibility that lymphocytosis in and around
tumors in patients with bladder cancer,
neuroblastoma, and seminoma may be
associated with improvement in their
prognosis is of some interest, and certainly is deserving of consideration in
patients with prostatic cancer.

On the basis of these studies and the
postulate that the balance between
thymic-dependent cytotoxic "killer"
lymphocytes (T-cells) and thymic-
independent lymphocytes (B-cells) producing blocking factors that may influence the course of the tumor-host relationship,[188] and additional evidence[189-192]
that patients with genitourinary cancer

may possess diminished cellular immunocompetence, Catalona and co-
workers have quantitated by the rosette-
forming cell assay, as a marker of
thymic-dependent lymphocytes, the level
of circulating T-cells in patients with
carcinoma of the bladder and prostate.[193]

In comparison with healthy controls,
they observed a significant reduction in
both groups of patients, with the level of
T-cells appearing to correlate inversely
with tumor stage in those with carcinoma
of the bladder, but not in patients with
prostatic cancer. They noted also that
their results paralleled their observations
of the evaluation of immunocompetence
by cutaneous hypersensitivity[189] and also
verified the earlier findings of Olsson et
al.[192]

As for the significance of the relationship between decreased levels of circulating T-cells and diminished immunocompetence favoring "tumor outgrowth,"[193]
this presupposes that T-cells are of overriding importance in the destruction of
malignant neoplasms. However, in some
instances macrophage function may be of
equal, if not greater, importance, e.g.,
Corynebacterium parvum, a stimulant of
reticuloendothelial activity, possesses
potent antitumor effects, but yet sup-
presses T-cell function (Castro, personal
communication).

Macrophage Function

Macrophages may participate specifically or nonspecifically in immunologic
reactions of the host. Studies demonstrate
that after increased mobilization of macrophages by stimulation with bacillus
Calmette-Guérin (BCG) experimental
animals possess increased resistance to
subsequent tumor challenge.[194,195] The
empiric observations by Dizon and
Southam[196] of the reduced capacity of
patients with malignancy to mobilize
macrophages following dermal abrasion
and the recent observations by Zbar et
al.[197] and others, suggest that aberrations

of tumor rejection may reside at the macrophage level. Preliminary observations of reduced chemotactic responsiveness of macrophages (in assay permitting one evaluation of macrophage function[198]) in patients with renal and transitional cell carcinoma of the bladder[199] may, as suggested by Brosman and Hausman,[199] be reflective of a reduced capacity of the host to mobilize macrophages to specific tumor foci.

In investigating the monocytic chemotactic response in patients with prostatic cancer, Brosman et al.[199a] observed depressed effector cell function in 41 patients evaluated as compared to a group of noncancer patients. Patients with metastatic disease possessed a greater defect than those with localized disease. Following radical prostatectomy, patients with localized disease showed an improvement in monocytic responsiveness.[199a]

Recent studies employing leukocyte adherence inhibition demonstrating antitumor-associated immunity and "blocking" factor(s),[173a] to be considered subsequently, are further suggestive of the significance of macrophage function in prostatic cancer.

Immune Cytolysis

Peripheral blood lymphocytes from patients with a variety of tumors have been observed to possess the capability to specifically "kill" autochthonous tumor cells. In several instances lymphocytes from patients with one type of malignancy are also cytotoxic to morphologically similar tumors from other patients. This lymphocyte-mediated destruction of tumor cells appears to be specific, as no cytotoxicity is observed with normal cells or with tumors of a different histologic type from those of the lymphocyte donors. This cytotoxic effect has been detected both when lymphocytes are obtained from tumor-bearing patients and when they are obtained from patients who have become

clinically symptom free. The former observation is analogous to observations made in experimentally induced animal neoplasms. That is, the finding that tumors could grow in vivo but were killed in vitro in the presence of autochthonous or allogeneic lymphocytes led to the identification of the presence of a factor in the serum of tumor-bearing individuals which could specifically block (abrogate) lymphocyte-mediated cytolysis. As such, blocking factors in the serum have been shown to play a major role in facilitating tumor growth in vivo and interfere with the host's natural or augmented resistance to malignancy.

Lymphocytic-mediated cytolysis has been observed in several genitourinary tumors, e.g., in renal cell carcinoma[200] and recently in patients with prostatic cancer.[200a] In a preliminary report, peripheral blood lymphocytes from patients with benign prostatic hypertrophy and carcinoma of the prostate were observed to be cytotoxic to tissue cultures of benign and malignant prostatic tissue.[200a] The observed cross-reactivity between benign and malignant prostatic tissue, suggestive of the sharing of antigens, is consistent with earlier humoral[56,131,148-149a] and recent cellular studies.[173a,245,246]

Delayed Type "Cutaneous" Hypersensitivity

The ability of an individual to manifest a delayed type hypersensitivity reaction to a variety of commonly encountered microbial antigens, e.g., purified protein derivative, streptokinase-streptodornase, and mumps virus, has proved useful as one criterion of evaluating one parameter of general, but not tumor-directed cell-mediated immunocompetence.[201] Suggested impairment of immunologic responsiveness, as indicated by the decreased ability to manifest delayed cutaneous hypersensitivity to these known antigens, has frequently been found in association with lymphoproliferative and advanced solid neoplasms.[202,203] Unfortunately, however, while some patients may manifest adequate responses to such antigens, they may be unable to do so when challenged with a "new" antigen. Recently, dinitrochlorobenzene (DNCB), an industrial chemical (which reacts with proteins in the keratin layer of the skin where it acts as a hapten, inducing contact sensitivity) has been widely used in evaluating immunocompetence.[204] The advantage of using DNCB is that it eliminates the often difficult problem of determining whether the patient has had prior exposure to some of the commonly used microbial antigens. Recent reports have demonstrated an excellent correlation between delayed cutaneous hypersensitivity to DNCB and prognosis in patients with malignancy.[204]

Other antigens, such as keyhole limpet hemocyanin[192] and schistosome eggs, have been recently evaluated as skin test reagents and, pending further study, loom as preferable choices. Preference of these reagents for skin testing lies in the fact that prior contact with these antigens is not expected in the general population, and thus a positive response — provided prior exposure may be ruled out — indicates that functions of cell-mediated competence are intact.

Evaluation of general delayed type cutaneous hypersensitivity in patients with prostatic cancer has recently been reported.

In the first of these,[205] cutaneous hypersensitivity to purified protein derivative in four patients with prostatic cancer was depressed in those with a poor clinical prognosis. One patient exhibited a pronounced Mantoux reaction following hormonal therapy — the significance of which remains to be determined. Particularly striking in this study was the observation that serum-suppressed tuberculin induced peripheral blood lymphocyte DNA synthesis prior to intravenous estrogen therapy but not following.[205] Whether this suppression was of a nonspecific variety often observed in rodent species during experimental tumor induction or was of a more specific nature, perhaps related to increased levels of certain serum proteins, e.g., alpha globulin, as has been hypothesized,[76-79] remains to be determined.

Cell-mediated immunocompetence to DNCB has recently been evaluated in 64 patients with genitourinary tumors, which included 24 with prostatic carcinoma.[189]

When grouped according to tumor type, varying degrees of host immunocompetence were observed. The highest incidence of impairment was among patients with transitional cell carcinoma followed in order of impairment by prostate, renal cell, and penile carcinoma, with those having testicular tumors possessing almost totally normal immunocompetence.[189]

When patients with transitional and renal cell carcinomas were categorized according to the extent of their tumor, i.e., whether they had clinically localized or known metastatic tumors, there was a higher incidence of impaired competence among patients with clinically localized disease. In contrast, in patients with prostatic cancer there was a greater degree of impairment in those patients with localized tumors than in those with metastatic tumors. No correlation was observed between host immunocompetence and the extent of tumor in patients with malignancy of the testis. Of the patients with penile carcinoma, one had localized disease and normal competence whereas the other, with lymph node metastases, was anergic.

Catalona et al.[189] suggest correlation of impairment of immunologic competence, as evaluated by reactivity to DNCB, with the clinical extent of tumor in patients with transitional and renal cell carcinomas but not in those patients with prostatic or testicular malignancy implies that different host-tumor relationships exist which are related to the histologic origin of these tumors and which may reflect important differences in their etiology.

In contrast to absence of a correlation between DNCB reactivity and the extent of tumor in patients with prostatic cancer,[189] Brosman et al.[199a] observed a correlation of responsiveness to DNCB, as well as to microbial "recall antigens," e.g., purified protein derivative, and the extent of tumor. In addition, evaluation of prostatic cancer patients' ability to elicit an inflammatory response, employing croton oil, further showed a correlation between their response and their stage and clinical course of disease.[199a] The inflammatory response to croton oil also correlated with the patient's response to DNCB.[199a]

In a subsequent study, Huus et al.[189a] similarly observed a correlation between the lack of DNCB reactivity and metastatic carcinoma. Huus et al.[189a] have suggested that this correlation may, compared to the absence of one in an earlier study,[189] be attributed to evaluation of DNCB reactivity after the diagnosis had been established thereby permitting a better and more accurate staging and better separation of their study groups.[189a]

Evaluation of tumor-directed cutaneous hypersensitivity in patients with prostatic cancer has recently been reported.[189b] Brannen et al.[189b] have observed a cutaneous delayed type hypersensitivity response to 3M KCl extracts of autologous and allogeneic malignant prostatic tissue in 3 and 1 of 7 patients with prostatic cancer, respectively. This response appeared to be specific, as no response to allogeneic extracts of benign prostatic tissue was observed. These preliminary observations suggest that malignant prostatic tissue possesses specific antigens to which the host may respond and provides in vivo demonstration suggestive of tumor-specific cell-mediated immunity in patients with prostatic cancer. These observations are in keeping with the in vitro demonstration of antitumor cell-mediated immunity in prostatic cancer patients by inhibition of leukocyte migration[245,246] and antigen-induced leukocyte adherence inhibition.[173a] Interestingly, the latter in vitro observations also employed 3M KCl extracts of prostatic tissue.

Lymphocyte Transformation

The ability of peripheral blood lymphocytes to undergo transformation (blastogenesis) and incorporate labeled thymidine (^{3}HTdR) following nonspecific stimulation with plant mitogens, e.g., phytohemagglutinin (PHA) and concanavalin A, has been suggested as an in vitro correlate of the activity of thymic-dependent lymphocytes and as one parameter for evaluating cell-mediated immunological responsiveness. Utilization of the blastogenic response of PHA-stimulated peripheral blood lymphocytes to evaluate cell-mediated immunologic responsiveness in patients with prostatic cancer has received, since the initial reports,[190,191,206] considerable attention, particularly from the standpoint of its usefulness in evaluating and distinguishing intrinsic (cellular) and extrinsic (extracellular) aberrations of lymphocytic function.

Robinson et al.,[190,191] in studies of patients with benign prostatic hypertrophy and prostatic cancer, observed a marked reduction in the blastogenic response of PHA-stimulated peripheral blood lymphocytes in patients with advanced metastatic disease and in patients with elevated levels of serum acid phosphatase. In contrast, there was a higher degree of blastogenesis in patients with small foci of cancer. On the basis of their observations, it was suggested that a high degree of blastogenesis following stimulation of peripheral blood lymphocytes with PHA may be associated with a favorable prognosis.[190,191] However, in contrast, recently completed studies, as illustrated in Table 4–4, by Mr. Gailon Bruns working in our laboratory,[81] and those of Catalona et al.[207] and McLaughlin et al.[208] have suggested that although there was a statistically significant reduction in the blastogenic response of PHA-stimulated peripheral blood lymphocytes as expressed by the Stimulation Index, in patients with prostatic cancer as compared with that of a control population, there was no statistically significant alteration in the Stimulation Index between any of the four stages of prostatic cancer evaluated.

It is of interest that the observations as noted in Table 4–4, as well as those of Catalona et al.[207] and McLaughlin et al.[208] of the suggested absence of a correlation between the blastogenic response to PHA and the clinical extent of disease are in agreement with results obtained following evaluation of patients with prostatic cancer by two other suggested parameters of cell-mediated immunity, i.e., delayed type hypersensitivity to DNCB[189] and

quantitation of thymic-dependent lymphocytes.[193]

One of the important features of the application of the blastogenic response of peripheral blood lymphocytes to the study of cell-mediated immunologic responsiveness is that it permits, by inclusion of appropriate controls—i.e., concurrent evaluation of the blastogenic response of stimulated peripheral blood lymphocytes cultured in autologous (the patient's serum) and homologous serum, e.g., pooled normal human AB positive serum—distinction between a proliferative response which may be attributable to an intrinsic aberration of the patient's lymphocytes vs that due to an extrinsic aberration or the concurrence of both. A Stimulation Index which is less in autologous serum than in homologous serum, e.g., 15 vs 60, suggests that this reduction is due to an extrinsic rather than to an intrinsic aberration of lymphocytic reactivity. However, the presence of one type of aberration does not preclude the presence or absence of the other, i.e., an individual may possess a

Table 4–4

Cellular reactivity of patients with prostatic cancer and its relationship to stage of malignancy as evaluated by incorporation of ^{3}H-thymidine by phytohemagglutinin-stimulated peripheral blood lymphocytes[a]

	Prostatic Cancer						
	Stage[b]				All		
	0(8)[e]	I(11)	II(11)	III(19)	Stages(49)	Controls(16)[c]	Significance[d]
Stimulation Index[f]	41.5	49.1	53.7	41.0	45.8	74.5	< 0.05

[a] Adapted from Bruns et al.[81]
[b] According to classification of Flocks.[74]
[c] Included 11 patients with benign prostatic hypertrophy and one each with condylomata, hypospadias, renal stone, urethral polyurethral stricture.
[d] As there was no statistically significant (P>0.05) alteration in Stimulation Index within each stage, only significance of difference in all stages compared with control is indicated.
[e] Number in parentheses = number of patients.
[f] Stimulation Index = peripheral blood lymphocytes + phytohemagglutinin/peripheral blood lymphocytes only.

low Stimulation Index in homologous serum, e.g., 30, suggesting an intrinsic defect. However, when his peripheral blood lymphocytes are cultured in autologous serum, this Stimulation Index may even be lower, e.g., 15, thus also pointing to an extrinsic aberration.

In this regard, observations that the Stimulation Index of patients with prostatic cancer,[81,82] while diminished, was even less in patients possessing an elevated level of serum α_2-globulin compared to a higher Stimulation Index, although low compared to a control group, in serum in which the level of α_2-globulin was within normal limits, suggested, on the basis of previous studies, the presence of plasma or serum inhibitory factors of lymphocytic reactivity in the α_2-globulin fraction[209-214] or "blocking" factor(s),[173a] i.e., diminished responsiveness was not entirely due to intrinsic aberrations but also to extrinsic. As such, it should be noted that the difference between the earlier studies of Robinson et al.[190,191] and those most recently reported,[81,82,207,208] may lie in the presence of plasma or serum inhibitory factors of lymphocytic reactivity rather than in intrinsic aberrations of the lymphocyte populations evaluated.

These initial observations,[81,82,190,191,206-208] prompted studies to evaluate the effect of serum from patients with prostatic cancer

on the in vitro reactivity of their lymphocytes by comparing their blastogenic response to PHA in the presence of autologous and homologous serum (Table 4–5). Evaluation in this manner of 17 patients disclosed that 14 (82%) possessed either an intrinsic [noted in two (12%)] or an extrinsic [noted in four (24%)] aberration, while eight (47%) possessed concomitant aberrations.[84] These observations appear to be in agreement with recently reported studies by others,[207,215] and offer further evidence of impaired cellular immunological responsiveness in patients with prostatic cancer which, as evidenced from this recent report,[84] are not entirely due to aberrant functions of the lymphocyte but rather concomitant aberrations.

Regarding further the possible relationship between the level of, an as yet unidentified component, in the α_2-globulin fraction of serum, contributing to the reduction in the proliferation of peripheral blood lymphocytes as observed in this study, the mean Stimulation Index and percent reduction of homologous vs autologous serum in the 17 patients evaluated are summarized in Table 4–6 according to whether they possessed an elevated level, i.e., ≥ 1.30 g/100 ml or normal level, i.e., < 1.30 g/100 ml of α_2-globulin.[72,73] While the Stimulation Indices of these patients in homologous serum were similar, i.e., 55 and 51,

Table 4–5

Method of determining effect of serum from patients with prostatic cancer on incorporation of ³H-thymidine by phytohemagglutinin-stimulated peripheral blood lymphocytes[a]

Peripheral blood lymphocytes cultured in	1 Peripheral blood lymphocytes + phytohemagglutinin (counts/minute)	2 Peripheral blood lymphocytes *only*	Stimulation Index = 1:2
Homologous serum	182,095[b]	3,119	58
Autologous serum	134,744	3,023	44
% reduction in Stimulation Index: homologous vs autologous serum			24

[a] From Ablin et al.[84]
[b] Mean of duplicate cultures.

Table 4-6

Effect of serum from patients with prostatic cancer possessing elevated and normal level of α_2-globulin on incorporation of ^{3}H-thymidine by phytohemagglutinin-stimulated peripheral blood lymphocytes[a]

Level of α_2-globulin	No. of patients	Mean level α_2-globulin (g/100 ml)	Stimulation index		% reduction homologous vs autologous
			Homologous serum	Autologous serum	
Elevated	8	1.42	55	36	40
Normal	9	0.96	51	41	20
All Sera	17	1.17	53	39	22

a From Ablin et al.[84]

when they were cultured in the presence of autologous serum, eight (47%) patients with a mean elevated level of α_2-globulin of 1.42 g/100 ml showed a 40% reduction in their proliferative response in comparison to the nine (53%) patients with a mean level of α_2-globulin within the range of normal 0.96 g/100 ml of only 20%.

Such observations suggest, that while a reduction was noted in patients possessing an elevated mean level of α_2-globulin as well as in those with a mean level of α_2-globulin within the range of normal, the patients with an elevated level of α_2-globulin possessed, by virtue of the observed two-fold reduction, a greater concentration of, an as yet unidentified component in the α_2-globulin fraction of serum. This, however, although supportive of the effect of an elevated "absolute" level of α_2-globulin on lymphocytic reactivity as put forth by several investigators, is at least in part misleading. (The terminology "absolute" level designates that only the total level of α_2-globulin and not that of specific components migrating in this fraction of serum, e.g., immunoregulatory α_2-globulin[211] or pregnancy-associated globulin[232f] was quantitated.) When the association between an elevated "absolute" level of α_2-globulin and the percent reduction in the Stimulation Index of homologous vs autologous serum of eight of the 17 (47%) patients possessing an elevated "absolute" level of α_2-globulin was evaluated, three (38%) showed reductions in their Stimulation Index when cultured in autologous serum. While, in contrast and particularly striking, was that of nine (53%) of the patients with a level of α_2-globulin within the range of normal, seven (78%) possessed a Stimulation Index which was lower in autologous than in homologous serum. Thus, observation of an aberration of the proliferative response of PHA in autologous serum was not always concomitantly associated with an elevated "absolute" level of α_2-globulin and vice versa.

An "absolute" level of α_2-globulin within the range of normal in a given patient does not preclude, as evident from this recent study, the possibility that this patient does not possess an elevated level of the particular, as yet unidentified, immunosuppressive or "immunoregulatory" component(s) which appears on the basis of several studies,[209-214] to be in the α_2-globulin fraction. Conversely an elevated "absolute" level of α_2-globulin in a given patient, possibly due to an elevation in other nonimmunoregulatory proteins, thereby, accounting for the "absolute" elevation, does not mean, as particularly so evidenced from these studies,[81,82,84] that this patient will have a reduced proliferative response.

The possibility that the reduction in lymphocytic reactivity observed in these recent reports[81,82,84,207,215] may not have been attributable to a component in the α_2-globulin fraction must also be considered. In this regard the possible presence in the sera studied of increased levels of prolactin shown to inhibit lymphocytic reactivity to PHA,[216] or of "blocking" factors,[173a] either of which were not evaluated in these reports must not be excluded. However, a possible reduction due to androgen-depleting therapy, as recently reported in patients with prostatic cancer receiving estrogen,[217-221] may be excluded as a contributing factor in the report by Ablin et al.,[84] as none of the patients (to my knowledge) evaluated had received estrogen prior to the time at which specimens for study were obtained.

The existence of a general diminution in immunocompetence, principally associated with aberrations of cell-mediated responsiveness in patients with prostatic cancer, would appear to be of more than academic interest. In this regard knowledge that various therapeutic modalities in themselves result in aberrations of host

resistance suggests they may reasonably lead to or enhance concomitant reduced surveillance of tumor in patients with prostatic cancer.

While, perhaps, premature to say of significance, I believe that brief comment of recent studies of the suggested immunosuppressive effects of androgen-depleting therapy, i.e., estrogenic therapy, in patients with prostatic cancer would be in order. In this regard I was initially struck by the possibility that as the administration of estrogen has been observed to result in a generalized stimulation of reticuloendothelial activity[222,223] leading to what appears to be enhancement of humoral antibody production,[224,225] and in selected instances, suppression of manifestations of delayed type hypersensitivity,[226-231] that the heretofore palliative effects of estrogenic therapy might be countered by a reduction in the surveillance efficiency of the patient's immunologic responsiveness to his tumor and to underlying infectious agents so prevalent and contributory to death in cancer patients,[232] particularly in those with prostatic cancer (Seal, personal communication). In more specific terms, estrogen might effect the proliferation and differentiation of thymic-dependent lymphocytes into effector immunocytes, leading to possible inhibition of specific immune cytolysis of autochthonous tumor cells and/or inhibition of the production or release of soluble lymphocyte factors, i.e., lymphokines.

Preliminary investigation of the effect of estrogen on cellular immunologic responsiveness has demonstrated that the blastogenic response of PHA-stimulated peripheral blood lymphocytes from healthy adult males was significantly suppressed when they were cultured in the presence of exogenous estrogen (diethylstilbestrol diphosphate).[217] Suppression of PHA-induced blastogenesis was also observed when peripheral blood lymphocytes from patients with prostatic cancer were cultured in the presence of autologous serum obtained following estrogen therapy, as compared with their response prior to the receipt of estrogen (Table 4–7).[218–221] Pertinent to the question of the therapeutic contribution and/or enhancement of reduced cellular responsiveness were observations that: (1) of seven patients with a normal response to PHA, i.e., a Stimulation Index of 50 to 110, prior to the receipt of estrogen, six (86%) showed reductions in responsiveness to a Stimulation Index <50 following receipt of estrogen and (2) of four patients with extrinsic aberrations of responsiveness with a Stimulation Index <50, prior to estrogen, three (75%) showed further reduction following receipt of estrogen. Particularly interesting was the finding that similar suppression was observed when peripheral blood lymphocytes from patients with Peyronie's disease and transsexuals receiving estrogen were cultured in autologous serum. Observation of suppression of blastogenesis in patients other than those with prostatic cancer and those without malignancy receiving estrogen suggests that the observed suppression was a result of an as yet unidentified alteration, resulting in

afferent blockage and as such would appear not to be associated with a specific pathologic state or malignancy but rather to a given mode of therapy.

In view of the association of increased levels of α_2-globulin with estrogen therapy (Cooper[232a] and Musa et al.[232b]) and of suppression of lymphocytes cultured in serum with elevated levels of α_2, levels of this protein were initially determined and compared to alterations in lymphocytic reactivity.[221] With exception of an increase in α_2 and accompanying decrease in lymphocytic responsiveness in one patient, alterations of α_2-globulin were negligible postestrogen remaining within the limits of normal.

The recent observations of Herr (personal communication) of suppression of PHA-induced blastogenesis by diethylstilbestrol diphosphate and of Wyle et al.[232c] demonstrating the suppressive effect of estradiol on purified protein derivative and PHA-stimulated peripheral blood lymphocytes are consistent with the observations in our laboratory.[217–221] In contrast to these observations and previous referred to effects of estrogen on immunologic responsiveness, studies by Bonney et al.[232d] demonstrated that estradiol failed to induce any reproducible

Table 4–7

Effect of serum from patients with prostatic cancer and patients without malignancy prior to and following estrogen therapy on incorporation ^{3}H-thymidine of autologous peripheral blood lymphocytes stimulated with phytohemagglutinin[a]

| Diagnosis | No. of patients | Stimulation Index[b] | | P[c] | No. (%) patients exhibiting reduction postestrogen |
		Preestrogen	Postestrogen		
Prostatic cancer	11	66.4	24.3	<0.05	10(91%)
Peyronie's disease	2	50.5	17.0	<0.05	2(100%)
Transsexual	5	——[d]	25.6	——[d]	4(80%)

[a] From Ablin et al.[221]
[b] Stimulation Index = peripheral blood lymphocytes + phytohemagglutinin/peripheral blood lymphocytes only.
[c] Probability that differences in Stimulation Index prior to and following receipt of estogen are not due to chance as determined by student's *t* test.
[d] Not measurable as patients received estrogen therapy prior to initiation of study.

immunosuppressive activity in inhibiting the rat popliteal node graft vs. host reaction. One wonders whether this absence of suppression may have been dose related. For example, we, as well as Herr (personal communication) and Wyle et al.,[232c] the latter with estradiol, have observed stimulation, i.e., increased lymphocytic blastogenesis, with concentrations of diethylstilbestrol diphosphate ≤10 μg/ml culture (Bruns and Ablin, unpublished observations).

Although the clinical significance of the immunologic effects of alterations in the hormonal milieu of the host requires further delineation, the implications of such effects as related to the prostate are clearly seen in the suppressive effect of estrogen on the immune response following experimental cryosurgery[50a,52a] and also perhaps in the suggested superior clinical response to cryotherapy and survival of patients who did not receive hormonal therapy vs. those patients who did.[28a] Earlier observations by Robinson et al.[232e] and Horne et al.,[232f] together with other studies of the relationship between hormonal therapy, protein synthesis, and immunocompetence, have been discussed in a more extensive consideration and review of the literature,[232g] to which the interested reader is referred.

Of further interest regarding the effect of androgen-depleting therapy on immunologic responsiveness, are recent studies by Castro et al.,[233] demonstrating that orchidectomy (in mice) is immunopotentiating. In patients with prostatic cancer, McLaughlin et al.[208] have observed increased responsiveness of PHA-induced blastogenesis following orchidectomy in four of six patients. Clinical remission correlated with increased responsiveness in one patient. Particularly striking are observations of a favorable clinical response, marked by remission of metastases, following perineal cryosurgery and orchidectomy (Tramoyeres, personal communication). However, results of immuno-

logic studies in these patients are as yet forthcoming.

In further consideration of the effects of therapy on immunologic responsiveness in patients with prostatic cancer, PHA-induced blastogenesis has been evaluated prior to and following cryosurgery and transurethral resection (TUR) of the prostate.[233a] In patients receiving TUR, the responsiveness of their lymphocytes to PHA was further reduced from preoperative levels when cultured in homologous and autologous serum up to one week postoperatively. In contrast, while lymphocytes from patients receiving cryosurgery also showed a reduction in responsiveness to PHA in autologous serum, they exhibited increased responsiveness when cultured in homologous serum. This increased responsiveness in homologous serum exceeded five- to seven-fold the level observed preoperatively, reaching a plateau four to six weeks postoperatively. Suppression in autologous serum following cryosurgery and in homologous and autologous serum post-TUR was characterized by a return ("rebound") of the patient's responsiveness. This return in responsiveness approximated or exceeded that observed prior to surgery. However, some TUR patients continued to show reduced responsiveness. As in previous reports employing PHA-induced lymphocytic blastogenesis no correlation between the degree of responsiveness and the patient's clinical stage of malignancy was observed.

Reduced responsiveness in autologous serum pointed to an extrinsic aberration of lymphocytic reactivity. As noted earlier, this was suggestive of the presence of as yet unidentified humoral inhibitory factor(s) associated with, among other factors considered elsewhere,[233a] an increased level of α_2-globulin.

Increased lymphocytic reactivity in homologous serum following cryosurgery, accompanied subsequently by a return in responsiveness of lymphocytes cultured in autologous serum and, perhaps, reduction of inhibitory (blocking) factor(s) may, however, have indicated a favorable response of the host reflective of the lowered tumor mass present following surgery. The latter response, i.e., "immunopotentiation," is in keeping with earlier studies suggestive of the development of humorally-mediated immunologic responsiveness[24,25] and to the recent report by Farraci et al.[69b] of augmented cell-mediated immunity following cryosurgery.

Observations of increased responsiveness and recent studies demonstrating a correlation of this with a reduction of serum inhibitory factor(s) and a favorable clinical response,[250a,250b] to be subsequently discussed (page 75), suggest that cryosurgery, rather than being solely immunopotentiating, may alternately be antigen depleting.

In studies of the effects of surgery on immunologic responsiveness, as well as those of hormonal therapy, attention is directed to the overall occurrence of a further reduction in the patient's responsiveness following therapy. Although transient, such depression, if involving tumor-cloned T-cells, may provide reduced surveillance to potential infectious agents and to metastatic tumor cells leading to an alteration of tumor-host homeostasis. While speculative, the potential of reduced tumor surveillance, at least in the case of TUR, appears to be supported by observations that patients expiring from prostatic cancer at our institution had an antecedent TUR.

The possibility of identifying those patients possessing aberrations of responsiveness prior to therapy, as well as those prone to develop or undergo further reductions in their responsiveness following therapy, would appear to be of real and relevant concern in the management of the patient with prostatic, as well as other types of, malignant neoplasms. The

possibility of pre- and/or postoperative immunotherapy in such patients may be indicated, pending further study.

The interpretation of the significance of the reduction of T-cells in patients with prostatic cancer and numerous studies of lymphocyte transformation pointing to either intrinsic or extrinsic suppression of the blastogenic response of peripheral blood lymphocytes and diminished cellular responsiveness in patients with prostatic cancer, as being perhaps contributory to malignancy resides with the assumption that T-cells are of overriding importance in the destruction of malignant neoplasms. However, in some situations macrophage function, which is stimulated by estrogen,[223,224,234] may be equally important.

Leukocyte Migration

Studies in laboratory animals have shown that the migration of immunologically competent mononuclear cells in culture may be inhibited by the presence of an antigen to which the cells are specifically sensitized.[235] The inhibition of migration has been shown to correlate with cutaneous delayed hypersensitivity reactions and has been suggested as its in vitro correlate.[236-238] However, a variety of technical problems involved in this assay, e.g., the extreme sensitivity of some of the cells of the migrating cell population to the toxicity of tissue antigen preparations, makes it imperative to be able to distinguish between inhibition simply due to cell death from that of specific inhibition by antigen.[239] Its use has been somewhat limited in the study of cellular immunity compared with that of the previously described assays. Successful reports of the use of inhibition of leukocyte migration have, however, been reported notably in patients with carcinoma of the breast,[240-244] and more recently in patients with prostatic cancer.[245,246]

Clinically significant specific reactivity to malignant prostatic tissue has been

Table 4–8

Method of determining specific reactivity of patient's leukocytes to pooled allogeneic extract of malignant prostatic tissue as evaluated by inhibition of leukocyte migration[a]

Patient	% Inhibition of leukocyte migration with pooled allogeneic prostatic tissue extracts of:			Specific % inhibition of migration of patient's leukocytes to malignant prostatic tissue extract[b]
	Normal	Benign	Malignant	
M.H.	23	15	28	0.26

Employing the following with the data given above:

Specific % ILM[c] for Malignant Prostatic Tissue Extract =

$$\frac{\left(\text{\% ILM with Normal Prostatic Tissue Extract} + \text{\% ILM with Benign Prostatic Tissue Extract}\right) - \text{\% ILM with Malignant Prostatic Tissue Extract}}{\text{\% ILM with Normal Prostatic Tissue Extract} + \text{\% ILM with Benign Prostatic Tissue Extract}}$$

$$= \frac{(23 + 15) - 28}{(23 + 15)}$$

$$= 0.26$$

[a]Adapted from Ablin et al.[246]

[b]On the basis of comparison with control data of a mean specific % ILM of 0.74 for malignant prostatic tissue obtained from evaluation of 13 controls (healthy adults and patients with diseases other than of the prostate) to allogeneic extracts of pooled normal and/or benign and malignant prostatic tissue, in accord with this method, a specific % ILM <0.74 was considered to indicate clinically significant reactivity of the patient's leukocytes to malignant prostatic tissue.

[c]% ILM = Per Cent Inhibition Leukocyte Migration.

observed in 13 (35%) of 37 patients with prostatic cancer by direct inhibition of leukocyte migration.[246] The method of determining the specific reactivity of a patient's leukocytes to malignant tissue was as illustrated in Table 4–8. As allogeneic extracts were employed, the results suggested that prostatic cancer patients possessed cell-mediated immunity to presumably common prostatic TAA.

Comparable clinically significant specific reactivity to malignant prostatic tissue was observed in only 1 (8%) of 13 control patients (11 healthy adults and two patients with carcinoma other than of the prostate: bladder and penis).

Further evaluation disclosed that the incidence of patients possessing clinically significant reactivity to malignant tissue was similar, regardless of the patient's stage of malignancy, histologic grade of tumor, or clinical status when these parameters were considered independently. The degree of sensitization of clinically significant reactivity to malignant tissue was however greater in patients with localized disease (Stages A and B), low grade tumor (I and II) and clinically inactive disease than in patients with advanced disease (Stages C and D), high grade tumor (III and IV) and clinically active disease.

Retrospective evaluation of the possible correlation of specific reactivity to malignant prostatic tissue as a prognostic index of clinical responsiveness revealed a positive correlation with the degree of in vitro sensitization in three of seven patients available for routine follow-up (Table 4–9). Correlation in four patients was questionable due to observations of "stimulation" of migration rather than inhibition. Stimulation of migration has been suggested by some to be reflective of weak sensitization to antigen.[237a] Weak sensitization due to posttherapy suppression of tumor-directed immunity in the four patients with questionable correla-

tion may be a reasonable explanation in light of observations of transient post-therapy suppression of PHA-induced lymphocytic reactivity in prostatic cancer patients[221,233a] and a reduction in the degree of inhibition of leukocyte migration in patients with melanoma and mammary carcinoma.[246a]

The absence of a correlation in the incidence of responsiveness to malignant prostatic tissue with the stage, grade, or clinical status of the patients evaluated is somewhat in keeping with studies of nonspecific lymphocytic responsiveness to PHA. However, occurrence of a more specific and greater cellular responsiveness in patients with localized disease, low grade tumor, and clinically inactive disease than in patients with advanced disease, high grade tumor, and clinically active disease and the suggestion of the possible prognostic significance of the degree of in vitro sensitization to malignant prostatic tissue provide the first evidence toward the possibility of distinguishing clinical reactivity in patients with prostatic cancer on the basis of their cellular responsiveness to tumor. Overall, the large variability in cellular responsiveness and the failure to identify clinically significant specific reactivity to malignant prostatic tissue in the majority (65%) of the patients evaluated raise considerable concern as to whether inhibition of leukocyte migration employing essentially crude saline extracts will provide the necessary in vitro assay of cellular responsiveness for the clinical evaluation of prostatic cancer patients.

In another approach, observations that peripheral blood lymphocytes of prostatic cancer patients possess diminished lymphocytic reactivity[81,82,190,191,206–208] which appears even less in the presence of serum possessing elevated levels of, as yet unidentified factors, migrating in the α_2-globulin fraction[81,82,84,207,215] or possibly, blocking factor(s),[173a] prompted further study of the capacity of such sera to effect

Table 4–9

Correlation of the degree of in vitro sensitization of specific reactivity to malignant prostatic tissue and clinical responsiveness in patients with prostatic cancer as evaluated by inhibition of leukocyte migration[a]

Patient	Stage of malignancy	Histologic grade of tumor	Clinical status	Specific % ILM to malignant prostatic tissue[b]	Clinical response	Correlation of specific % ILM to clinical response
E.B.	A	I	Inactive	−2.13[c]	Good	Questionable[d]
O.G.	D	III	Active	−5.25	Expired	Questionable
D.Gr.	D	III	Active	2.40	Expired	Positive
R.H.	D	III	Active	−0.48	Expired	Questionable
M.H.	A	I	Inactive	0.26	Stable	Positive
N.M.	C	II	Inactive	−0.60	Good	Questionable
P.P.	C	III	Inactive	0.54	Stable	Positive

[a] From Ablin et al.[246] By permission of S. Karger AG, Basel.
[b] Specific % ILM which was >0, but <0.74 was considered on the basis of comparison of reactivity of leukocytes from controls with that of prostatic cancer patients to indicate clinically significant specific reactivity to malignant prostatic tissue.
[c] Negative number designates "stimulation," i.e., the leukocytes were not inhibited from migrating but rather migrated further than control.
[d] Questionable due to the occurrence of "stimulation."

other suggested in vitro parameters of cellular responsiveness.

The effect of sera from seven patients with prostatic cancer, on their ability to inhibit the migration of allogeneic leukocytes, has recently been evaluated by a modification of the direct leukocyte migration test.[80,83,84,246] An example of a typical experiment illustrating this method is presented in Table 4-10. Slight inhibition was observed with normal human serum as determined by comparing the area of migration of 10.0 cm^2 of leukocytes cultured in the presence of medium, plus normal human serum to the area of migration of 10.6 cm^2 of leukocytes cultured in medium plus phosphate buffered saline. As such, the percent inhibition of leukocyte migration for normal human serum was 5.7, i.e.,

$\frac{10.6 - 10.0}{10.0} \times 100 = 5.7\%$; the percent inhibition of leukocyte migration of the prostatic cancer serum in comparison with that obtained with normal human serum was 30.0, i.e., $\frac{10.0 - 7.0}{10.0} \times 100 = 30.0\%$.

As summarized in Table 4-11, sera from the seven patients evaluated with a mean level of α_2-globulin of 1.81 g/100 ml possessed a mean percent inhibition of leukocyte migration of 17.7. When viewed with respect to whether these patients possessed a significant elevation of α_2-globulin, four patients with a mean level of 2.41 g/100 ml had a mean percent inhibition of leukocyte migration of 24.8. In contrast, the mean percent inhibition of leukocyte migration for three patients with a mean level of α_2-globulin of 1.03 g/100 ml, i.e. <1.30 g/100 ml, was 8.3.

Table 4–10

Method of determining effect of serum from patients with prostatic cancer on migration of leukocytes[a]

	Leukocytes cultured in medium plus:		
	Phosphate-buffered Saline	Normal Serum	Prostatic Cancer Serum
Mean Area of migration[b] (cm^2)	10.6	10.0	7.0
% inhibition of leukocyte migration	0	5.7	30.0

[a] Adapted from Ablin et al.[84]
[b] Mean from three capillary tubes run in duplicate.

Table 4–11

Effect of serum from patients with prostatic cancer possessing elevated and normal level of α_2-globulin on migration of leukocytes[a]

Level of α_2-Globulin	No. of Patients	Mean Level α_2-Globulin (g/100 ml)	% Inhibition of Leukocyte Migration
Elevated	4	2.41	24.8
Normal	3	1.03	8.3
All Sera	7	1.81	17.7

[a] From Ablin et al.[84] By permission of S. Karger AG, Basel.

The possibility that the observed inhibition of leukocyte migration was attributable to the presence of cytotoxic or leukoagglutinating antibodies was excluded, as these sera were observed to be devoid of such activity. The further possibility of a nonantibody cytotoxic effect due to toxic factors present was excluded by evaluating the viability of cell preparations prior to and during the procedure, by trypan blue dye exclusion.

The observation of the occurrence of maximum inhibitory activity with serum from patients possessing an elevation of, an as yet unidentified factor(s) migrating in the α_2-globulin fraction, suggested that this factor(s) may possess either: 1.) migration–inhibitory-like capacity as previously observed in the sera of patients with lymphoproliferative diseases[247,248] and in the plasma of patients with neoplasms (the type of which were not identified) and aged individuals[249]; 2.) migration-inhibition stimulatory capacity,[250] or 3.) migration-inhibition inhibitory capacity. The relationship of these factor(s) to, as yet unidentified components present in the α_2-globulin fraction of serum, remains to be determined.

The prognostic potential of alterations in α_2-globulin in association with a favorable clinical response following cryotherapy (Table 4–1) and studies demonstrating the suppressive effect of as yet unidentified factor(s) migrating in the α_2-globulin fraction of serum on in vitro parameters of cellular responsiveness in prostatic cancer (Tables 4–1, 4–6, 4–11), as previously alluded to, prompted investigation of the correlation of alterations in the level of α_2-globulin and suppressive properties of sera prior to and following cryoprostatectomy with clinical responsiveness.

In a preliminary study employing PHA-induced lymphocytic blastogenesis and inhibition of leukocyte migration, evidence of a reduction in the suppressive properties of serum from six of eight patients was observed following cryosurgery. As shown in Table 4–12, six patients with a reduction in the suppressive effect of their serum postoperatively showed a concomitant reduction in α_2. Clinically, four patients had a favorable response and two had poor responses. In two patients developing suppressive properties in their serum, one showed an increase in α_2-globulin. The level in the remaining patient remained essentially unchanged. Both of these patients had a favorable clinical response.

While these, as well as the previous observations described, are interesting, they are equally tenuous. The preliminary, as well as the nonspecific nature of the suppressive factors identified, reflecting general rather than specific immunoresponsiveness of the host cannot be overemphasized. In this regard, if the approaches herein described are to be of value, we must rely on the subsequent isolation and identification of specific immunoregulatory components and/or the identification of blocking factor(s) of tumor-specific or TA immunity and not on the measurement of "absolute" levels of α_2-globulin which may be skewed by the presence of nonimmunoregulatory proteins, e.g., disclosed from studies of inhibition of PHA-induced blastogenesis by serum from patients with prostatic cancer.[84]

Preliminary physicochemical studies in our laboratory have thus far shown that this inhibitory factor does not appear to be associated with the α_2-macroglobulin, α_2HS-glycoprotein, or the ceruloplasmic fraction of the sera evaluated. Recently, however, significant correlation between elevated levels of serum ribonuclease, an immunosuppressive protein (present in the α_2-globulin fraction[250c]) and impaired responsiveness to DNCB was observed.[250d] In addition, a significant correlation between levels of ribonuclease and the extent of prostatic malignancy has been noted.[250d] The biologic and clinical sig-

Table 4–12

Alterations in the level of α_2-globulin, PHA-induced lymphocytic blastogenesis and inhibition of leukocyte migration before and after cryoprostatectomy as related to clinical responsiveness[a]

Patient	Stage of malignancy	Level of α_2-globulin (g/100 ml)		Lymphocytic blastogenesis Stimulation Index		Clinical response[b]
		Precryo	Postcryo	Precryo	Postcryo	
C.J. (2)[c]	III	4.46	1.21	6	24	Favorable (A, B, C)
S.K. (2)	III	2.38	0.92	14	42	Favorable (A, B, C)

				Leukocyte migration % inhibition		
				Precryo	Postcryo	
R.B. (3)	III	2.49	1.46	36	23	Poor
D.C. (1)	II	2.19	1.41	24	11	Poor
M.G. (1)	III	1.28	0.50	33	17	Favorable (A, B)
H.P. (2)	III	1.47	0.73	18	12	Favorable (A, B, C)
J.S. (1)	II	0.85	0.84	-3[d]	3	Favorable (A)
C.W. (2)	II	0.90	1.28	-5	19	Favorable (A, B)

[a] Adapted from Ablin.[250a]

[b] Evaluation of clinical response indicated, was made following completion of the patient's total course of cryotherapy, i.e., in a patient receiving two freezing treatments, clinical response indicated was that obtained following second freeze and was judged as: *Favorable—A*, Symptomatic improvement, feeling of well being and palliation of pain as expressed by the patient; *B*, Diminution in the size of the patient's initial primary prostatic tumor; *C*, Regression of metastases. *None*—No change in patient's disease from preoperative status. *Poor*—Progression of the patient's disease from preoperative status.

[c] Number in parentheses indicates number of freezing treatments patient received.

[d] Negative number indicates "stimulation," i.e., the leukocytes were not inhibited from migrating but rather migrated further than the control.

nificance of this association of the immunosuppressive effect of increased levels
of ribonuclease on cutaneous hypersensitivity and the extent of tumor is worthy of
further investigation.

Equally interesting regarding the origin
of immunosuppressive factor(s) are observations of suppression of leukocyte migration by factors elaborated from tumor
cells[243] and of lymphocytic reactivity by
human seminal plasma[250e,250f] and rabbit
CPF (Ablin, unpublished observations).
Together with observations of a reduction
of the immunosuppressive properties of
serum from prostatic cancer patients following cryoprostatectomy,[250a,250b] these
observations provide some rationale for
the feasibility of the elaboration of suppressive factors from malignant prostatic
tissue and their reduction following
cryosurgical destruction of viable tumor.
That is, suppression and its resultant
reduction following cryosurgical destruction of tumor may be attributed to a
reduction in soluble prostatic TAA shed
into the circulation by previously viable
tumor. While not at a sufficient concentration to engender an immune response in
the aging and tumor-burdened host, this
antigen may, however, have been
sufficient to pre-empt the effector limb of
cell-mediated responsiveness contributing to the observed suppression of lymphocytic reactivity. Cryosurgery, resulting in necrosis and cell death with
depletion of the primary source of antigen
may thereby have permitted a previously
overwhelmed host to respond, viz., the
favorable clinical response observed. It is
tempting in this regard to draw a corollary
to electrophoretic studies of serum from
animals following cryosurgery of the
prostate (Ablin, unpublished observations). In these studies elevated levels of
macromolecular components migrating in
the α- and β-globulin fractions were
observed to decline with the detection of
circulating antibodies to prostate.

A factor or factors in the serum of
patients with prostatic cancer have been
shown to have an effect on two suggested
in vitro correlates of cell-mediated immunologic responsiveness–lymphocytic
reactivity to PHA and leukocyte migration. The existence of humoral inhibitory
factor(s) emphasizes the importance, as
previously suggested,[73] of identifying the
presence of abnormal serum proteins,
particularly in view of their possible
effect on the degree to which a patient
with malignancy may respond to his
tumor. Such factor(s) may explain, in part
why, in the face of "surveillance," malignant cells in many instances avoid destruction. That is, they may prevent interaction between leukocyte–inhibitory
factor-sensitive cells and tumor cells. The
possible occurrence of such interaction
emphasizes further the role of humoral
inhibitory or "immunoregulatory" factors, such as those as yet to be identified
in the α_2-globulin fraction of serum, on
immunologic responses (e.g., on inhibition of leukocyte migration and lymphocytic reactivity) as potential ab-
rogators of mechanisms of host resistance,
e.g., immunological surveillance.

Leukocyte Adherence Inhibition

Interest in further elucidation of the
association of immunobiologic phenomena as adjunctive means in the diagnosis,
prognosis, and therapeutic management
of patients with prostatic cancer has been
directed, as apparent from the foregoing,
in the main toward evaluation at the cellular level. Such studies have, with exception of evaluation of the degree of in vitro
sensitization to tumor by inhibition of
leukocyte immigration,[245,246] relied principally upon nonspecific parameters.

Other than demonstrating that prostatic
cancer patients possess aberrations of
immunocompetence which become
further depressed following therapy (the
exception being, as discussed previously,
cryosurgery, which appears to possess a
biphasic effect), results derived from

evaluation of nonspecific parameters of cellular responsiveness, as herein reviewed, not only show no correlation with the clinical extent of disease but do not provide a means for determining host responsiveness to tumor.

Inhibition of leukocyte migration, while providing initial evidence suggestive of antitumor cell-mediated immunity, as well as correlation of this immunity with the clinical course of disease, is beset with varying technical difficulties.[246] These difficulties have detracted from its potential usefulness on a sufficiently large enough scale to permit extensive clinical application. On this basis, modification of the recently described leukocyte adherence inhibition test[250g] has been employed as a possible alternative to evaluate antitumor immunity in patients with prostatic cancer.[173a]

Suppression of cellular responsiveness by serum from prostatic cancer patients, although observed through evaluation of nonspecific parameters and the concomitant abrogation or reduction of this suppression following cryoprostatectomy, also prompted study of the interference (blocking) of antitumor immunity by serum of the patients evaluated.

In a study employing leukocyte adherence inhibition, peripheral blood lymphocytes from patients with prostatic cancer were observed to react to varying degrees with 3M KCl extracts of autologous and allogeneic prostatic tumors when cultured in homologous serum as a source of normal serum. When sensitized peripheral blood lymphocytes and tumor extract were cultured in autologous serum, inhibition (blocking) of the interaction of lymphocytes and antigen was observed.

An example illustrating these reactions obtained through application of leukocyte adherence inhibition is presented in Table 4–13. In light of the recent introduction of this test, brief explanation of its basic format and interpretation of the results presented in the example given appear appropriate.

Based principally on the concept that

Table 4–13

Application of Leukocyte Adherence Inhibition Test for detection of antitumor cell-mediated immunity, serum "blocking" factor (antibody), antigenic cross-reactivity and specificity of serum "blocking" factor (antibody) in patient with prostatic cancer[a]

Patient's leukocytes plus:	Mean % adherence	Explanation
Homologous serum	65	Normal adherence (control)
Homologous serum + Autologous[b] tumor extract	8	Cells reactive with autologous extract, indicating immunity
Autologous serum + Autologous tumor extract	60	Serum "blocking"
Autologous serum + Allogeneic tumor extract	17	Cells reactive with allogeneic extract, indicating cross-reactive immunity but absence of "blocking" by autologous serum and demonstrating specificity of serum "blocking" factor for autologous tumor

[a]From Ablin et al.[173a]
[b]*Autologous* and *allogeneic* designate the relationship of tumor extract and serum to the source of leukocytes used.

interaction of antigen with sensitized, peripheral blood lymphocytes results in liberation of "lymphokines" which alter the inherent adhering properties ("stickiness") of indicator macrophages or leukocytes, a baseline of normal % adherence as a control was initially determined by culturing the patient's peripheral blood lymphocytes in medium and homologous serum in the absence of tumor extract. The patient's lymphocytes were then cultured with homologous serum and autologous tumor extract. As shown in the example (Table 4–13), 8% adherence in such cultures was reduced compared to the normal baseline of 65% obtained in the absence of tumor extract. This difference in % adherence suggested that an interaction of extract (antigen) with presumably sensitized lymphocytes had occurred. In contrast to interaction of antigen and lymphocytes in the presence of homologous serum, culturing of the patient's lymphocytes with autologous serum and tumor extract resulted in an increase in the % adherence from 8 to 60, the latter approximating the % adherence obtained in the absence of extract. This difference in % adherence suggested the absence of the interaction of antigen and

sensitized cells. Absence of a detectable reaction between tumor extract and autologous lymphocytes, presumed to be sensitized on the basis of their interaction with extract, in the absence of autologous serum, has been suggested to be due to the presence of factor(s) in the patient's serum interfering (blocking) with this interaction. This effect of autologous serum may be analogous to "blocking" observed in colony inhibition and lymphocyte cytotoxicity tests[173] and may be indicative of one means by which the potential effects of sensitized "killer" lymphocytes are inhibited in vivo.

As further shown (Table 4–13), blocking was not observed when the tumor extract was allogeneic with respect to the origin of lymphocytes and serum. Rather, cross-reactivity, indicating that the patient's lymphocytes were also sensitized to antigens apparently shared in common within tumors of the same type, was observed.

Antigenic cross-reactivity between individual tumors within a given tumor type is in keeping with observations of antitumor immunity in patients with other tumors, e.g., breast, colon, and melanoma.[250g] Observation, however

Table 4–14

Antitumor immunity, serum "blocking" factor (antibody), antigenic cross-reactivity and specificity of "blocking" factor (antibody) in patients with prostatic cancer[a]

Patient's leukocytes plus:	Mean % adherence obtained with patient:							
	R.C.	G.E.	J.F.	W.G.	W.H.	T.R.	J.T.	S.T.
Homologous serum	50	65	47	35	66	53	27	72
Homologous serum + Autologous tumor extract	—[b]	8	31	10	17	34	7	—
Autologous serum + Autologous tumor extract	—	60	70	23	72	57	15	—
Autologous serum + Allogeneic tumor extract	27	23,17[c]	17	12	5	—	13,28	21

[a] From Ablin et al.[173a]
[b] Not evaluated.
[c] Evaluated with two different extracts.

suggestive, of a specificity of blocking for autologous tumor *only* is somewhat unique and will require further confirmation.

Results obtained thus far employing this assay in the evaluation of eight patients with prostatic cancer are presented in Table 4–14.

Studies of the tissue-specificity of antitumor immunity have disclosed reactivity of sensitized lymphocytes from patients with prostatic cancer with benign prostatic tissue (two patients) and with normal bladder (one patient). No reactivity was observed in one patient evaluated with kidney prepared from a patient with renal cell carcinoma.

In the two patients showing cross-reactivity of their lymphocytes with benign prostatic tissue, it should be mentioned that the % adherence was greater than that observed when the same lymphocytes were reacted with malignant prostatic tissue. This has suggested that, although reactivity was observed with benign tissue, the degree of sensitization and immunity was greater to malignant tissue.

Similar cross-reactivity has been observed, however, at the humoral level. In one study antisera from animals immunized with extracts of carcinomatous prostatic tissue reacted with benign prostatic tissue extracts.[131] In other studies sera from patients with benign prostatic hypertrophy and carcinoma of the bladder yielded immunofluorescent staining patterns similar to those observed with prostatic cancer patients on tissue sections[149a] and cell cultures[165a] of malignant prostatic tissue. In studies to evaluate the disease-specificity of the observed immunity, cross-reactivity to malignant prostatic tissue was not observed with lymphocytes from patients with breast carcinoma, renal cyst, or prostatitis or from healthy adults.

In view of the small patient population evaluated, the preliminary nature of observations suggestive of antitumor immunity and "blocking" factor(s) has been emphasized.[173a] Evidence of some degree of reactivity with tissues other than malignant prostate, however slight, suggests that this immunity might best be referred to as "antitumor associated immunity."

Immunotherapy

Experimental and clinical evidence of the possible participation of immunobiologic factors in the pathogenesis of diseases of the prostate and the possible utilization of parameters of cellular and humoral immunologic responsiveness employed to evaluate these factors certainly are suggestive for indicating a possible role for immunotherapy as a therapeutic modality in patients with prostatic cancer. However, in spite of this evidence, and the fact that cancer of the prostate is the second-ranking cause of death from cancer in the male,[251] attempts at immunotherapy have been sorely neglected.

We may, in consideration of the application of immunotherapy in prostatic cancer, view three possible approaches, including (1) active, (2) passive, and (3) nonspecific stimulation.

Active

In an attempt to provide a sufficient antigenic stimulus to induce the formation of antitumor antibodies, Czajkowski et al.[252] coupled extracts of autologous tumors by bisdiazobenzidine to Cohn Fraction II rabbit gamma globulin. Of 14 patients included in this study, one had adenocarcinoma of the prostate. Evaluation of immunologic responsiveness was by immediate hypersensitivity, gel precipitation, and immunofluorescence. While no skin test reactivity was noted, this patient developed antibodies which precipitated with autologous tumor extract and were observed by immunofluorescence to be IgG antibodies, which reacted with the cell membrane of autologous prostatic tissue. This patient survived 11 months following initial immunization.

Following the approach of Czajkowski et al.,[252] Cunningham et al.[253] have reported on a series of 42 patients with advanced malignancy, including a patient with "anaplastic prostatic carcinoma." These patients were evaluated by a variety of immunologic procedures, which included: immediate and delayed type hypersensitivity, hemagglutination, gel-precipitation, and leukocyte migration. Unfortunately the one patient with prostatic cancer was one of four receiving multiple therapies and was not evaluated.

Perhaps the vital impetus directing attention to the potential use of active immunotherapy in prostatic cancer was reports[22,24,25] suggesting that observations of regression of metastatic lesions in patients following multiple in situ freezing of their primary prostatic tumor, were primarily on the basis of the development of prostatic tissue-specific antibodies following experimental cryosurgery,[33,34] attributable in part to augmentation of host resistance, possibly of an immunological nature.

The procedure as initially suggested entailed freezing a sufficiently large portion of the primary prostatic tumor in an effort to relieve lower urinary tract symptoms and to elicit an initial immunologic response.[22,24,25] The tumor site was then refrozen at a later date in an attempt to boost the production of prostatic tissue (tumor?)-specific or TAA.

Subsequent reports of the favorable clinical response obtained following cryotherapy, which have offered indirect evidence suggestive of the participation of factors of host resistance in achieving these results, include those of Flocks et al.[28,28a] and Gursel et al.[27,30]

In their initial report, Gursel et al.[27] observed palliation of pain owing to metastases previously refractory to hormonal therapy in eight of 11 patients, with regression of bone metastases in one. On autopsy, two of five patients showed no evidence of residual disease. In a subsequent report,[30] Gursel et al. observed a favorable response in 20 of 39 patients.

Employing an open perineal exposure and direct cryosurgical destruction of the prostate in 11 patients, Flocks et al.[28] have reported palliation of pain with no evidence of local recurrence. Regression of metastases was not clinically evident, although no metastatic disease occurred in Stage 3 (C) carcinoma. In a subsequent study of 123 patients following cryosurgery,[28a] rectal examination within the first three months revealed no evidence of tumor in 106 (86%) On follow-up, only five of these patients presented evidence of local recurrence.[28a]

At the second International Symposium on Cryosurgery and Endoscopy in Urology (Stuttgart, Germany, 1973)[30a] and the recent International Congress of Cryosurgery (Torino, Italy, 1974),[30b] there were innumerable reports of the successful application of cryotherapy in the treatment of prostatic cancer. In many of these reports, reference was made to subjective as well as to objective clinical indications of factors other than in situ tumor destruction by freezing as contributing to the favorable clinical responses obtained. Unfortunately, few if any, immunological studies were done in these patients. These recent reports, together with those cited earlier,[14-32] appear to provide a formidable body of direct evidence suggestive of the palliative effects of cryosurgery and indirect evidence of the participation of factors of host resistance as being contributory to this effect.

Further particulars of the clinical application of cryosurgery will be dealt with in another chapter. It would seem appropriate at this point to summarize those factors that appear to support the initial hypothesis[22,24,25] that cryosurgery constitutes an antigenic stimulus of sufficient magnitude to augment host resistance directly through the development of an immunologic response and/or indirectly by modifying factors that may have interfered with the host's ability to manifest an immunologic response of sufficient magnitude to destroy aberrant cell lines.

Direct
1. Development of prostatic tissue-specific antibodies following experimental cryosurgery[33-37]
2. Freeze-thaw induced molecular alteration of CPF[51] and of γ-globulin following cryosurgery[38]
3. Regression and development of tumor specific transplantation immunity following cryosurgery of chemically and virally induced neoplasms[39,68-69c]
4. Identification of: a) prostatic tissue (tumor?)-specific antigens[56] and b) in vivo-bound immunoglobulins[116-118,123,124]
5. Elution of cell-bound prostatic antibody reactive with autologous prostatic tissue following cryotherapy[150]
6. Development of antibodies following cryotherapy which cross-react with CPF[47]
7. Histopathologic alterations in the monkey prostate following cryosurgery characterized by mononuclear infiltrates; separation of the basal lamina and destruction of acinar epithelial cells by lymphocytic infiltrates[57a]

Indirect
1. Correlation of alterations in the level of as yet unidentified immunosuppressive factors(s), migrating in the α_2-globulin fraction of serum[76-84] with the clinical response following cryosurgery[85]
2. Increase in IgM in patients in whom disappearance or decrease of bone pain[96] and regression of metastases was associated following cryotherapy[91,94b]

3. Suggested correlation of preoperative levels of TAA (CEA-like antigen) <2.5 ng/ml with an "excellent" clinical response following cryotherapy[30]
4. Suggestion of depressed cell-mediated[81,82,189,189a,190,191,193,199a,207,208] and normal, or at least functioning humoral[148-149a] immunologic responsiveness, facilitating the development of tolerance to metastatic prostatic tumor cells to which following their release due to freezing damage, prostatic tissue (tumor?)-specific or TAA induced the development of cytotoxic antibodies.

Further discussion of the development of the experimental and clinical aspects of the immune response following cryosurgery has been the subject of a recent review.[38]

Other salient factors pertinent to the utilization of cryosurgery in terms of immunopotentiation shall be considered under "Prospective Considerations."

Passive

Reasonably successful in the treatment of other malignancies, through the use of transfer factor and immune RNA, there is at this writing no indication as to the report of passive immunotherapy in prostatic cancer.

Nonspecific

In a reevaluation of several reports of the earlier success in the treatment of renal and testicular tumors by the administration of endotoxins, e.g., Coley's toxin[254] and of the coincidental observation of the regression of the primary prostatic tumor following toxin therapy for a nonmalignant disease (Nauts, personal communication), Johnston[255] treated a large series of patients with various malignancies, including one patient with cancer of the prostate with Coley's toxin. This patient had had a prostatectomy (suprapubic) and at the time of injection possessed bony metastases with severe pain. He received 49 intravenous injections of toxin over 14½ weeks with an end result of partial palliation of pain, and died one year following the initiation of toxin therapy. Treatment of four other patients with prostatic cancer with typhoid vaccine showed no favorable effect.

Using BCG as a nonspecific stimulant, Villosor[256] reported a favorable result in the treatment of a patient with advanced prostatic cancer.

Merrin et al.[257] and Guinan et al.[258,259] have reported the use of purified protein derivative and BCG in two and BCG in seven patients with prostatic cancer, respectively. A subsequent study of 17 patients receiving BCG by Merrin et al.[257a] has recently been reported.

Merrin et al.[257] administered multiple injections of first strength purified protein derivative into the prostate transperineally, followed by multiple transperineal injection of BCG (Connaught) into the prostate and soft tissue metastases. Of two patients so treated, one showed no response; the second showed necrosis of tumor. Among several immunologic parameters evaluated, an increase in IgG was observed in the patient with tumor necrosis. In their subsequent study,[257a] 17 patients, based on their skin test reactivity to purified protein derivative, were divided into two groups. Three of seven purified protein derivative-positive patients (Group I) receiving intraprostatic injections of BCG showed necrosis of tumor. None of the patients negative to purified protein derivative (Group 2) receiving BCG orally converted to purified protein derivative-positive or showed tumor necrosis. Immunologic evaluation in these patients, although by essentially nonspecific parameters, indicated improvement in three receiving BCG intraprostatically.

In the reports by Guinan et al.,[258,259] no significant changes were noted in the clinical status of seven patients following a single deltoid intradermal vaccination of BCG (Tice). Of several immunological parameters evaluated, three purified protein derivative-negative patients became positive post-BCG; mean monocyte counts, notably of the macrophage population, tripled, and variable alterations were noted in the percent inhibition of leukocyte migration with saline and perchloric acid extracts of carcinomatous prostatic tissue.

PROSPECTIVE CONSIDERATIONS

In spite of the foregoing, our knowledge of the participation of mechanisms of immunobiologic factors, as well as the participation of other as yet to be identified factors of host resistance in prostatic disease, is far from complete. We may, however, from the rather broad base of experimental and clinical observations made thus far consider briefly those areas worthy of further endeavor. In so doing, we may also recognize, as alluded to some extent in discussion of "Clinical Consideration," "pitfalls" of present areas of pursuit. These studies, despite their limitations, also provide us with a rational basis for further consideration of immunotherapy in prostatic cancer.

Experimental

Implications that alterations of the endocrine environment have profound effects on immunologic responsiveness, particularly forms of androgen-depleting therapy (i.e., estrogen, orchidectomy), at present widely employed in the treatment of prostatic cancer, emphasizes the need for further investigation. The identification of specific receptors, e.g., for corticosteroid hormones on thymocytes, suggests that identification of receptors for other hormones on recirculating lymphocytes, or tumor cells themselves, would not be untenable. Such receptors may be of significance to the capacity of lymphocytes to recirculate as well as their capacity for secretion of lymphokines. When hormonal receptors are present on tumor cells, e.g., as recently shown by Acevedo et al. for chorionic gonadotropin, "they may due to their immunosuppressive properties contribute to the immunologic inertness of the host to tumor."[260]

Although a great deal of our present knowledge of the prostate—including one of the most successful forms of therapy, cryosurgery, for the treatment of prostatic cancer—has been derived from studies of cryostimulation, there remain several areas associated with this modality which are in need of further study, e.g.:

1. Studies of the relationship of the autoimmune response to low temperature stimulation should be pursued. The correlation of freeze-thaw velocities and the intensity of the immune response is of significance not only for the possible establishment of a reliable model for the study of autoimmunity, but could be of immediate clinical value in view of preliminary data suggesting that there may be an optimal freeze-thaw regimen as evidenced by the remission of metastatic lesions in patients so treated. Such an approach would offer a distinct therapeutic refinement over present cryosurgical techniques which for the most do not define a specific temperature regime but rather utilize freeze damage to effect tissue destruction.

2. Cryotherapy can be effective as a means of controlling malignant growth in a variety of viral and chemically-induced neoplasms in murine hosts. Such neoplasms could be surgically "seeded" in the prostate gland and subsequently be subjected to freezing insult. Perhaps utilization of a larger animal such as a subhuman primate like the rhesus monkey, in which the details of the methodology and necessary modifications of existing cryosurgical equipment have already been established, would be a reasonable choice.

3. Results of tumor specific transplantation experiments demonstrating that in situ freezing of tumors provides greater immunity to subsequent tumor challenge than does the removal by conventional surgical excision are worthy of further study. In this regard, the effect of parameters considered to constitute the "cryosensitivity" of the host should be evaluated in relationship to the intensity of the immune response engendered. Here, particularly in light of the occurrence of an immune response at the cellular level following cryosurgery, evaluation must include a more thorough investigation of the cellular response, e.g., suggested in vitro correlates of delayed hypersensitivity such as migration inhibitory factor(s) and the possible formation of in situ immune complexes. Further study of the interaction of cellular responsiveness with the earlier elucidated humoral response, including delineation of homocytotropic antibodies recently observed following cryosurgery of the rabbit prostate,[261] should also be pursued.

Clinical

Identification of prostatic tissue-specific antigens, notably those characterized as acid phosphatase and their suggested absence or reduced concentration (deficiency) in malignant tissue are of interest because of their possible associated deficiencies with specific stages and grades of growth patterns of prostatic malignancy. In light of this earlier identification of prostatic tissue-specific acid phosphatase antigens,[56] the recently reported radioimmunoassay for the quantitative measurement of prostatic acid phosphatase could provide a useful assay for investigation of this possibility.[137]

Confirmation and extension of studies suggestive of the identification of the presence rather than loss, of specific tumor antigens, or TA would be most welcome.

The ability to evaluate, not necessarily the number of T- and B-cells, but rather to quantitate those cells which are antigen-sensitive would appear to provide a more specific measure of an individual's immunocompetence than quantitation of a given population, which most reasonably so may contain "anergic" cells.

The blastogenic response of peripheral blood lymphocytes to PHA and other nonspecific mitogens has been widely employed as one criteria of evaluating the cellular responsiveness of patients with malignancy. It should be pointed out that the ability of a given patient's peripheral blood lymphocytes to undergo nonspecific blastogenesis does not mean that they will also respond and at a similar level of reactivity, to specific antigens. Therefore to evaluate the capacity of specific recognition of an antigen, peripheral blood lymphocytes should possibly be reacted with a variety of known antigens in addition to prostatic tissue (tumor?)-specific or TAA. Specific identification and isolation of humoral immunoregulatory factors and their effect on the blastogenic response to these tissue (tumor?)-specific or TAA, as well as on other suggested in vitro correlates of cellular responsiveness, should also possibly be evaluated.

Although further studies are recommended, in vitro parameters other than lymphocytic blastogenesis should be used. Even with the use of specific antigen(s), blastogenesis does not appear to be related to the degree of sensitization or resistance. At least that was the indication from preliminary studies in our laboratory in which prostatic tissue extracts were the source of antigen. In addition, it is possible for peripheral blood lymphocytes to possess specific recognition function (e.g., the ability to undergo blastogenesis) without having effector function.

Knowledge that the development and intensity of the immune response following experimental cryosurgery of the prostate may be attributed to CPF, a prostatic specific androgenically and ontogenically dependent secretory product, implies that factors altering the synthesis of this component will affect its antigenicity. These factors have been suggested to constitute what may be referred to as the "cryosensitivity" of the target organ and of the subject at the time of application of the freezing insult, i.e., 1.) concentration of glandular secretions (autoantigens); and 2.) physiological state i.e., the elaboration of androgen.

Androgen-depleting therapy employed in the treatment of prostatic cancer leads to prostatic atrophy. If the human prostate possesses an analog of CPF in the form of tumor-specific or TAA, the resulting atrophic gland in patients receiving androgen-depleting therapy is protein (antigen) depleted. Thus, if cryotherapy, as one form of active immunotherapy is to be employed, one does not deplete the source of antigen and also suppress the immune responsiveness of the patient. For example, the patient who has previously received estrogenic and/or surgically ablative hormonal therapy may not be an appropriate candidate for cryotherapy. Previous application of cryosurgery in patients so treated may offer one explanation for reports of unfavorable results as well as of the failure to engender an immune response. A patient must possess the capacity to respond, if one is to expect cryosurgery to be immunopotentiating. As logical and reasonable as this statement is, many unfortu-

Table 4–15

Possible approaches to immunotherapy in patients with prostatic cancer[a]

---

1. ACTIVE
   A. Parenteral immunization with whole cells or suspensions of cellular components[b] which may be:
      (i) Killed or inactivated autologous or allogeneic (from histologically identical tumor) tumor cells, e.g., irradiated
      (ii) Modified in order to render them more antigenic, e.g., with neuraminadase, or incorporated with adjuvants, e.g., BCG
   B. Cryoimmunization
2. PASSIVE
   A. Antitumour sera
   B. Antiplasma cell sera
   C. Lymphocytes
      (i) Nonactivated
         (a) Allogeneic (from histologically identical tumor)
         (b) Autologous grown in vitro
         (c) Normal (from identical twins or HL-A identical siblings)
      (ii) Activated in vitro with:
         (a) PHA
         (b) Tumor-specific or TAA
   D. Extracts of sensitized lymphocytes
      (i) Transfer factor
      (ii) Immune RNA
   E. Plasmapheresis
3. NONSPECIFIC
   A. BCG
   B. *Corynebacterium parvum*
   C. poly I: C

---

[a]From Ablin.[262] By permission of S. Karger AG, Basel.
[b]Avoidance of the use of soluble tumor antigens is suggested on the basis of studies indicating that in vivo liberation of soluble antigens may lead to the development of "blocking" factor(s).[151]

nately have paid no heed to this simple fact. The recent observations of the significantly higher survival rate in patients not receiving hormonal therapy prior to cryosurgery compared with those who did,[28a] may exemplify one aspect of this phenomenon.

The suitability of hormonally treated prostatic cancer patients for other possible approaches to immunotherapy, as recently considered,[262] and summarized in the interest of brevity in Table 4–15, also becomes of concern.

With the variable clinical response observed following cryotherapy of the primary prostatic tumor in man, and observations pointing to aberrations of immunologic responsiveness, predominantly at the cellular level, it would appear that there is a third factor—immunocompetence, which must be given strong consideration not only in the selection of cryosurgery as the modality of treatment but also in selections of other therapeutic forms which are potentially "immunopotentiating." In the therapeutic management of the patient with prostatic cancer, we are faced with the prospect of treating an individual who, in the fifth or higher decades of life, possesses, in the majority of cases, waning immunocompetence. This, together with the knowledge that immunotherapy may actually act in an antagonistic manner through the development of antibodies that abrogate existing or possibly augmented cell-mediated mechanisms, possibly causing acceleration of the patient's disease, emphasizes the critical issue of the selection of a given mode of therapy. Therefore, the modality of selected therapy must be that which will not only appear to be palliative in the management of the patient's disease, but which will in view of that patient's hormonal, ontogenic and immunologic status also not lead to further debilitation.

An effort has been made in this regard, at least from the point of implementation of cryotherapy, through organization of a study group for the purpose of attempting to provide a rational approach to determining the acceptability of a given patient for cryosurgery. When this is the treatment of choice, it should be altered or combined with other modalities, if necessary.[263]

It would seem only reasonable that in addition to judging a patient's malignancy in accordance with his clinical stage and pathologic grade of tumor, we must in view of the implications of immunobiologic factors in prostatic cancer and of the inevitable utilization in numerous instances of combined therapies (surgery, radiation, chemotherapy

and immunotherapy) also assess the patient immunologically. The immunologic history and the present cellular and humoral immunologic responsiveness should be evaluated. An outline for a possible working scheme representing not necessarily the end result of the collation of such an evaluation, but rather a preliminary step in this direction through what has been referred to as "immunostaging" of patients with malignancy,[264] as recently revised,[265] is presented in Table 4–16. Once evaluated, a given mode of therapy may be selected which, on the basis of pretherapy evaluation of several parameters of immunologic responsiveness, permits subsequent correlation of changes in these parameters with the patient's clinical course during and following therapy. Such "immuno-monitoring" during the patient's clinical management may also permit identification of an earlier point in a particular treatment regimen in the individual who, not progressing favorably, perhaps should be treated in a different manner.

Preliminary evaluation of the applicability of "immunostaging" has shown a correlation ($p < 0.01$) between the "immunostage" and clinical stage in 21 (75%) of 28 patients with prostatic cancer.[266] Paradoxically, the parameters of im-

Table 4–16

Preliminary scheme for the "immunostaging" of patients with malignancy[a]

"Immunostage"	Status	Immunity[b]		
		Humoral		Cellular
1	Strong	IgM		Present
2	Moderate	IgM	or	Present
3	Poor	IgG		Absent
4	Anergic	"Blocking" Factor(s)		Absent

[a] From Ablin[265]
[b] It should be noted in evaluation of humoral immunity that the immunoglobulin class refers to the identification of specific antibody, e.g., complement-dependent cytotoxic antibody, and *not* merely to the level (mg%) of the immunoglobulin class indicated. Similarly, the presence or absence of cellular immunity refers to that responsiveness of the host to tumor-specific or tumor-associated antigen(s).

munologic responsiveness evaluated in this study were comprised essentially of a broad spectrum of nonspecific factors reflecting more or less general immunocompetence rather than tumor-specific immunity. As such these observations exemplify all too well the dilemma in attempting to select what parameters of responsiveness are the most significant.

Obviously any potential utilization of "immunostaging" will depend upon a concerted effort by other investigators. Eventually, with adequate modification, "immunostaging" may provide us with some indication as to whether a patient should be given conservative or aggressive therapy as well as an indication of whether the selected therapy should be altered or combined with other modalities, once initiated.

The hypothesis proposed by some investigators[41b,267] that the prostate is an immunologically privileged site may explain the diverse behavior of the natural history of prostatic cancer[12] and the rationale for using cryosurgery in the treatment of prostatic cancer. In the rabbit development of the immune response appears to follow the release of a highly potent sequestered immunogen, CPF, whose content of IgG is altered.[38] Membranal damage induced by freezing and thawing may permit the liberation of the previously sequestered (and now altered) prostatic tissue (tumor?)-specific or TAA into the circulation leading to the production of an immune response.

Further support comes from: 1.) the identification of serum antibodies to prostatic tissue in patients with prostatitis[174] and prostatic cancer[148–149a]; 2.) the elution of cell-bound antibodies following cryotherapy demonstrating the actual liberation of prostatic tissue (tumor?)-specific or TAA due to freezing damage[150]; and 3.) recent observations by Danielsson and Molin (Eliasson, personal communication) of patients with gonorrhea, who one year post-penicillin therapy, possessed

gonococci in their prostatic fluid as demonstrable by the fluorescent antibody method *and* of observations of previous gonorrhea patients who, although symptom-free, induced following coitus, gonorrhea in their sexual partners.

Suppression of in vitro immunologic responsiveness by: 1.) accessory sexual gland secretions,[250e,250f] 2.) tumor-elaborated factors,[243] and 3.) serum from patients with prostatic and other malignant neoplasms has been noted. The latter may be due to normal or tumorogenic cell suppressive secretions (antigen?) liberated (shed) in the circulation following membranal damage pre-empting the effector limb of cellular responsiveness (numerous reports of which may be cited) and substances elaborated from malignant cells toxic to macrophages (shown to be present in the prostate[268]) and inhibitors of inflammation.[269] Because of a reduction or loss of the suppressive properties of serum following regression or extirpation of experimentally induced tumors[270,271] and the eradication of prostatic tumor in man,[250a,250b] I would hypothesize that the immunologic "privilegedness" of the prostate is *alternately* attributable to normal or tumor-elaborated immunosuppressive factors. In addition one may well envisage, on the basis of experiments demonstrating the impermeability of tumor vessels to cellular elements, that deposition of these substances on the muscle fibers of venules may impair the diapedesis of leukocytes (Stein-Werblowsky, personal communication), contributing further to the patient's inability to respond to tumor. If such is the case, cryosurgery, as a means of achieving necrosis and cell death with depletion of the primary source of suppressive factors (antigen), may be antigen depleting rather than solely immunopotentiating. If undertaken in the early course of the disease, the combined use of cryosurgery and plasmapheresis for the removal of tumor-elaborated suppressive factors could prove most useful. Prospective consideration of other possible approaches of immunotherapy, as summarized in Table 4–15, have been discussed elsewhere.[262] Since our knowledge of the participation of the host's response to cancer is far from complete, these prospective considerations must in the final analysis be judged in the light of this ignorance.

ACKNOWLEDGEMENTS

Special acknowledgement is made to the late distinguished Professor Doctor Ernest Witebsky who introduced me to the present subject and provided much of the necessary initial guidance and encouragement. Grateful acknowledgement is made to Mrs. Arlene Sullivan for secretarial assistance.

References

1. Mathé, G., et al.: Active immunotherapy for acute lymphoblastic leukaemia. Lancet 1:697, 1969.
2. Morton, D., et al.: Demonstration of antibodies against human malignant melanoma by immunofluorescence. Surgery 64:233, 1968.
3. Eilber, F. R., and Morton, D. L.: Sarcoma-specific antigens: Detection by complement fixation with serum from sarcoma patients. J. Natl. Cancer Inst. 44:651, 1970.
4. Ehrlich, P.: Immunology and cancer research. In The Collected Papers of Paul Ehrlich. Edited by F. Himmelweit. London, Pergamon Press, 1957, Vol. II.
5. Foley, E. J.: Antigenic properties of methylcholanthrene-induced tumors in mice of the strain of origin. Cancer Res., 13:835, 1953.
6. Prehn, R. T., and Main, J. M.; Immunity to methylcholanthrene-induced sarcomas. J. Natl. Cancer Inst. 18:769, 1957.
7. Burnet, F. M.: Immunological aspects of malignant disease. Lancet 1:1171, 1967.
8. Ablin, R. J.: Immunologic properties of sex accessory tissue components. In Male Accessory Sex Organs. Structure and Function in Mammals. Edited by D. Brandes. New York, Academic Press, 1974.
9. Bellanti, J. A.: Immunology. Philadelphia, W. B. Saunders, 1971.
10. Gell, P. G. H., and Coombs, R. R. A.: Clinical Aspects of Immunology. Oxford, Edinburgh, Blackwell Scientific, 1968.
11. Good, R. A., and Fisher, D. W.: Immunobiology. Stamford, Sinauer Associates, Inc., 1971.

12. Ashley, D. J. B.: On the incidence of carcinoma of the prostate. J. Pathol. Bacteriol. 90:217, 1965.
13. Gonder, M. J., et al.: Experimental prostate cryosurgery. Invest. Urol. 1:610, 1964.
14. Soanes, W. A., et al.: Apparatus and technique for cryosurgery of the prostate. J. Urol. 96:508, 1966.
15. Gonder, M. J. et al.: Cryosurgical treatment of the prostate. Invest. Urol. 3:372, 1966.
16. Jordan, W. P., Jr., et al.: Cryotherapy of benign and neoplastic tumors of the prostate. Surg. Gynecol. Obstet. 125:1265, 1967.
17. Sesia, G., et al.: Follow-up results in cryotherapy of prostate obstruction. J. Cryosurgery 1:254, 1968.
18. Soanes, W. A., and Gonder, M. J.: Use of cryosurgery in prostatic cancer. J. Urol. 99:793, 1968.
19. Hansen, R. I., et al.: Cryosurgery of the prostate. Urol. Int. 24:160, 1969.
20. Ortved, W. E.: Transurethral resection of the prostate with cryosurgery. J. Cryosurgery 2:143, 1969.
21. Rouvalis, P.: Cryosurgery of the prostate under local anesthesia. J. Urol. 102:244, 1969.
22. Soanes, W. A., et al.: Clinical and experimental aspects of prostatic cryosurgery. J. Cryosurgery 2:23, 1969.
23. Green, N. A.; Cryosurgery of the prostate gland in the unfit subject. Br. J. Urol. 42:10, 1970.
24. Soanes, W. A., et al.: Remission of metastatic lesions following cryosurgery in prostatic cancer: Immunologic considerations. J. Urol. 104:154, 1970.
25. Ablin, R. J., et al.: Prospects for cryoimmunotherapy in cases of metastasizing carcinoma of the prostate. Cryobiology 8:271, 1971.
26. Reuter, H. J.: Endoscopic cryosurgery of prostate and bladder tumors. J. Urol. 107:389, 1972.
27. Gursel, E., et al.: Regression of prostatic cancer following sequential cryotherapy to the prostate. J. Urol. 108:928, 1972.
28. Flocks, R. H., et al.: Perineal cryosurgery for prostatic carcinoma. J. Urol. 108:933, 1972.
28a. Flocks, R. H., et al.: Management of Stage C Prostatic Carcinoma. In Symposium on the Prostate. Edited by R. H. Flocks and W. W. Scott. Urol. Clin. North Am. 2:163, 1975. Philadelphia, W. B. Saunders.
29. Haschek, H.: Die kältechirurgie der prostatahypertrophie. Langenbecks Arch. Chir. 332:457, 1972.
30. Gursel, E. O., et al.: Cryotherapy in advanced prostatic cancer. Urology 1:392, 1973.
30a. Reuter, H. J.: Cryosurgery in Urology. International Symposium in Stuttgart. Stuttgart, Georg Thieme, 1973.
30b. Oliaro, T.: International Congress of Cryosurgery, Second Session. Min. Med. 65:3679, 1974.
31. Schmidt, J. D.: Cryosurgical prostatectomy. Cancer 32:1141, 1973.

32. Megalli, M. R., et al.: Closed perineal cryosurgery in prostatic cancer. New probe and technique. Urology 4:220, 1974.

33. Jagodzinski, R., et al.: An experimental system for the production of antibodies in response to cryosurgical procedures. Cryobiology 3:456, 1967.

33a.Shulman, S.: Experimental cryosurgery and antibody response. J. Cryosurgery 2:90, 1969.

34. Ablin, R. J., et al.: Secondary immunologic response as a consequence of the in situ freezing of rabbit male adnexal glands tissues of reproduction. Exp. Med. Surg. 29:72, 1971.

35. Zappi, E., et al.: Cryoimmunization. Antibody responses after selective and repeated cryostimulations of the coagulating gland and the seminal vesicle of the male rabbit. Invest. Urol. 10:171, 1972.

36. Stoll, H. W., et al.: The autoimmune response to male reproductive tissues of rabbits. I. Simplified cryosurgical procedures for inducing antibody to accessory tissue. Invest. Urol. 12:108, 1974.

37. Stoll, H. W., et al.: The autoimmune response to male reproductive tissues of rabbits. II. The secondary response as an indicator of cryosensitization to accessory tissue. Invest. Urol. 12:116, 1974.

38. Ablin, R. J.: Cryo-immunotherapy: Clinical and experimental considerations of the nature of the immune response. In Symposium on the Normal and Abnormal growth of the Prostate. Edited by E. R. Axelrod, Springfield, Ill., C C Thomas, 1975.

39. Neel, H. B., III, et al.: Cryosurgery of SV40 prostatic transplant tumors. Int. Surg. 57:61, 1972.

39a.Abdalla, A. M., and Oliver, J. A.: Prostatic carcinoma of human origin transplanted in the golden hamster. J. Urol. 106:590, 1971.

39b.Bruns, G. R., et al.: Transformation and propagation of prostatic tissue in vivo (Abstract). Clin. Res. 23:489A, 1975.

40. Richman, A. V., et al.: Heterotransplantation of human prostatic adenoma cells, MA 160, into nonimmunosuppressed hamsters. Cancer Res. 32:2186, 1972.

41. Javadpour, N., et al.: Fetal antigens' cross-reactivity with transformed prostatic tissue. Surg. Forum 25:98, 1974.

41a.Lande, I. J., et al.: Apparent absence of tumor-specific antigens of a rat methylcholanthrene (MCA)-induced prostatic tumor (Abstract). Fed. Proc. 35:3429, 1976.

41b.Bishop, D. W.: Discussion on experimental tumors: The immune state involved in subcutaneous implants of prostatic tissue. Nat'l Cancer Inst. Monogr. 12:409, 1963.

42. Paulson, D. F., et al.: SV40-transformed hamster prostatic tissue: A model of human prostatic malignancy. Surgery 64:241, 1968.

43. Ablin, R. J., et al.: Fluorescent studies of antibodies to rabbit male urogenital tissue. Experientia 25:993, 1969.

44. Ablin, R. J., et al.: Immunoglobulin G.: Identification of rabbit IgG in coagulo-prostatic fluid by gel diffusion precipitation and immunoelectrophoresis. Indian J. Exp. Biol. 8:185, 1970.

45. Ablin, R. J.: Distribution of rabbit IgG in the accessory sexual gland tissues of the male rabbit. J. Reprod. Fertil. 30:201, 1972.

46. Ablin, R. J.: Immunologic studies of the rabbit coagulating gland and its secretions. Biol. Reprod. 8:327, 1973.

47. Ablin, R. J., et al.: Precipitating antibody in the sera of patients treated cryosurgically for carcinoma of the prostate. Exp. Med. Surg. 27:406, 1969.

48. Camus, L., and Gley, E.: Action coagulante de liquide de la prostate extreme du herisson sur le contenu des vésicules séminales. C.r. hebd. Séanc. Acad. Sci. (Paris) 128:1417, 1899.

49. Freund, J., and Thompson, G. E.: Toxic effects of fluid from the coagulating gland of the guinea pig. Proc. Soc. Exp. Biol. Med. 94:350, 1957.

50. Barnes, G. W.: The antigenic nature of male accessory glands of reproduction. Biol. Reprod. 6:384, 1972.

50a.Stoll, H. W., et al.: The autoimmune response to male reproductive tissues of rabbits. III. Effects of testosterone and estrogen on cryoimmunogenic and immunochemical expressions of the central accessory glands. Invest. Urol. 12:236, 1975.

51. Bronson, P., et al.: Evaluation of the freeze-thaw alteration of rabbit male urogenital tissue antigens by double diffusion gel precipitation. Cryobiology 6:401, 1970.

52. Ablin, R. J.: Cryostimulation—An explanation of the mechanism of in situ autosensitization (Abstract). Biol. Reprod. 9:100, 1973.

52a.Ablin, R. J., et al.: Cryostimulation. Androgenic and ontogenic dependence of the immune response following in situ autosensitization (Abstract). Cryobiology 12:571, 1975.

53. Barnes, G. W., and El-Mofty, S.: Immunofluorescent and immunodiffusion study of male rat reproductive glands VI. Cong. Intern. Reprod. Anim. Insem. Artif. (Paris) 1:511, 1968.

53a.Barnes, G. W., et al.: Autoimmunization by the intra-abdominal release of rabbit male accessory glands secretions (Abstract). Cryobiology 12:572, 1975.

54. Ablin, R. J.: Cryosurgery of the rabbit prostate. Comparison of the immune response of immature and mature bucks. Cryobiology 11:416, 1974.

54a.Vottero-Cima, E., et al.: Tissue-specific antigens and autoantibodies in the early developing rabbit male reproductive glands. Ann. Immunol. (Inst. Pasteur) 126C:629, 1975.

54b.Ablin, R. J., and the Cryoimmunotherapeutic Study Group: Cryosensitivity: Factors influencing the development of an immunologic response following cryosurgery of the prostate. Urology 5:317, 1975.

55. Jagodzinski, R. V., et al.: Modifications of the

Linde CE-4 cryosurgical unit for clinical and experimental cryosurgery. Cryog. Technol. 6:6, 1970.

56. Ablin, R. J., et al.: Tissue and species-specific antigens of normal human prostatic tissue. J. Immunol. 104:1329, 1970.

57. Ablin, R. J., et al.: Cryosurgery of the monkey (Macaque) prostate. I. Humoral immunologic responsiveness following cryostimulation.. Cryobiology, 13:47, 1976.

57a. Ablin, R. J., and Reddy, K. P.: Cryosurgery of the monkey (Macaque) prostate. II. Apparent immunopathologic alterations following cryostimulation. Cryobiology, In press.

58. Flocks, R. H., et al.: Studies on the antigenic properties of prostatic tissue I. J. Urol. 84:134, 1960.

59. Peel, S.: An immunologic study of dog prostate and the effects of injecting antidog prostate serum. Invest. Urol. 5:427, 1968.

60. Macalalag, E. V., Jr., and Prout, G. R., Jr.: Anti-canine prostatic fluid serum and prostatic degeneration. Invest. Urol. 4:321, 1967.

61. Yantorno, C., et al.: Autoimmune orchitis induced by autoimmunization with seminal plasma in the rabbit. J. Reprod. Fertil. 27:311, 1971.

62. Orsini, F., and Shulman, S.: The antigens and autoantigens of the seminal vesicle. I. Immunochemical studies on guinea pig vesicular fluid. J. Exp. Med. 134:120, 1971.

63. Ablin, R. J., et al.: The effect on reproduction in female rabbits of antibodies to a specific autoantigen in the secretions of the male accessory sex glands. J. Reprod. Fertil. 39:359, 1974.

64. Rosenmann, E., et al.: Humoral antibody response in female rats to antigens of male accessory sex glands. Effects of circulating antibodies on fertility. Int. J. Fertil. 16:113, 1971.

65. Flocks, R. H., et al.: Studies on spermagglutinating antibodies in antihuman prostate sera. J. Urol. 87:475, 1962.

66. Nagakubo, I.: A study on autoimmune antigen of the prostatic tissue. Jpn. J. Urol. 61:485, 1970.

67. Yantorno, C., et al.: Experimental autoimmune damage to rabbit male accessory glands. Invest. Urol. 10:397, 1973.

67a. Ablin, R. J., and Soanes, W. A.: Experimental production of autoimmune aspermatogenic orchitis in the rabbit in consequence of in situ freezing of the testis. Eur. Surg. Res. 4:98, 1972.

67b. Zappi, E., et al.: Cellular and humoral responses of autosensitized rabbits to a testis cryo-injury. Immunology 26:477, 1974.

67c. Zappi, E., et al.: Contralateral epididymoorchitis after cryo-injury to the male gonad. Immunology 25:891, 1973.

67d. Hansen, R. I., and Wanstrup, J.: Cryoprostatectomy: Histological changes elucidated by serial biopsies. Scand. J. Nephrol. 7:100, 1973.

68. Myers, R. S., et al.: Tumor-specific transplanta-

tion immunity after cryosurgery. J. Surg. Oncol. 1:241, 1969.

69. Blackwood, C. E., and Cooper, I. S.: Response of experimental tumor systems to cryosurgery. Cryobiology 9:508, 1972.

69a. Schweizer, K., et al.: Immunological studies after cryosurgical tumor treatment. Minn. Med. 65:3658, 1974.

69b. Farraci, R. P., et al.: In vitro demonstration of cryosurgical augmentation of tumor immunity. Surgery 77:433, 1975.

69c. Riggi, G.: The Effect of Cryonecrosis on Immunitary Resistance to Syngeneic Tumors. In Antibody Response to Cryotherapy. Edited by R. J. Ablin. To be Published.

70. Sunderman, F. W., and Sunderman, F. W., Jr.: Serum Proteins and Dysproteinemias. Philadelphia, Lippincott, 1964.

71. Sandor, G.: Serum Proteins in Health and Disease. London, Chapman & Hall, 1966.

71a. Szendröi, Z.: Die Bedeutung der Elektrophorese bei urologischen Erkrankungen. Acta Med. 5:93, 1954.

71b. Scott, L. S., and Chalmers, J. C.: An electrophoretic study of the serum globulins in vesical and prostatic cancer. Br. J. Urol. 30:8, 1958.

72. Ablin, R. J., et al.: Serum proteins in patients with benign and malignant diseases of the prostate. Neoplasma 18:271, 1971.

73. Ablin, R. J., et al.: Serum proteins in prostatic cancer. I. Relationship between clinical stage and level. J. Urol. 110:238, 1973.

74. Flocks, R. H.: Carcinoma of the prostate. J. Urol. 101:741, 1969.

75. Lynch, W. J., and Joske, R. A.: The occurrence of abnormal serum proteins in patients with epithelial neoplasms. J. Clin. Pathol. 19:461, 1966.

76. Ablin, R. J.: Discussion. Immunosuppression Workshop. 4th International Congress of the Transplantation Society, San Francisco, California, 24–29 September, 1972.

77. Ablin, R. J.: Cancer, immunological surveillance, and α_2-globulin (Letter). Lancet 2:874, 1972.

78. Ablin, R. J.: Immunological surveillance and α-globulin. Isr. J. Med. Sci. 9:480, 1973.

79. Ablin, R. J.: Interference of immunologic surveillance by immunoregulatory alpha globulin. A hypothesis. Neoplasma 20:159, 1973.

80. Ablin, R. J.: Migration-inhibitory activity in the serum of patients with prostatic cancer (Abstract). Clin. Res. 22:609A, 1974.

81. Bruns, G. R., et al.: Reduced lymphocytic blastogenesis in prostatic cancer (Abstract). Clin. Res. 22:610A, 1974.

82. Ablin, R. J., et al.: Evaluation of cellular immunologic responsiveness in the clinical management of patients with prostatic cancer. I. Thymic dependent lymphocytic blastogenesis. Urol. Int. In press.

83. Ablin, R. J., et al.: Migration-inhibitory effect of serum from patients with prostatic cancer. Oncology 30:423, 1974.

84. Ablin, R. J., et al.: Serum proteins in prostatic cancer. II. Effect on in vitro cell-mediated immunologic responsiveness. Urology 6:22, 1975.

85. Ablin, R. J., et al.: Alterations of alpha$_2$-globulin and the clinical response in patients with prostatic cancer following cryotherapy. Oncology 32:127, 1975.

86. Juret, P., and Frayssinet, C.: Bull. Cancer (Paris) 44:156, 1957. (As cited by Sandor, G.: Serum Proteins in Health and Disease. London, Chapman & Hall, 1966.)

87. Minton, J. P., and Bianco, M. A.: Serum α_2-globulins in breast carcinoma. Arch. Surg. 109:238, 1974.

87a. Stimson, W. H.: Correlation of the blood-level of a pregnancy-associated α-macroglobulin with the clinical course of cancer patients. Lancet 1:777, 1975.

87b. Suga, S., and Tamura, Z.: Analysis of serum protein changes in patients with advanced gastric cancer with special reference to α-globulin fractions. Cancer Res. 32:426, 1972.

87c. Gerber, J., et al.: Biochemical blood studies in patients with carcinoma of the ovaries during treatment with preparation C-283. I. Behavior of serum protein fractions. Arch. Immunol. Ther. Exp. 19:861, 1971.

87d. McPhedran, P., et al.: Alpha$_2$-globulin "spike" in renal carcinoma. Ann. Intern. Med. 76:439, 1972.

88. Zacharia, T. P., and Pollard, M.: Elevated levels of α-globulins of sera from germfree rats with 3-methylcholanthrene-induced tumors. J. Natl. Cancer Inst. 42:35, 1969.

89. Bogden, A. E. et al.: Primary (methyl-cholanthrene-induced) fibrosarcomas and glycoprotein synthesis. Cancer Res. 27:230, 1967.

90. Hinrichs, D. J., et al.: Serum globulin changes in tumor-bearing hamsters. Oncology 27:64, 1973.

91. Ablin, R. J., et al.: Alterations of serum proteins in patients with prostatic cancer following cryoprostatectomy (Abstract). Clin. Res. 20:882, 1972.

92. Ablin, R. J., et al.: Serum proteins in prostatic cancer. IV. Alterations following cryoprostatectomy. Urol. Int. In press.

93. Drylie, D. M., et al.: Immunologic consequences of cryosurgery. I. Serum Proteins. Invest. Urol. 5:619, 1968.

94. Ablin, R. J., et al.: Levels of immunoglobulins in the serum of patients with carcinoma of the prostate. Neoplasma 19:57, 1972.

94a. Ablin, R. J.: Serum proteins in prostatic cancer. III. Relationship of levels of immunoglobulins and complement to clinical stage of disease. Urology 7:39, 1976.

94b. Ablin, R. J., et al.: Serum proteins in prostatic cancer. V. Alterations in immunoglobulins and clinical responsiveness following cryoprostatectomy. Urol. Int. In press.

95. Gursel, E. O., et al.: Serum immunoglobulins in patients with prostate cancer. Urol. Res. 1:145, 1973.

96. Gursel, E., et al.: Effects of cryotherapy on serum immunoglobulins in patients with prostate cancer. XVI Congress International Society Urology. 2:286, 1973.

97. Guinan, A., et al.: Urinary excretion of immunoglobulins in prostatic cancer (Abstract). Clin. Res. 22:490A, 1974.

98. Ablin, R. J., et al.: Levels of C'3 in the serum of patients with benign and malignant diseases of the prostate. Neoplasma 19:61, 1972.

98a. Schmidt, J. D., et al.: Serum immunoglobulins in genitourinary malignancies. J. Urol. 115:293, 1976.

99. Buckley, C. E., III, et al.: Longitudinal changes in serum immunoglobulin levels in older humans. Fed. Proc. 33:2036, 1974.

99a. McKenzie, D., et al.: Complement reactivity of cancer patients: Measurements by immune hemolysis and immune adherence. Cancer Res. 27:2386, 1967.

100. Abelev, G. I.: Alpha-fetoprotein in ontogenesis and its association with malignant tumours. Adv. Cancer Res. 14:295, 1971.

101. Zamcheck, N., et al.: Immunologic diagnosis and prognosis of human digestive-tract cancer: Carcinoembryonic antigens. N. Eng. J. Med. 286:83, 1972.

102. Kraft, S. C.: "Humors from tumors:" Carcinoembryonic antigen, alpha-fetoprotein, and digestive system cancer. Ann. Intern. Med. 76:502, 1972.

103. Alexander, P.: Fetal "antigens" in cancer. Nature 236:137, 1972.

104. Gold, P., and Freedman, S. O.: Demonstration of tumor-specific antigens in human colonic carcinomata by immunological tolerance and absorption techniques. J. Exp. Med. 121:439, 1965.

105. Lo Gerfo, P., et al.: Demonstration of an antigen common to several varieties of neoplasia. Assay using zirconyl phosphate gel. N. Engl. J. Med. 285:138, 1971.

106. Reynoso, G., et al.: Carcinoembryonic antigen in patients with different cancers. J.A.M.A. 220:361, 1972.

107. Laurence, D. J. R., et al.: Role of plasma carcinoembryonic antigen in diagnosis of gastrointestinal, mammary, and bronchial carcinoma. Br. Med. J. 3:605, 1972.

108. Reynoso, G., et al.: Carcinoembryonic antigen in patients with tumors of the urogenital tract. Cancer 30:1, 1972.

109. Guinan, P., et al.: Carcinoembryonic antigen in patients with urologic cancers. Urol. Res. 1:101, 1973.

110. Neufeld, L., et al.: Carcinoembryonic antigen in the diagnosis of prostate carcinoma. Oncology 29:376, 1974.

111. Guinan, P. D., et al.: Carcinoembryonic-like antigen and acid phosphatase in the diagnosis of carcinoma of the prostate (Abstract). Clin. Res. 22:715A, 1974.

112. Hsu, C. C. S., and Lo Gerfo, P.: Correlation between serum alpha-globulin and plasma inhibitory effect on PHA-stimulated lymphocytes in colon cancer patients. Proc. Soc. Exp. Biol. Med. 139:575, 1972.

113. Al Sheik, H. I., et al.: Carcinoembryonic-like antigen and alpha$_2$-globulin in prostatic cancer (Abstract). Clin. Res. 22:714A, 1974.

114. Thitipraserth, A., et al.: Carcinoembryonic antigen in the plasma and urine of patients with urologic cancer (Abstract). Proc. Inst. Med. Chicago 29:323, 1973.

115. Guinan, P., et al.: The prognostic value of carcinoembryonic antigen in prostatic cancer. 2nd Midwest Fall Immunology Conference, Chicago, Illinois, 1973.

116. Tannenbaum, M., and Lattimer, J. K.: Immunopathology of prostate—benign and malignant (Abstract). XVI Congress International Society Urology, Amsterdam, The Netherlands. 1973.

117. Tannenbaum, M., et al.: Immunopathology of the prostate, benign and malignant (Abstract). American Urological Association, Inc., 69th Annual Meeting, St. Louis, Missouri, 1974.

118. Tannenbaum, M., et al.: Biology of the prostate. II. An immunofluorescent study of benign prostatic hypertrophy and carcinoma. Urology (To be published).

119. Wechsler, M., et al.: The cancer associated antigen test as an index to failure of complete removal of urological cancers. J. Urol. 109:699, 1973.

120. Abelev, G. I., et al.: Production of embryonal alpha-globulin by transplantable mouse hepatoma. Transplantation 1:174, 1963.

121. Mehlman, D. J., et al.: Serum alpha$_1$-fetoglobulin with gastric and prostatic carcinomas. N. Engl. J. Med. 285:1060, 1971.

121a. Guinan, P. D., et al.: Alpha-feto-protein in prostate cancer (Abstract). Clin. Res. 23:339A, 1975.

122. Tal, C., and Halperin, M.: Presence of serologically distinct protein in serum of cancer patients and pregnant women. An attempt to develop a diagnostic cancer test. Isr. J. Med. Sci. 6:708, 1970.

123. Ablin, R. J., et al.: Localization of immunoglobulins in human prostatic tissue. J. Immunol. 107:603, 1971.

124. Ablin, R. J., et al.: In vivo bound immunoglobulins in the human prostate. Their identification and possible significance. Z. Immunitaetsforsch 144:233, 1972.

125. Hirzfeld, L., et al.: Über die serologische Spezifität der Krebszellen. Klin. Wochenschr. 8:1563, 1929.

126. Davidsohn, I.: Early immunologic diagnosis and prognosis of carcinoma. Am. J. Clin. Pathol. 57:715, 1972.

127. Gupta, R. K., et al.: Loss of isoantigens A, B and H in prostate. Am. J. Pathol. 70:439, 1973.

128. Shulman, S.: Antigenicity and autoimmunity in sexual reproduction: A review. Clin. Exp. Immunol. 9:267, 1971.

129. Ablin, R. J., et al.: Precipitating antigens of the normal human prostate. J. Reprod. Fertil. 22:573, 1970.

130. Kramer, H. J., et al.: Studies of human kidney and urine acid phosphatase. I. Biochemical characteristics and in vitro factors influencing measurement. Enzym. Biol. Clin. 11:435, 1970.

131. Ablin, R. J.: Immunologic studies of normal, benign, and malignant human prostatic tissue. Cancer 29:1570, 1972.

132. Kirchheim, D., et al.: Histochemistry of the normal, hyperplastic, and neoplastic human prostate gland. Invest. Urol. 1:403, 1964.

133. Parkin, L., et al.: Acid phosphatase in carcinoma of the prostate in man. J. Histochem. Cytochem. 12:288, 1964.

134. Kent, J. R., et al.: Acid phosphatase content of prostatic exprimate from patients with advanced prostatic carcinoma: A potential prognostic and therapeutic index. Cancer 25:858, 1970.

135. Nilsson, T.: On Some Histochemical and Biochemical Aspects of the Human Prostate. Thesis. University of Lund, 1973.

136. Nairn, R. C., et al.: Immunological differences between normal and malignant cells. Br. Med. J. 2:1335, 1960.

137. Cooper, J. F., and Foti, A.: A radioimmunoassay for prostatic acid phosphatase. I. Methodology and range of normal male serum values. Invest. Urol. 12:98, 1974.

138. Mattila, S.: Proteins of the human prostate tissue as characterized by electrophoresis, immunodiffusion and immunoelectrophoresis in agar gel, combined with histochemical staining methods. Ann. Chir. Gynaecol. Fenn. 56 (Suppl. 149):7, 1967.

139. Mattila, S.: Detection of two molecular forms of the human prostatic acid phosphatase. Invest. Urol. 6:337, 1969.

140. Mattila, S.: Further studies on the prostatic tissue antigens. Separation of two molecular forms of aminopeptidase. Invest. Urol. 7:1, 1969.

141. Reif, A. E., et al.: Acid phosphatase isozymes in cancer of the prostate. Cancer 31:689, 1973.

142. Bubenik, J.: Tumour immunity and prostate carcinoma (Abstract). XVI Congress International Society Urology. Amsterdam, The Netherlands, 1973.

143. Ablin, R. J., and Soanes, W. A.; Immunohistologic studies of carcinoma of the prostate. I. Human IgG antibodies to structural components of rabbit liver. Ann. Clin. Res. 3:226, 1971.

144. Burnham, T. K.: Antinuclear antibodies in patients with malignancies. (Letter) Lancet 2:436, 1972.

145. Zeromski, J. O., et al.: Malignancy associated with antinuclear antibodies. (Letter) Lancet 2:1035, 1972.

146. Ablin, R. J., et al.: Bile canaliculi antibodies: Benign or pathological? (Letter). Lancet 1:33, 1974.

147. Yunis, E. J., and Greenberg, L. J.: Immunopathology of aging. Fed. Proc. 33:2017, 1974.

148. Ablin, R. J., et al.: Immunohistologic studies of carcinoma of the prostate II. Antibodies to prostatic tissue. Z. Immunitaetsforsch. 142:432, 1972.

149. Ablin, R. J., et al.: Antibodies reactive with autologous prostatic tissue in adenocarcinoma of prostate. Urology 3:491, 1974.

149a. Ablin, R. J.: Serum antibody in patients with prostatic cancer. Br. J. Urol. 48:355, 1976.

150. Ablin, R. J., et al.: Elution of in vivo bound antiprostatic epithelial antibodies following multiple cryotherapy of carcinoma of prostate. Urology 2:276, 1973.

151. Sjögren, H. O., et al.: Elution of "blocking factors" from human tumors capable of abrogating tumor-cell destruction by specifically immune lymphocytes. Int. J. Cancer 9:274, 1972.

152. Ablin, R. J.: Antiepithelial antibodies in prostatic cancer (Letter). Arch. Dermatol. 105:759, 1972.

153. Beutner, E. H., and Jordon, R. E.: Demonstration of skin antibodies in sera of pemphigus vulgaris patients by indirect immunofluorescent staining. Proc. Soc. Exp. Biol. Med. 117:505, 1964.

154. Burnham, T. K., and Fine, G.: Indirect cutaneous immunofluorescence. I. Morphologic observations in bullous diseases, malignancies and connective tissue diseases. Arch. Dermatol. 105:52, 1972.

155. Ablin, R. J.: Antiepithelial antibodies in the serum of patients with benign and malignant diseases of the prostate. Z. Immunitaetsforsch. 146:8, 1973.

156. Ablin, R. J.: Demonstration of intercellular and basement-membrane zone antibodies in benign prostatic hypertrophy. Dermatologica 146:163, 1973.

157. Bystryn, J-C., et al.: Antibodies against the cytoplasm of human epidermal cells. Arch. Dermatol. 108:241, 1973.

158. Willis, R. A.: Carcinoma of the Prostate. In Pathology of Tumors. St. Louis, Mosby, 1948.

159. Schellhammer, P. F., et al.: Prostatic carcinoma with cutaneous metastases. Br. J. Urol. 45:169, 1973.

160. Bogrow, S. L.: Zur kasuistik der Dermatitis herperiformis Duhring. Arch. Dermatol. Syph. 98:327, 1909.

161. Jordon, R. E., et al.: The concurrence of bullous pemphigoid with malignancies and immunologic disturbances. In Autosensitization in Pemphigus and Bullous Pemphigoid. Edited by E. H. Beutner et al. C C Thomas, Springfield, Ill., 1971.

162. Saikia, N. K.: Pemphigus and malignancy. Br. J. Dermatol. 88:407, 1973.

163. Saikia, N. K., et al.: A case of bullous pem-

phigoid and figurate erythemia in association with metastatic spread of carcinoma. Br. J. Dermatol. 88:331, 1973.

164. Cormia, F. E., and Domonkos, A. N.: Cutaneous reactions to internal malignancy. Med. Clin. North Am. 49:655, 1972.

165. Ablin, R. J.: Antiepithelial antibodies: A possible clue to malignant neoplasms (Letter). Arch. Dermatol. 109:911, 1974.

165a. Dmochowski, L., et al.: Virologic and immunologic studies of human prostatic carcinoma. Cancer Chemother. Rep. 59:17, 1975.

166. Ablin, R. J., and Baird, W. M.: Lymphocytotoxic antibodies in the sera of patients with prostatic cancer (Letter). J.A.M.A. 216:2015, 1971.

167. Ablin, R. J., and Baird, W. W.: Cytotoxic antibodies to allogenic lymphocytes in prostatic cancer (Letter). J.A.M.A. 219:87, 1972.

168. Stjernholm, R. L., et al.: A lymphotoxic factor in multiple sclerosis serum. J. Reticuloendothel. Soc. 8:334, 1970.

169. Yagoda, A.: Non-hormonal cytotoxic agents in the treatment of prostatic adenocarcinoma. Cancer 32:1131, 1973.

170. Hellström, I. E., et al.: Demonstration of cell-bound and humoral immunity against neuroblastoma cells. Proc. Natl. Acad. Sci., USA 60:1231, 1968.

171. Hellström, I., et al.: Studies on cellular immunity to human neuroblastoma cells. Int. J. Cancer 6:172, 1970.

172. Hellström, I. and Hellström, K. E.: Colony inhibition studies on blocking and nonblocking serum effects on cellular immunity to Moloney sarcomas. Int. J. Cancer 5:195, 1970.

173. Hellström, I., et al.: Blocking of cell-mediated tumor immunity by sera from patients with growing neoplasms. Int. J. Cancer 7:226, 1971.

173a. Ablin R. J., et al.: Anti-tumour cell mediated immunity and 'blocking' factor (antibody) in prostatic cancer. In Proceedings Third International Symposium on the Detection and Prevention of Cancer. Edited by H. E. Nieburgs. New York, Marcel Dekker, Inc., 1976.

174. Grimble, A., and Lessof, M. H.: Anti-prostate antibodies in arthritis. Br. Med. J. 2:263, 1965.

175. Tannenbaum, M., et al.: Biology of the prostate gland: The electron microscopy of cytoplasmic filamentous bodies in human benign prostatic cancer cells adjacent to cancerous cells. Cancer Res. 27:1415, 1967.

176. Tannenbaum, M., and Lattimer, J.: Similar virus-like particles found in cancers of the prostate and breast. J. Urol. 103:471, 1970.

177. Shah, K. V., et al.: The occurrence of SV40-neutralizing antibodies in sera of patients with genitourinary carcinoma. J. Surg. Oncol. 3:443, 1971.

178. Farnsworth, W. E.: Human prostatic reverse transcriptase and RNA-virus. Urol. Res. 1:106, 1973.

178a. Seal, E., et al.: Oncornavirus-like protein expression in human prostatic tissue. Urol. Res. 4:23, 1976.

178b.Silk, M.: Stilbestrol antibodies in prostatic cancer. In Urology Research. New York, Plenum Press, 1972.

179. Hurri, L., and Perttala, Y.: Observations on non-specific Waaler-Rose and latex reactions in cancer patients. Ann. Med. Int. Fenn. 54:181, 1965.

180. Bartfeld, H.: Incidence and significance of seropositive tests for rheumatoid factor in nonrheumatoid diseases. Ann. Intern. Med. 52:1059, 1960.

181. Thunold, S., et al.: Anti γ-globulin factors in serum and tissue of cancer patients. Int. Arch. Allergy Appl. Immunol. 38:260, 1970.

182. Waller, M., et al.: Study of rheumatoid factor in a normal population. Arthritis Rheum. 7:513, 1964.

183. Martin, R. F., and Bekwith, J. B.: Lymphoid infiltrates in neuroblastomas: Their occurrence and prognostic significance. J. Pediatr. Surg. 3:161, 1968.

184. Bill, A. H., and Morgan, A.: Evidence for immune reactions to neuroblastoma and future possibilities for investigation. J. Pediatr. Surg. 5:111, 1970.

185. Swan, H. T., and Knowelden, J.: Prognosis in Hodgkin's disease related to the lymphocyte count. Br. J. Haematol. 21:343, 1971.

186. Sarma, K. P.: The role of lymphoid reaction in bladder cancer. J. Urol. 104:843, 1970.

187. Amin, M., and Lich, R., Jr.: Lymphocytes and bladder cancer. J. Urol. 111:165, 1974.

188. Good, R. A.: Critique of surveillance hypothesis. In Immune Surveillance. Edited by R. T. Smith, and M. Landy. New York, Academic Press, 1970.

189. Catalona, W. J., et al.: Abnormalities of cell-mediated immunocompetence in genitourinary cancer. J. Urol. 111:229, 1974.

189a.Huus, J. C., et al.: Delayed cutaneous hypersensitivity in patients with prostatic adenocarcinoma. J. Urol. 114:86, 1975.

189b.Brannen, G. E., et al.: Specificity of cell membrane antigens in prostatic cancer. Cancer Chemother. Rep. 59:127, 1975.

190. Robinson, M. R. G., et al.: Lymphocyte transformation in carcinoma of the prostate. Br. J. Urol. 43:480, 1971.

191. Robinson, M. R. G., et al.: A new concept in the management of carcinoma of the prostate. Br. J. Urol. 43:728, 1971.

192. Olsson, C. A., et al.: Immunologic unreactivity in bladder cancer patients. J. Urol. 107:607, 1972.

193. Catalona, W. J., et al.: T lymphocytes in bladder and prostatic cancer patients. J. Urol. 112:378, 1974.

194. Halpern, B. N., et al.: Effet de la stimulation du systeme reticuloendothelial par l'innoculation du bacille de calmette-guérin sur le developpement d'epithelioma atypique t-8 de guerin chez le rat. C.R.Soc. Biol. 153:919, 1959.

195. Old, L. J., et al.: The role of the reticuloendothelial system in the host reaction to neoplasia. Cancer Res. 21:1281, 1961.

196. Dizon, S., and Southam, C. M.: Abnormal cellular response to skin abrasion in cancer patients. Cancer 16:1288, 1963.

197. Zbar, B., et al.: Tumor-graft rejection in syngeneic guinea pigs: Evidence for a two-step mechanism. J. Natl. Cancer Inst. 44:473, 1970.

198. Snyderman, R., et al.: Human mononuclear leukocyte chemotaxis: A quantitative assay for humoral and cellular chemotactic factors. J. Immunol. 108:857, 1972.

199. Brosman, S., and Hausman, M. S.: Defective monocyte chemotactic response in genitourinary carcinoma. Urology 4:129, 1974.

199a.Brosman, S., et al.: Immunologic alteration in patients with prostatic cancer. J. Urol. 113:841, 1975.

200. Cummings, K. B., et al.: Cell-mediated immunity to tumor antigens in patients with renal cell carcinoma. J. Urol. 110:31, 1973.

200a.Avis, F., et al.: Antigenic cross reactivity between benign prostatic hyperplasia and adenocarcinoma of prostate. Urology 5:122, 1975.

201. Ablin, R. J.: Immunologic deficiency diseases—V. Bull. Sangamon County Med. Soc. 36:182, 1971.

202. Gross, L.: Immunological defect in aged population and its relationship to cancer. Cancer 18:201, 1965.

203. Hughes, L. E., and MacKay, W. D.: Suppression of the tuberculin response in malignant disease. Br. Med. J. 2:1346, 1965.

204. Eilber, F. R., and Morton, D. L.: Impaired immunologic reactivity and recurrence following cancer surgery. Cancer 25:362, 1970.

205. Steward, A. M.: Tuberculin reaction in cancer patients, "Mantoux release," and lymphosuppressive-stimulatory factors. J. Natl. Cancer Inst. 50:625, 1973.

206. Silk, M.: Effect of plasma from patients with carcinoma on in vitro lymphocyte transformation. Cancer 20:2088, 1967.

207. Catalona, W. J., et al.: Lymphocyte stimulation in urologic cancer patients. J. Urol. 112:373, 1974.

208. McLaughlin, A. P., III, et al.: Immunologic competence in patients with urologic cancer. J. Urol. 111:233, 1974.

209. Kamrin, B. B.: The use of globulins as a means of inducing acquired tolerance to parabiotic union. Ann. N.Y. Acad. Sci. 73:848, 1958.

210. Mowbray, J. F.: Effect of large doses of an α-glycoprotein fraction on the survival of rat skin homografts. Transplantation 1:15, 1963.

211. Cooperband, S. R., et al.: Transformation of human lymphocytes: Inhibition by homologous alpha globulin. Science 159:1243, 1968.

212. Glaser, M., et al.: Inhibition of plaque formation, rosette formation and phagocytosis by alpha globulin. Immunology 23:205, 1972.

213. Glasgow, A. H., et al.: Immunoregulatory α-globulin: Failure to inhibit antibody response when administered after antigen exposure. J. Immunol. 111:272, 1973.

214. Glasgow, A. H., et al.: An immunosuppressive peptide fraction in the serum of cancer patients. Surgery 76:35, 1974.

215. McLaughlin, A. P., III, and Brooks, J. D.: A plasma factor inhibiting lymphocyte reactivity in urologic cancer patients. J. Urol. 112:366, 1974.

216. Karmali, R. A., et al.: Prolactin and the immune response. (Letter) Lancet 2:106, 1974.

217. Ablin, R. J., et al.: The effect of estrogen on the incorporation of ^{3}H-thymidine by PHA-stimulated human peripheral blood lymphocytes. J. Immunol. 113:705, 1974.

218. Ablin, R. J., et al.: Diethylstilbestrol exposure and lymphocytic impairment (Letter). J.A.M.A. 229:1863, 1974.

219. Ablin, R. J., et al.: Suppression of lymphocytic blastogenesis in patients with prostatic cancer following estrogenic therapy (Abstract). Ninth Leukocyte Culture Conference, December, 1974.

220. Ablin, R. J., et al.: Antiandrogenic suppression of lymphocyte blastogenesis: In vitro and in vivo observations. Experientia. 30:1351, 1974.

221. Ablin, R. J., et al.: Hormonal therapy and alteration of lymphocyte proliferation. J. Lab. Clin. Med. 87:227, 1976.

222. Halpern, B. N., et al.: Influence of sex hormones on the stimulation of the phagocytic function of the reticuloendothelial system induced by inoculation of BCG in the mouse. C.R. Soc. Biol. 154:1994, 1960.

223. Nicol, T., et al.: Oestrogen: The natural stimulant of body defence. J. Endocrinol. 30:277, 1964.

224. Von Haam, E., and Rosenfeld, I.: The effect of estrone on antibody-production. J. Immunol. 43: 109, 1942.

225. Stern, K., and Davidsohn, I.: Effect of estrogen and cortisone on immune hemoantibodies in mice of inbred strains. J. Immunol. 74:479, 1955.

226. Lurie, M. B., et al.: Constitutional factors in resistance to infection. I. The effect of estrogen and chorionic gonadotropin on the course of tuberculosis in highly inbred rabbits. Am. Rev. Tuberc. Pulm. Dis. 59:168, 1949.

227. Lurie, M. B., et al.: Constitutional factors in resistance to infection. II. The effect of estrogen on tuberculin skin sensitivity and on the allergy of the internal tissues. Am. Rev. Tuberc. Pulm. Dis. 59:186, 1949.

228. Lajos, L., and Görcs, J.: Pathological proliferation of the trophoblast homograft in women. Nature 196:178, 1962.

229. Kappas, A., et al.: Effects of steroid sex hormones on immunological phenomena. Nature 198:902, 1963.

230. Thompson, J. S., et al.: The effect of estrogenic hormones on immune responses in normal and irradiated mice. J. Immunol. 98:331, 1967.

231. Waltman, S. R., et al.: Prevention of corneal graft rejection by estrogens. Transplantation 11:194, 1971.

232. Inagaki, J., et al.: Causes of death in cancer patients. Cancer 33:568, 1974.

232a. Cooper, D. W.: A serum protein present in pregnant women. Nature 200:892, 1963.

232b. Musa, B. U., et al.: Elevation of certain plasma proteins in man following estrogen administration: A dose response relationship. J. Clin. Endocrinol. 25:1163, 1965.

232c. Wyle, F. A., et al: The effect of steroid hormones on PPD and PHA stimulated lymphocytes (Abstract). Clin. Res. 23:96A, 1975.

232d. Bonney, W. W., et al.: Effectiveness and toxicity of immunosuppressive agents: Inhibition of the rat popliteal node graft-vs-host reaction. J. Pharmacol. Exp. Ther. 190:576, 1974.

232e. Robinson, M. R. G., et al.: Lymphocyte transformation and the prognosis of prostatic cancer. XVI Congress International Society Urology, Vol. 2, p. 177–188, 1973.

232f. Horne, C. H. W., et al.: Studies on pregnancy-associated globulin. Clin. Exp. Immunol. 13:603, 1973.

232g. Ablin, R. J., et al.: Modulatory effects of oestrogen therapy on immunologic responsiveness. J. Cancer Detection and Prevention, In press.

233. Castro, J. E., et al.: Orchidectomy as a method of immunopotentiation in mice. In Immunopotentiation. Edited by E. E. W. Wolstenholme, and J. Knight. Amsterdam, Elsevier, 1973.

233a. Ablin, R. J., et al.: Perturbations of host resistance in patients with prostatic cancer following cryosurgery and transurethral resection. Am. Surg. In press.

234. Margery, C. J., and Baum, M.: Oestrogen as a reticuloendothelial stimulant in patients with cancer. Br. Med. J. 2:367, 1971.

235. George, M., and Vaughan, J. H.: In vitro cell migration as a model for delayed hypersensitivity. Proc. Soc. Exp. Biol. Med. 111:514, 1962.

236. Søborg, M., and Bendixen, G.: Human lymphocyte migration as a parameter of hypersensitivity. Acta Med. Scand. 181:247, 1967.

237. Søborg, M.: In vitro detection of cellular hypersensitivity in man. Specific migration inhibition of white blood cells from brucella-positive persons. Acta Med. Scand. 182:167, 1967.

237a. Søborg, M.: In vitro migration of peripheral human leukocytes in cellular hypersensitivity. Acta Med. Scand. 184:135, 1968.

238. Bendixen, G., and Søborg, M.: A leucocyte migration technique for in vitro detection of cellular (delayed type) hypersensitivity in man. Dan. Med. Bull. 16:1, 1969.

239. Rosenberg, S. A.: Problems with the leukocyte migration inhibition technique in the study of human tumor immunity. J. Natl. Cancer Inst. Monogr. 37:139, 1973.

240. Andersen, V., et al.: Effect of autologous mammary tumour extracts on human leukocyte migration in vitro. Int. J. Cancer 5:357, 1970.

241. Rosenberg, S. A., et al.: In vitro assay for detecting cellular immunity in man: Application to the study of human cancer immunity (Abstract). Proc. Am. Assoc. Cancer Res. 12:324, 1971.

242. Wolberg, W. H., and Goelzer, M. L.: In vitro assay of cell mediated immunity in human cancer: Definition of leukocyte migration inhibitory factor. Nature 229:632, 1971.

243. Wolberg, W. H.: Inhibition of migration of human autogenous and allogeneic leukocytes by extracts of patients' cancers. Cancer Res. 31:798, 1971.

244. Wolberg, W. H.: Inhibition of leukocyte migration by human tumors. Arch. Surg. 109:211, 1974.

245. Ablin, R. J., et al.: Evaluation of cellular immunologic responsiveness in the clinical management of patients with prostatic cancer (Abstract). American Urological Association, Inc., 69th Annual Meeting. St. Louis, Missouri, 1974.

246. Ablin, R. J., et al.: Evaluation of cellular immunologic responsiveness in the clinical management of patients with prostatic cancer. III. Inhibition of leukocyte migration. Urol. Int. In press.

246a.Cochran, A. J., et al.: Postoperative depression of tumor-directed cell-mediated immunity in patients with malignant disease. Br. Med. J. 4:67, 1972.

247. Cochran, A. J., et al.: Migration-inhibiting effect of sera from patients with Burkitts' lymphoma. J. Nat. Cancer Inst. 51:1431, 1973.

248. Cohen, S., et al.: Serum migration-inhibitory activity in patients with lymphoproliferative diseases. N. Engl. J. Med. 290:882, 1974.

249. Bice, D., et al.: Inhibition of macrophage migration by plasma from patients with neoplasms and aged individuals. (Abstract). Clin. Res. 22:27A, 1974.

250. Davis, R. C., et al.: The effect of immunoregulatory α-globulin (IRA) on antigen-mediated macrophage immobilization in vitro. J. Immunol. 106:755, 1971.

250a.Ablin, R. J.: Alpha₂-globulin and prostatic cancer: Alteration in level and immunosuppressive properties prior to and following cryoprostatectomy. IRCS Med. Sci. 4:60, 1976.

250b.Ablin, R. J.: Serum proteins in prostatic cancer. VI. Reduction of the suppressive ('Blocking'?) properties of serum on in vitro parameters of cell-mediated immunologic responsiveness following cryosurgery. Urol. Int. In press.

250c.Mobray, J. F.: Immunosuppressive action of ribonucleases. J. Clin. Pathol. 20(Suppl.):499, 1967.

250d.Catalona, W. J., et al.: Serum ribonuclease in urologic cancer. Relation to host immunocompetence. Urology 2:577, 1973.

250e.Stites, D. P. and Erickson, R. P.: Suppressive effect of seminal plasma on lymphocyte activation. Nature 253:727, 1975.

250f. Prakash, C., et al.: Inhibition of in vitro immune responses by a fraction from seminal plasma. Scand. J. Immunol. 5:77, 1976.

250g.Halliday, W. J., et al.: Detection of anti-tumour cell mediated immunity and serum blocking factors in cancer patients by the leukocyte adherence inhibition test. Br. J. Cancer 29:31, 1974.

251. Vital Statistics of the United States, 1968, Vol. II—Mortality, part A. National Center for Health Statistics, DHEW, 1972.

252. Czajkowski, N. P., et al.: A new method of active immunisation to autologous human tumour tissue. Lancet 2:905, 1967.

253. Cunningham, T. J., et al.: Treatment of advanced cancer with active immunization. Cancer 24:932, 1969.

254. Nauts, H. C.: Enhancement of Natural Resistance to Renal Cancer: Beneficial Effects of Concurrections and Immunotherapy with Bacterial Vaccines. Monograph #12, New York Cancer Research Institute, Inc. New York, 1973.

255. Johnston, B. J.: Clinical effects of Coley's toxin I. A controlled study. Cancer Chemother. Rep. 21:19, 1962.

256. Villosor, R. P.: The clinical use of BCG vaccine in stimulating host resistance to cancer. J. Phil. Med. Assoc. 41:619, 1965.

257. Merrin, C., et al.: Immunotherapy of prostatic cancer with bacillus Calmette-Guérin and purified protein derivative. Preliminary results. Urology 2:651, 1973.

257a.Merrin, C., et al.: Immunotherapy of prostatic carcinoma with bacillus Calmette-Guerin. Cancer Chemother. Rep. 59:157, 1975.

258. Guinan, P., et al.: BCG immunotherapy in carcinoma of prostate. Lancet 2:443, 1973.

259. Guinan, P., et al.: BCG immunotherapy in carcinoma of the prostate. In Neoplasm Immunity: BCG Vaccination. A Chicago Symposium, 1973. Edited by R. G. Crispen, Institute for Tuberculosis Research, University of Illinois, 1974.

260. Acevedo, H. F., et al.: Human chorionic gonadotropin in cancer cells. I. Identification in in vitro and in vivo cancer systems. In Proceedings Third International Symposium on the Detection and Prevention of Cancer. Edited by H. E. Nieburgs. New York, Marcel Dekker, Inc., 1976.

261. Riera, C. M., et al.: Homocytotropic autoantibodies in rabbits sensitized by cryosurgery. J Immunol. 111:647, 1973.

262. Ablin, R. J.: Immunotherapy for prostatic cancer. Previous and prospective considerations. Oncology 31:177, 1975.

263. Ablin, R. J. and The Cryoimmunotherapeutic Study Group.: A rational approach toward determining the candidacy of the prostatic cancer patient for cryoimmunotherapy. An interim report. Europ. Surg. Res., 1976.

264. Ablin, R. J., et al.: "Immunostaging" as a

guideline to immunotherapy in malignancy. Curr. Ther. Res. 16:765-768, 1974.

265. Ablin, R. J.: Immunologic aspects of malignancy. Factors of concern in the prospective candidate for immunotherapy. Allergol. Immunopathol. 3:105, 1975.

266. Ablin, R. J., et al.: Immunologic aspects of malignancy. II. Host immunocompetence and relationship to the clinical stage in patients with prostatic cancer. Allergol. Immunopathol. In press.

267. Gittes, R. F., and McCullough, D. L.: Occult carcinoma of the prostate: An oversight of immune surveillance—a working hypothesis. J. Urol. 112:241, 1974.

268. Gupta, R. K.: Mast cell variations in prostate and urinary bladder. Arch. Pathol. 89:302, 1970.

269. Fauve, R. M., et al.: Antiinflammatory effects of murine malignant cells. Proc. Natl. Acad. Sci. (USA) 71:4052, 1974.

270. Ashikawa, K., et al.: An increase of serum alpha-globulin in tumor-bearing hosts and its immunological significance. Jpn. J. Exp. Med. 41:339, 1971.

271. Lilley, D. P., et al.: Tumor growth in the guinea pig: Alpha globulin changes associated with lymphocyte suppression. J. Natl. Cancer Inst. 55:701, 1974.

Chapter 5

Histochemistry of the Prostate

DAVID BRANDES and DIETER KIRCHHEIM

The human prostate is formed by tubuloalveolar glands which open into the urethra through a series of excretory ducts. The glandular elements are embedded in an abundant stroma with a predominantly smooth muscular component.

The glands are lined by tall columnar secretory cells which rest on a basement membrane. Many chemical components of these cells, especially enzymes, have been demonstrated by histochemical methods at the light and electron microscopic levels.[1-3] The substances thus demonstrated reflect the metabolic and secretory activities of the cells, which in turn are indicators of the status of androgenic stimulus in the host.[4,5] Furthermore, some of these histochemical tests are altered in the neoplastic glands[6,7] and also show significant changes following antiandrogenic treatments such as gonadectomy, or treatment with estrogens and antiandrogenic compounds such as cyproterone. In a similar context the

ultrastructural organization of prostatic cells is altered in malignant neoplasia, and the various organelles undergo marked rearrangements after antiandrogenic treatment.

Histochemical tests and fine structural observations are therefore of diagnostic value and have a place in the evaluation of the effectiveness of antiandrogenic and possible chemotherapeutic treatments of prostatic carcinoma. Only those histochemical tests and ultrastructural studies that may have diagnostic or prognostic application will be considered in this chapter. Extensive references to the histochemistry and ultrastructure of this organ are available in a recent publication.[4]

HISTOCHEMICAL CHANGES IN PROSTATIC CARCINOMA

Histochemical tests for various enzymes have indicated changes in intensity of the reaction when comparing normal and malignant prostatic glands. The content of zinc, as shown by histochemical methods, is also altered in prostatic carcinoma.

Supported in part by Grants 1 PO1 HD–06323, NICHD, HD–00042, NICHD, and CA–08518, NCI, USPHS.

99

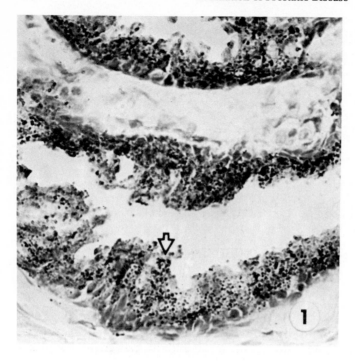

Figure 5–1. Normal prostate, human. Acid phosphatase reaction, positive in cytoplasmic granules (arrow). (×400).

Acid Phosphatase

Normal Prostate

Histochemically, this enzyme shows an intracytoplasmic distribution, and the reaction products appear in particulate form (Figure 5–1). A dual localization of this enzyme in secretory granules or vacuoles and in lysosomes has been shown cytochemically by electron microscopy, in various species.[4] Lysosomal acid phosphatase is tartrate- and NaFl-sensitive and is markedly inhibited by these two chemical compounds, but their inhibitory effect on secretory acid phosphatase is less obvious. These findings suggest that lysosomal acid phosphatase is responsible for the increase of this enzyme in the serum of patients with metastatic cancer of the prostate.

Prostatic Carcinoma

Acid phosphatase is elevated in the serum of patients with metastatic cancer of the prostate. This has led to the erroneous belief that it can be linked to an increase of this enzyme in the pathologic gland. Contrary to this belief, the content of acid phosphatase is decreased in prostatic cancer glands according to quantitative and histochemical studies.[8] This apparent contradiction between decrease of the enzyme in the malignant gland and its increase in the blood of the patient is discussed subsequently in greater detail.

Aminopeptidase

Normal Prostate

This enzyme is very abundant in the normal gland as a strong positive reaction. Histochemical studies have revealed the secetory nature of this enzyme, which can be detected in the apical border and in the lumen of the gland.[6]

Prostatic Carcinoma

Histochemical tests for this enzyme have shown striking changes when comparing normal and malignant glands. Whole coronal sections of glands with focal areas of carcinoma show a marked

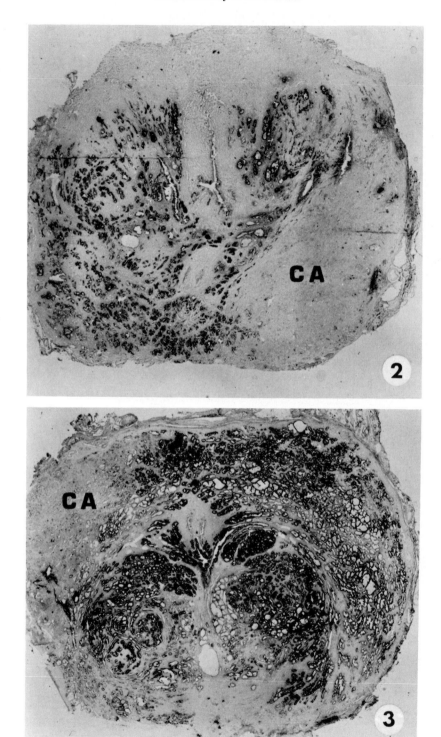

Figures 5-2 and 5-3. Human prostatic carcinoma, coronal section. Aminopeptidase stain. Normal glands show a positive reaction. Area with carcinoma (CA) is negative for this enzyme. (×2.5).

decrease or even absence of histochemically demonstrable aminopeptidase, clearly indicating its value in the detection of early prostatic carcinomas (Figures 5–2 and 3). The striking difference in aminopeptidase activity between strongly positive normal and negative malignant glands is illustrated in more detail in Figures 5–4 and 5. A thorough description of differences in various cell compo-

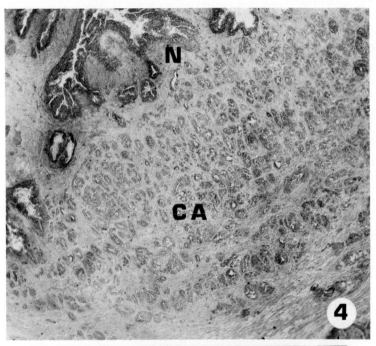

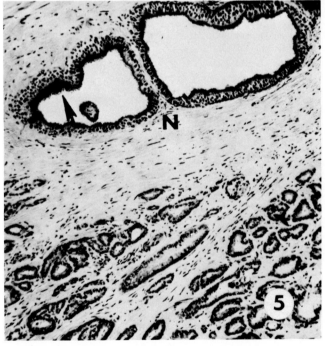

Figures 5–4 and 5–5. Details of two preceding figures. Aminopeptidase reaction is intense in normal glands (N), especially in the secretory border (arrow in Figure 5–5). (×350).

nents between normal and neoplastic prostate glands, both by biochemical and histochemical methods, is provided in an article by Grayhack and Wendel.[8]

Histochemical Changes and Malignant Growth

In most instances the changes in the chemical composition of malignant cells are in the nature of either a decrease or deletion of a given substance, in particular, intracellular enzymes.[8] Furthermore, these enzymatic deficiencies are accentuated with the degree of cell dedifferentiation of the neoplasia and can also be detected in distant metastasis.

The functional significance of these deficiencies of chemical components in malignant cells is not completely understood. Many of these substances are secretory products, and their decrement may reflect partial loss of functional activities in malignant cells. In addition, substances such as organic acids and trace metals, which are of importance in the metabolism of these cells, are also decreased in the malignant state.[8]

FINE STRUCTURAL CHANGES IN PROSTATIC CARCINOMA

Marked alterations have been detected in the ultrastructural characteristics of prostatic cancer cells.[7] These changes not only include alterations in the architecture and mutual relationships between cells but also apply to the fine structural appearance of the various cell organelles. As in the case of histochemical reactions, ultrastructural changes in prostatic cancer cells become accentuated with increasing degree of dedifferentiation.

Ultrastructure of Normal Prostatic Glands

The tall cuboidal cells lining prostatic acini rest on a well-defined basement membrane (Figures 5–6 and 7). The secretory nature of these cells is reflected in their fine structural architecture. Well-

defined regional differentiation and polarization of cell organelles are an expression of functional specialization of the various zones and of the predominant synthetic and secretory activities in these cells (Figures 5–6 and 7). The glandular cells contain a moderately well-developed rough endoplasmic reticulum and abundant free polysomes where synthesis of secretory proteins takes place. Abundant mitochondria are scattered throughout the entire cytoplasm. Secretory products are stored in secretory vacuoles, which predominate in the apical pole toward the lumen (Figure 5–8). The apical pole and in particular the supranuclear region are occupied by a well-developed Golgi apparatus (Figure 5–8) where the sugar molecules of secretory glycoproteins are synthesized. Secretion of products from the cells into the lumen is accomplished through apocrine and merocrine mechanisms.[1] In the first case, secretory vacuoles in the apical pole fuse with the plasma membrane and subsequently open into the lumen where they discharge their contents. In other instances, apocrine secretion tends to prevail. The apical portion of the cells becomes homogeneous and expands into a bleb that is finally extruded into the lumen.[1]

Ultrastructural Alterations in Prostatic Carcinoma

The shift from normal to malignant in prostatic cells is characterized by the loss of polarization of cytoplasmic organelles and their structural alteration. These changes become accentuated with increasing dedifferentiation or anaplasia and reflect the loss of normal function. As proliferating prostatic cancer cells fail to form adequate terminal units, communication between these defective acini and larger ducts becomes interrupted, which is particularly true in the case of infiltrating tumors and distant metastasis. Residual secretory products elaborated in

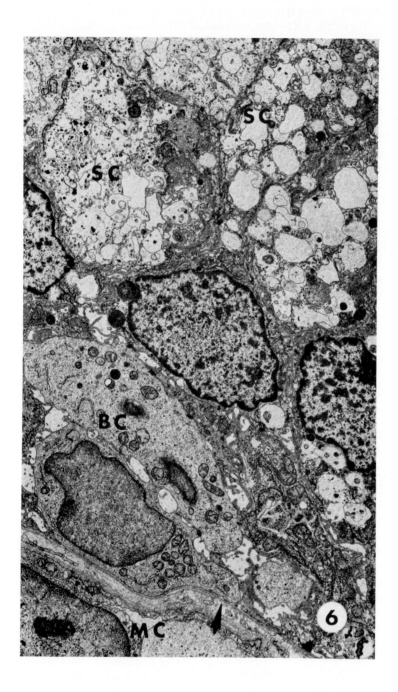

Figure 5–6. Human prostate, normal. Accumulation of secretory vacuoles in apical pole of secretory cells (SC). Basal cells (BC) are interposed between secretory cells and basement membrane (arrow). Mesenchymal cells (MC) surround acinus. (×7000).

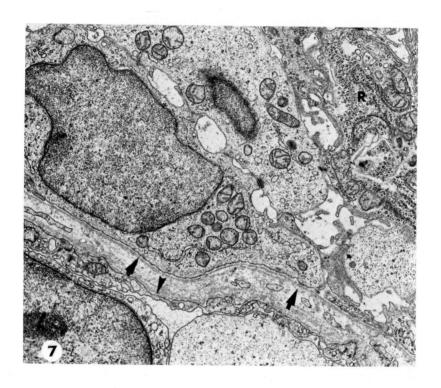

Figure 5–7. Detail of acinar basement membrane (arrows) and basement membrane-like matrix at surface of fibroblasts (arrow-head). Abundant polysomes (R) are seen in secretory cells. (×10,500).

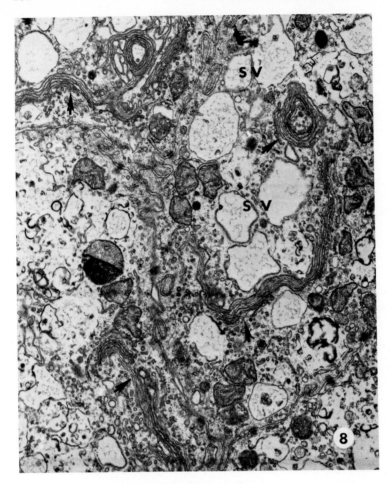

Figure 5–8. Detail of secretory vacuoles (SV) and profuse Golgi elements (arrows), polarized in the apical pole. (×10,500).

the undifferentiated tumor cells can no longer be channeled into excretory ducts. They tend to accumulate inside the cells but eventually will leak into the surrounding interstitial connective tissue. This may presumably occur through diffusion, but actual breakage in degenerating cells that overgrow their blood supply most likely represents the frequent mechanism whereby intracellular substances reach the interstitium and eventually the bloodstream.

The progression in the alteration of cell organelles and in the loss of ultrastructural organization can be recognized when examining specimens from tumors graded 1 through 4, which covers the range from well-differentiated through anaplastic carcinoma. In grade 1, well-differentiated carcinoma (Figure 5–9), ultrastructural organization is preserved and deviation from the normal can hardly be detected. The apical deposition of secretory vacuoles and the development and localization of the Golgi apparatus are similar to that seen in normal glandular cells. Here, the difference with the normal is strictly histologic, consisting of loss of basement membrane and basal cells and crowding of the acinar glands with a back-to-back arrangement due to marked reduction of interacinar stromal elements (Figure 5–10). These changes do not affect all neoplastic acini uniformly.

In grades 2 through 4, histologic dearrangement becomes accentuated. Loss of

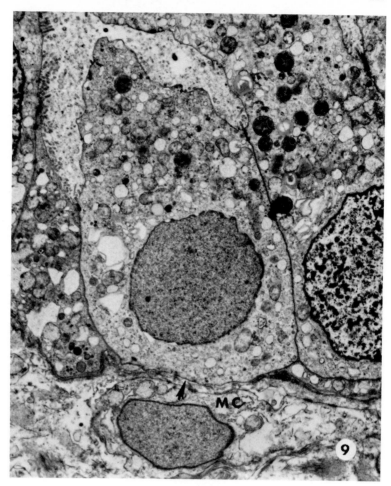

Figure 5–9. Well-differentiated (grade 1) human prostatic carcinoma. Note poorly defined basement membrane (arrow) and absence of basal cells. A mesenchymal cell (MC) lies between this acinus and a contiguous one not shown. (× 10,500).

basement membrane and basal cells and back-to-back arrangement of acini are more frequently seen. Failure to form proper glandular structures results in the appearance of rudimentary acini.

The anaplastic change culminates with the presence of isolated groups of cells which show no attempt at glandular formation, as can be readily observed in grade 4 carcinoma. Ultrastructural changes are also accentuated with increasing degree of dedifferentiation and affect the arrangement and structure of every organelle in the cells.

Loss of Basement Membrane and Basal Cells, Back-to-Back Acini

These changes can be detected even in some of the well-differentiated grade 1 carcinomas (Figure 5–9) and become accentuated in poorly differentiated and undifferentiated carcinomas. As a rule, rudimentary acini and infiltrating anaplastic tumor cells are invariably devoid of basement membrane and lack the layer of basal cells.

The back-to-back arrangement seen in light microscopy reflects the loss of mesenchymal cells, mainly smooth mus-

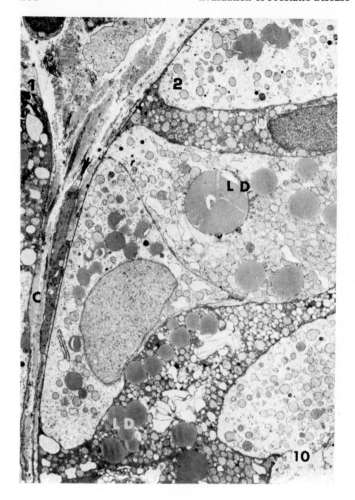

Figure 5–10. Prostatic carcinoma, grade 3. Back-to-back acini (1 and 2), with only single muscle fiber (arrow) and scanty collagen (C) interposed between them. Lipid droplets (LD). (×4,200).

cle and fibroblasts, which are usually interposed between adjacent acini. In electron microscopy preparations, a layer of collagen fibers and sometimes a single smooth muscle fiber can still be seen between the back-to-back acini (Figure 5–10).

Loss of Organelle Polarization

Loss of cytoplasmic organelle polarization is a reflection of impairment of the orderly process of secretory product synthesis and subsequent accumulation of these products in the apical pole for final extrusion into the excretory system of ducts.

The series of events that may lead to this alteration of the secretory process can be reconstructed from the electron microscopic observations. The excessive cellular proliferation in the neoplastic acini and small ducts leads to compression of the lumina, which acquire a slit-like configuration (Figure 5–11) and eventually become obliterated. As a result, increasing numbers of cells lose contact with the lumen, and the stimulus for orderly arrangement of cell organelles—whatever its nature may be—is apparently lost. The Golgi apparatus and secretory vacuoles are primarily affected in this process and become randomly scattered throughout the entire cytoplasm (Figures 5–12 and 13).

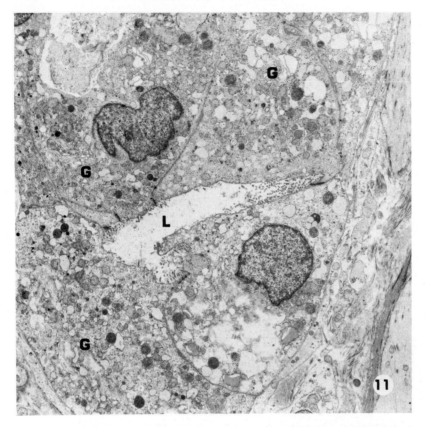

Figure 5–11. Prostatic carcinoma, intermediate degree of differentiation. Slit-like lumen (L) and depolarization of cytoplasmic organelles. Golgi elements (G) and secretory vacuoles are dispersed throughout entire cell body. (×8,400).

Luminal Changes

Concurrent with the compression and obliteration of the glandular lumen, a system of intracytoplasmic luminal spaces can be detected in many cells (Figures 5–13 and 14). This is particularly apparent in the poorly differentiated and in the extremely anaplastic glands, as well as in neoplastic single cells infiltrating the interstitium. The presence of microvilli and a tendency for secretory vacuoles to concentrate around these intracytoplasmic cavities reveal their luminal nature (Figure 5–14).

As to its functional significance, intracytoplasmic luminal formation most likely represents a compensatory attempt of the cells to develop an alternative pathway for discharge of materials ac-cumulated in the cytoplasm. It is interesting that intracellular luminal spaces occur frequently in fetal cells of secretory organs and that the definite acinar lumina of adult glands are formed by the fusion of the intracelluar spaces of adjacent cells.[9,10] In this context, the development of intracytoplasmic lumina would indicate that anaplastic tumor cells tend to revert to a fetal type of situation in an attempt to reconstitute their altered ex-cretory mechanisms.

Structural Alterations of Cellular Organelles (Golgi elements, mitochondria, nucleus, and accumulation of lipid droplets)

Readily detectable changes are man-ifested in many of the organelles, which

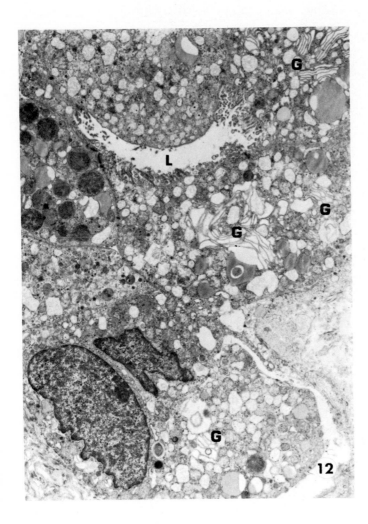

Figure 5–12. Prostatic carcinoma. Accentuated anaplasia with rudimentary lumen (L) and dispersed hypertrophic Golgi components (G). (×8,400).

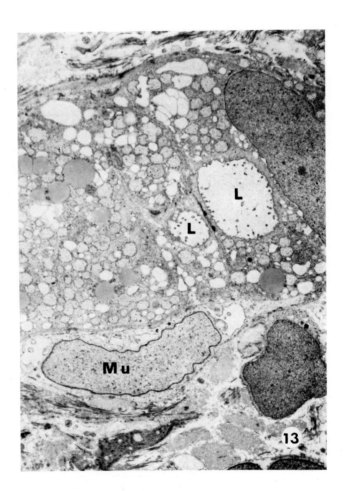

Figure 5–13. Prostatic carcinoma. Group of anaplastic cells with intracytoplasmic lumina (L). Remaining muscle fiber (Mu) is next to tumor cells (×8,400).

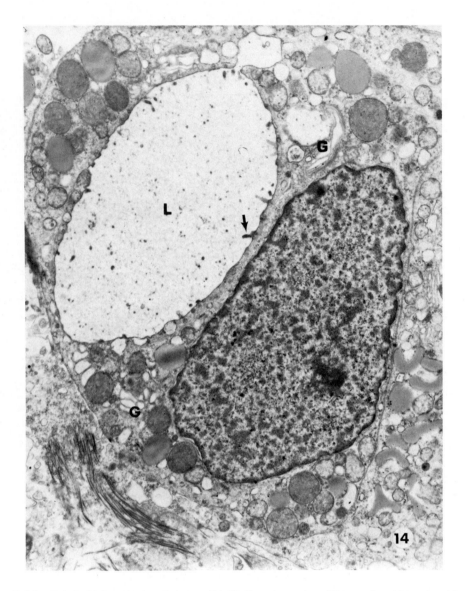

Figure 5–14.   Detail of intracytoplasmic lumen (L). Rudimentary microvilli (arrow) and hypertrophic Golgi elements (G) are seen. (×14,000).

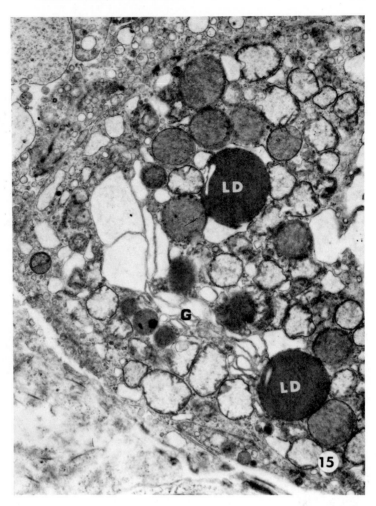

Figure 5–15. Details of hypertrophy of the Golgi (G) and lipid droplet deposition (LD) seen in cancer cells. (×17,500).

may correspond to functional or biochemical abnormalities of the malignant cells.

The Golgi elements not only lose their polarity and become dispersed but also show a considerable hypertrophy and dilation of the various types of membrane-bound constituents (Figures 5–12 and 15). In view of the role of this cellular component in the packing and storage of secretory products prior to extrusion into the lumen, the hypertrophy and dilation of Golgi cisternae are not surprising. In great probability this results from the accumulation of secretory material which cannot be extruded owing to narrowing or obliteration of the lumen in the poorly differentiated or anaplastic acini.

Mitochondrial changes in prostatic cancer cells include an increase in number as well as marked alteration of the cristae, which appear as closely packed filaments arranged in a disorderly fashion (Figure 5–16). It is possible that these morphologic changes relate to the biochemical abnormalities described in tumor cell mitochondria.[11–13]

Lipid droplets are markedly increased in the neoplastic cells but the functional or pathologic significance of their accumulation is not clear. It is suggested that the lipid droplets may contain andro-

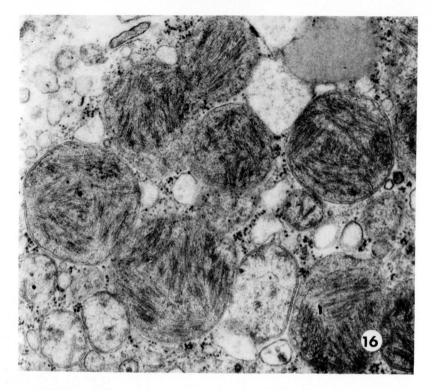

Figure 5–16. Mitochondrial alterations in cancer cells. Filamentous cristae are closely packed and appear disarranged. (×35,000).

gens or their metabolites or that they may be derived from the retention of substances that are normally extruded into the lumen.[14,15]

Nuclear Changes

As in many other tumors, prostatic cancer cells—especially in the anaplastic varieties—show atypical alterations including pleomorphism, hyperchromasia, and markedly irregular shapes. Some of these changes are illustrated in Figures 5–17 and 18 and include elongation and multilobulation, fibrous appearance of the chromatin, and extensive invagination occupied by cytoplasmic protrusions containing a variety of cell organelles.

Invasiveness

Groups of cells forming abortive acini, but mostly isolated single cells, can be seen penetrating interstitial spaces (Figures 5–19–22). Occupancy of foreign territory by the tumor cells takes place at the expense of preexisting stromal elements, such as collagen and smooth muscle fibers. Infiltrating tumor cells expand their domain by exerting a deleterious effect on the various stromal components. Smooth muscle fibers and collagen undergo degeneration and breakdown in the areas of tumor cell invasion (Figures 5–20–22).

The exact mechanism whereby tumor cells can destroy stromal elements or other cells and occupy their spaces is not well understood. This had been initially attributed to atrophy provoked by compression of normal elements by expanding tumor cells, but consideration has also been given to the possibility that more complex biochemical mechanisms play a

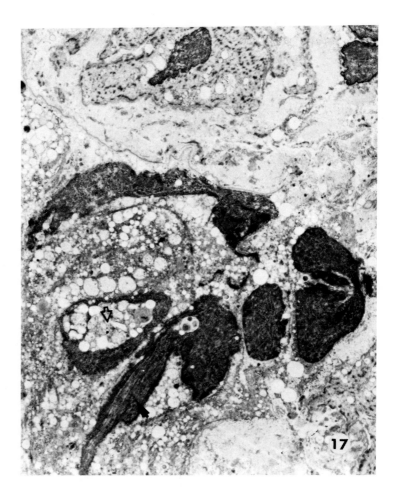

Figure 5–17. Anaplastic prostatic carcinoma. Atypical nucleus, showing multilobulation, fibrous deposition of chromatin (arrow), and intranuclear invagination (open arrow). (×10,500).

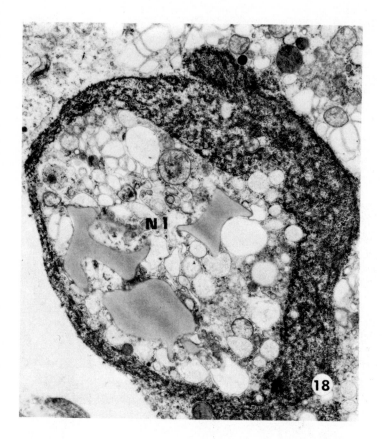

Figure 5–18. Detail of anaplastic nucleus with voluminous cytoplasmic invagination (NI). Variety of cytoplasmic organelles, including lipid droplets, can be seen in invagination. (×28,000).

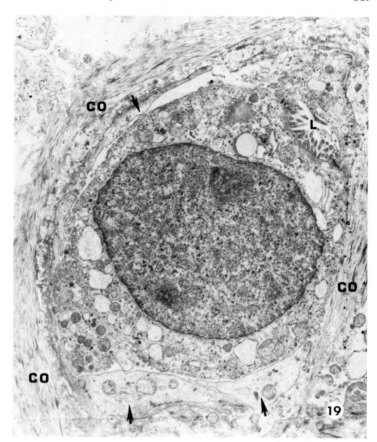

Figure 5–19. Isolated anaplastic cancer cell with intracytoplasmic lumen (L). Tumor cell has permeated a space between collagen fibers (CO), which are still intact. (×12,000).

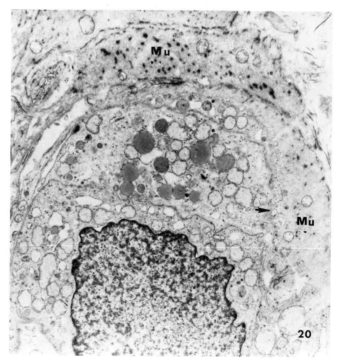

Figure 5–20. Isolated anaplastic cells pushing their way between muscle fibers (Mu). Muscle is still intact, but in some areas tumor cells and smooth muscle seem to fuse (arrow). (×7,500).

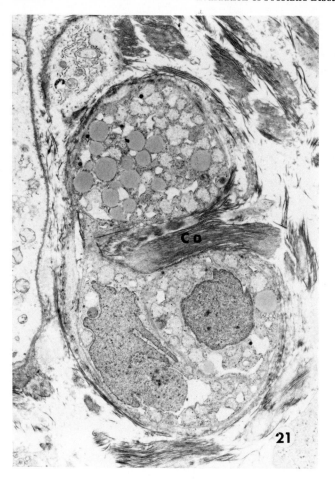

Figure 5–21. Anaplastic cancer cell bending against "resisting" collagen bundle (Co). Disintegrating collagen fibers surround tumor cell. (×9,100).

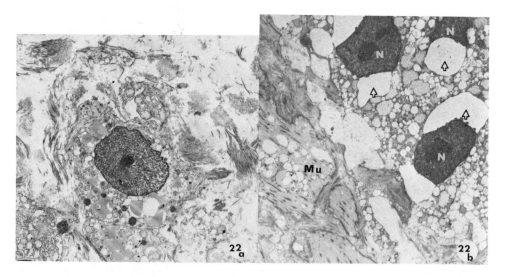

Figure 5–22. A, Invasive tumor cell amid disintegrating collagen fibers. (×5,850). B, Tumor cell with atypical nuclei (N), which show extremely dilated perinuclear cisternae (open arrows). Adjacent muscle fibers (Mu) are undergoing vacuolar degeneration. (×9,000).

role in this process. Studies have indicated that dissolution of stromal elements and parenchymal cells of invaded organs may be mediated by release of lytic enzymes into the areas of contact between malignant cells and normal elements.[16] More recently, great emphasis has been placed on the study of changes in the surface properties of malignant cells in relation to invasiveness and metastasis.[17]

In studies using animal transplantable tumors,[18] evidence has been presented that suggests that some of the invading tumor cells may interchange cellular substances and even cytoplasmic organelles with normal cells with which they come in contact. Of particular interest, in connection with invasiveness, is the possibility that products from disintegrating tumor cells may have toxic effects and promote destruction of normal structures, thus creating space for tumor cell propagation. Such a possibility to account for invasiveness of prostatic cancer cells is illustrated in Figures 5–19 to 22. The tumor cells gain access into the interstitial spaces and appear first surrounded by healthy looking collagen bundles and

smooth muscle fibers. In what is interpreted as progressive stages in the invasive process, tumor cells seem to come into close contact with surrounding normal components, and apparently, as a consequence of some deleterious effect of the tumor cells, muscle fibers and collagen undergo degeneration and breakdown. Presumably this will provide the space for multiplication and expansion of the tumor cell population at the expense of normal structures.

ANTIANDROGENIC TREATMENT OF PROSTATIC GLANDS

Castration and the use of estrogens induce a temporary regression of the clinical and anatomic symptoms of prostatic carcinoma. Although much information has accumulated on biochemical and metabolic deviations pertaining to the effects of orchiectomy and estrogens on prostatic biology,[4,5] the cellular mechanisms involved in regression are less well understood.

Because of the lack of suitable animal tumor models and the inability to obtain frequent biopsies in man, much of the

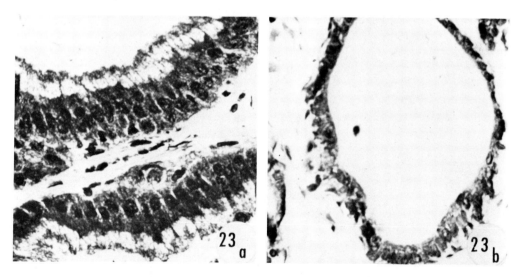

Figure 5–23. Rat ventral prostate. A, Intact rat. Tall columnar epithelial cells with intense basophilia due to abundant ribonucleic acid in endoplasmic reticulum. Clear supranuclear halo corresponds to Golgi area. (×315). B, Castrated rat. Atrophy of epithelial cells and decreased basophilia due to loss of endoplasmic reticulum. (×315).

information in the field has been obtained by the use of normal prostatic glands of rodents, especially the rat.

Following castration or estrogen treatment, the glandular cells of the rat prostate undergo marked reduction in size and appear as low cuboidal, as opposed to the tall cylindrical configuration seen in the untreated rats (Figure 5–23). Marked alteration in cell organelles, which are reflected in loss of function, can be detected by simple histochemical methods. In toluidine blue preparations (Figure 5–23), the atrophic prostate cells of the castrated rats reveal a marked decrease in cytoplasmic basophilia. Ultrastructurally this corresponds to loss of endoplasmic reticulum and ribosomes and biochemically to impaired protein synthesis.[4,5]

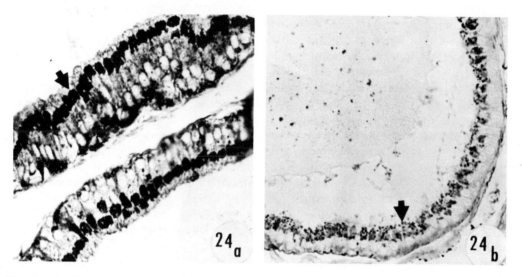

Figure 5–24. Rat ventral prostate. A, Intact rat. Silver impregnation of Golgi apparatus. Supranuclear, compact staining of highly developed Golgi (arrow). (×315). B, Castrated rat. Loss of silver deposits and granular disperse appearance of Golgi (arrow). (×315).

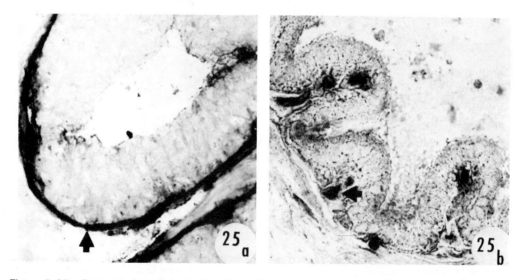

Figure 5–25. Rat ventral prostate. A, Intact rat. Alkaline phosphatase reaction is markedly intense at basal area of acinus and in periacinar blood vessels (arrow). (×315). B, Castrated rat. Disappearance of alkaline phosphatase from base of acini, but persistent in blood vessels (arrow). (×315).

Also the staining intensity of the Golgi apparatus, concerned with synthesis of complex polysaccharides and secretion in general, is markedly reduced after castration (Figure 5–24), which is in close agreement with the loss of secretory function under these conditions. Alkaline phosphatase, an enzyme normally present in the basal areas of the acini, is greatly reduced or absent in the castrated animal (Figure 5–25). It is of interest that alkaline phosphatase activity in the small blood vessels in the same areas is not affected by castration, indicating the presence of hormone-dependent and hormone-independent forms of the enzyme in structures intimately related to the acinus. Patterns of intracellular distribution of hydrolytic enzymes and some peptidases undergo remarkable changes after castra-

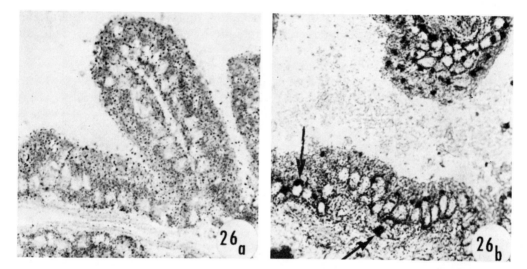

Figure 5–26. Rat ventral prostate. A, Intact rat. Aminopeptidase reaction in the form of granules evenly distributed in the cytoplasm (×315). B, Castrated rat. Aminopeptidase reaction is present in large cytoplasmic clumps (arrows). (×315).

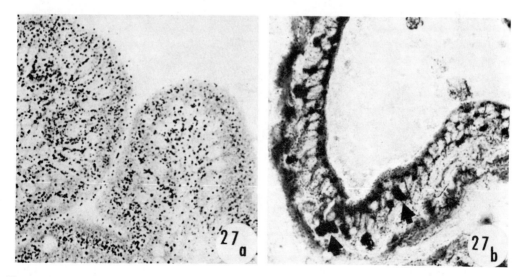

Figure 5–27. Rat ventral prostate. A, Intact rat. Acid phosphatase stain. Fine granular deposits dispersed in cytoplasm. (×315). B, Castrated rat. Acid phosphatase reaction present in large clumps (arrows). (×315).

tion. The localization of these enzymes occurs in the form of discrete granules in the prostatic cells of intact animals, whereas they tend to form large conglomerates in the castrated animal (Figures 5–26–28). These histochemical changes, which reflect involvement of lysosomes in prostatic involution in the hormone deprived animal, have been confirmed by electron microscopy and biochemical studies.

As mentioned earlier, rat prostatic epithelial cells undergo marked reduction in size after castration or estrogen therapy. In the case of human prostatic carcinoma, these treatments apparently also induce cell death, as judged by the disappearance of established metastasis.

Elimination of the androgenic stimulus by castration or by other antiandrogenic measures leads to sequestration and autodigestion of cytoplasmic organelles mediated by lysosomal enzymes. As a result of the inhibition of synthesis of secretory proteins, the rough endoplasmic reticulum markedly developed in the

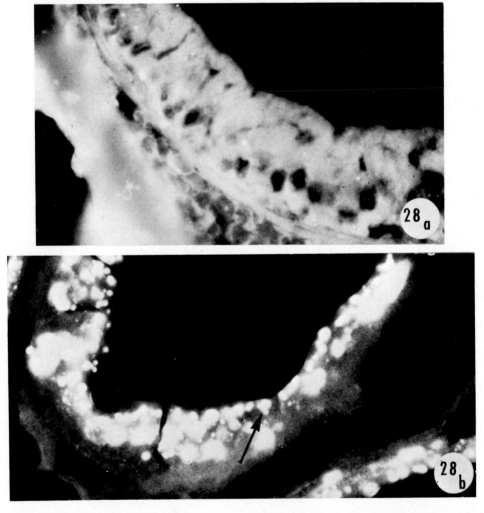

Figure 5–28. Autofluorescence of lysosomes. A, Intact rat, showing minor autofluorescence. In B, from a castrated rat, prostatic epithelium reveals marked autofluorescence in large conglomerates. These correspond to the large acid phosphatase-positive clumps seen in castrated rats. This confirms the lysosomal nature of the acid phosphatase-positive bodies seen in the castrate (×300).

normal model (Figure 5–29) becomes depleted, and the flattened cisternae acquire a coiled configuration (Figure 5–30). These flattened cisternae and other cytoplasmic organelles such as mitochondria, ribosomes, and Golgi elements become sequestered within autophagic vacuoles (Figure 5–31) where they undergo degradation catalyzed by lysosomal hydrolyses.[3,4,19] As a result of this process, the concentration of organelles shows marked reduction, and from two weeks postcastration onward the prostatic cells become greatly depleted of the various cytoplasmic components (Figure 5–32). This and the decreased protein synthesis due to lack of hormonal stimulation are responsible for the marked shrinkage in cell volume.

Similar changes have been detected in human prostatic carcinomas treated by orchiectomy and estrogens. Figure 5–33 illustrates a well-differentiated prostatic acinus in a patient treated by orchiectomy

and estrogens, in which many of the epithelial cells are almost completely devoid of cytoplasmic organelles. This can be seen in great detail in Figure 5–34. It is of interest that some of the cells lining the same acinus are less drastically affected by androgen deprivation and estrogen treatment and preserve a certain degree of their complement of cytoplasmic organelles (Figure 5–35). In the rat, a similar lack of uniformity in the degree of cellular atrophy throughout the same acinus and in different acini of a given gland following castration suggests variations in sensitivity of individual cells to androgenic deprivation. This raises the important question as to whether these cells, which appear to be less hormone dependent, represent an autonomous cell population capable, at a later time, of resuming growth in the absence of androgens as seen in orchiectomized and estrogen-treated patients.

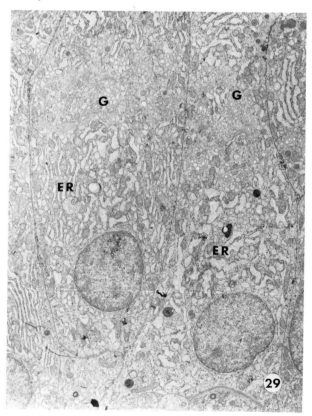

Figure 5–29. Rat ventral prostate, intact animal. Epithelial cells showing abundant endoplasmic reticulum (ER) and highly developed Golgi complexes (G). (×9,000).

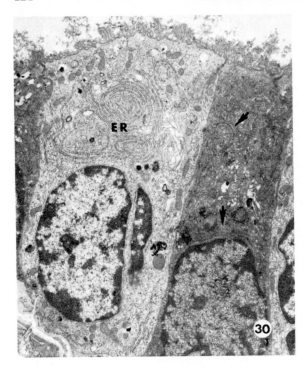

Figure 5–30. Castrated rat, ventral prostate. Coiling (ER) and collapse (arrows) of endoplasmic reticulum. (×9,000).

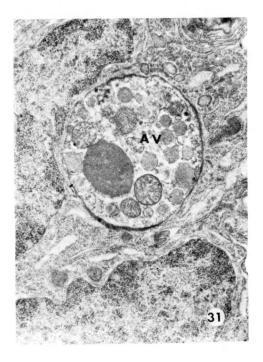

Figure 5–31. Castrated rat, ventral prostate. Autophagic vacuole (AV), where cytoplasmic organelles, including mitochondria, are being degraded. (×18,000).

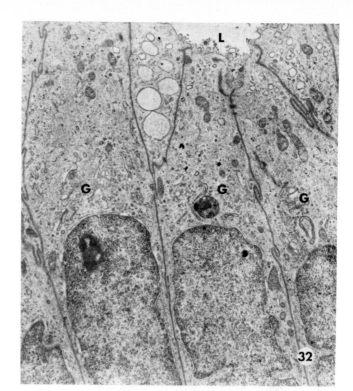

Figure 5–32. Castrated rat, ventral prostate. Degradation of cytoplasmic organelles, as seen in Figure 5–31, results in marked loss of cytoplasmic organelles. Remaining components of Golgi apparatus are still visible (G). (×15,000).

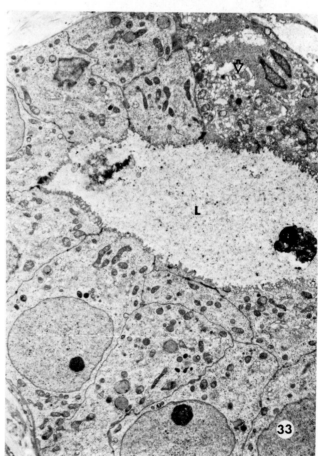

Figure 5–33. Human prostatic carcinoma, in patient treated by orchiectomy and estrogen. Well-differentiated acinus showing effects of androgenic deprivation, reflected in paucity of cytoplasmic organelles in most of cells. Group of cells (open arrow), however, has escaped effect of antiandrogenic treatment and shows signs of adequate stimulation. Lumen (L) contains secretory material. (×3,600).

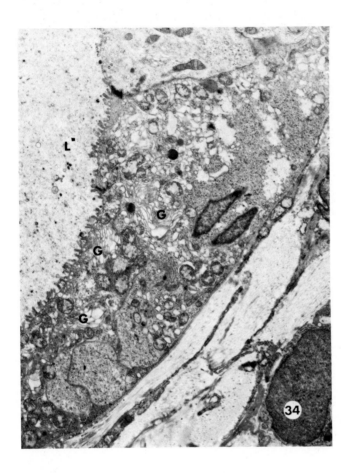

Figure 5–34. Detail of cells marked with arrow in Figure 5–33. Well-developed Golgi complex (G), abundance of secretory vacuoles, and secretion in lumen (L) in absence of adequate androgen stimulation (orchiectomy and estrogen therapy) strongly suggest hormonal independence or lower threshold for this group of cells. (×3,600).

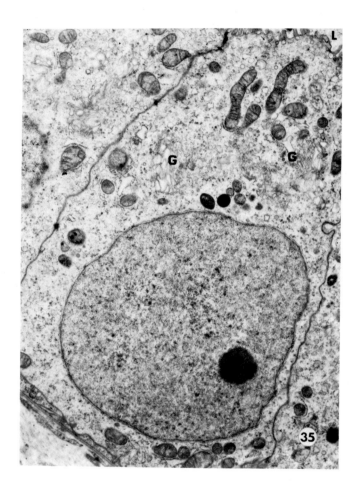

Figure 5–35. In contrast to cells in Figure 5–34, hormone-dependent cells in same acinus show loss of secretory vacuoles and paucity of Golgi (G). (×21,000).

References

1. Brandes, D.: The fine structure and histochemistry of prostatic glands in relation to sex hormones. *In* International Review of Cytology. Edited by G. H. Bourne and J. F. Danielli. New York, Academic Press, 1966, Vol. 20.

2. Brandes, D.: Fine structure and cytochemistry of male sex accessory organs. *In* Male Accessory Sex Organs: Structure and Function in Mammals. Edited by D. Brandes. New York, Academic Press, 1974.

3. Brandes, D.: Hormonal regulation of fine structure. *In* Male Accessory Sex Organs: Structure and Function in Mammals. Edited by D. Brandes. New York, Academic Press, 1974.

4. Brandes, D.: Male Accessory Sex Organs: Structure and Function in Mammals. New York, Academic Press, 1974.

5. Williams-Ashman, H. G., and Reddi A. H.: Androgenic regulation of tissue growth and function. *In* Biochemical Actions of Hormones. Edited by G. Litwak. New York, Academic Press, 1972, Vol. II.

6. Kirchheim, D., et al.: Histochemistry of the normal, hyperplastic and neoplastic human prostate gland. Invest. Urol. 1:403, 1964.

7. Kirchheim, D., et al.: Fine structure and cytochemistry of human prostatic carcinoma. *In* Male Accessory Sex Organs: Structure and Function in Mammals. Edited by D. Brandes. New York, Academic Press, 1974.

8. Grayhack, J. T., and Wendel, E. F.: Hormone dependence of carcinoma of the prostate. *In* Male Accessory Sex Organs: Structure and Function in Mammals. Edited by D. Brandes. New York, Academic Press, 1974.

9. Olin, P., et al.: Biosynthesis of thyroglobulin related to the ultrastructure of the human fetal thyroid gland. Endocrinology 87:1000, 1970.

10. Shepard, T H.: Development of the human fetal thyroid. Gen. Comp. Endocrinol. 10:174, 1968.

11. Emmelot, P., and Bos, C. J.: The effect of thyroxin on the swelling of mitochondria isolated from normal and neoplastic livers. Exp. Cell Res. 12: 191, 1957.

12. LeBreton, E., and Moulé, Y.: Biochemistry and physiology of the cancer cell. *In* The Cell: Biochemistry, Physiology, Morphology. Edited by J. Brachet and A. E. Mirsky. New York, Academic Press, 1961, Vol. V.

13. Lenta, M. P., and Riehl, M. A.: The coenzyme I oxidase system in normal and tumor tissues. Cancer Res. 12:498, 1952.

14. Braunstein, H.: Staining lipid in carcinoma of the prostate gland. Am. J. Clin. Pathol. 41:44, 1964.

15. Mao, P., et al.: Human prostatic carcinoma: An electron microscope study. Cancer Res. 26:955, 1966.

16. Sylven, B. E. G. V.: The host-tumor interzone and tumor invasion. *In* Biological Interactions in Normal and Neoplastic Growth. A Contribution to the Host-Tumor Problem. Henry Ford International Symposium. Edited by M. J. Brennan and W. L. Simpson. Boston, Little, Brown, 1962.

17. Rapin, A. M. C., and Burger, M. M.: Tumor cell surfaces: General alterations detected by agglutinins. *In* Advances in Cancer Research. Edited by G. Klein and S. Weinhouse. New York, Academic Press, 1974, Vol. 20.

18. Brandes, D., et al.: Invasion of skeletal and smooth muscle by L 1210 Leukemia. Cancer Res. 27:2159, 1967.

19. Helminen, H. J., and Ericcson, J. L. E.: On the mechanism of lysosomal enzyme secretion. Electron microscopic and histochemical studies on the epithelial cells of the rat's ventral prostate lobe. J. Ultrastruc. Res. 33:528, 1970.

Chapter 6

Acid Phosphatase

THOMAS M. SODEMAN and JOHN G. BATSAKIS

The acid phosphatases (orthophosphoric monoester phosphohydrolase, E.C. 3.1.3.2) hydrolyze esters of orthophosphoric acid at an acidic pH. Enzyme hydrolysis results in the splitting of the O-P bond by the following mechanism:

$$\underset{\overset{|}{OH}}{\overset{\overset{O}{\|}}{R\text{-}O\text{-}P\text{-}OH}} \underset{\pm H_2O}{\overset{[H^+]}{\rightleftharpoons}} R\text{-}OH + \underset{\overset{|}{OH}}{\overset{\overset{O}{\|}}{HO\text{-}P\text{-}OH}}$$

The entire class of acid phosphatases manifests a rather flat pH activity curve, 4–7, with the pH of most reactions being measured in the range of 4.8–6.0. The pH optimum varies with the *source* of the enzyme and the substrate used for the measurement of the enzyme activity.[1]

While the activity of acid phosphatase has been described in highest amounts in the cells and the secretions of the prostate gland, acid phosphatase activity has a rather wide tissue distribution. Activity is present in serum, erythrocytes, platelets, leukocytes, liver, spleen, kidney, and other tissues.[2] Most of these tissues, including the prostate gland, contain two or more molecular variants (isoenzymes) of the acid phosphatase.[3] At least six

genetically determined isoenzymes have been reported within the erythrocytes, with the other tissues exhibiting lesser numbers of molecular variants.[4]

Histochemical studies have indicated that the tissue acid phosphatases are located mainly in epithelia.[5] Reticuloendothelial cells contain some enzyme activity, but little or none is associated with the stroma or supporting tissues. Some of the apparent variability in tissue distribution is owing to the high dependence on the substrate used and additional test conditions that vary with specific tissue acid phosphatases or molecular variants, or both.[1,3,4]

Within these tissues, the hydrolytic acid phosphatases are found mainly in the lysosomes[6] and require disruption of the lysosomal membrane for their release. Multiple forms present with the lysosomes are apparently released at a variable rate. Ultrastructural examination suggests that acid phosphatase is transferred from the ribosomes on the endoplasmic reticulum to Golgi saccules and vesicles and from there to the lysosomes (dense bodies).[7]

Similar to our lack of knowledge of the

function of the alkaline phosphatases, very little is known of the metabolic significance of the acid phosphatases. In the prostatic cell, they apparently do not have a major metabolic role. Extracellularly, however, in prostatic fluid, the phosphatases are concerned with the metabolic activity of the spermatozoa by their catalyzing transfer of phosphates.[1,2]

Except for a rather high acid phosphatase activity in urine and the high activity in the secretions of the male urogenital tract, acid phosphatase in other normal body fluids is limited. Acid phosphatase of *prostatic* origin is not usually detectable in the normal systemic circulation, and the activity found in normal serum or plasma probably comes in large part from platelets.[1,2,8] The amount contributed to "normal" serum by the platelets varies from investigator to investigator and its quantitation is hampered by the varying substrate affinities of several different acid phosphatases in the tissues.[9] Certainly studies dealing with the marked differences in activity between platelet-rich and platelet-poor plasma strongly implicate the platelets as a major source of plasma enrichment. Additional circumstantial evidence is obtained by observations of acid phosphatase activity in patients with thrombocytopenia, in whom the contribution from platelets is slight vs patients with high platelet counts, in whom increases of five times normal were seen.[10]

The measurable serum acid phosphatase fluctuates considerably with the age of the subject. Newborns manifest an activity approximately two to two and one-half times normal adult levels. Greater-than-adult normal levels of activity persist (with a gradual yet progressive decline) until puberty and cessation of body growth. From that time, serum activity is stable except upon the intervention of disease. Normal activity levels for all ages are expressed in units unique to the assay system.[1] This relates primarily to substrate and buffer qualifications, i.e., using phenyl phosphate as the substrate, the total enzyme activity in a normal adult is 2.5 to 4 King-Armstrong or Gutman units, and the tartrate-labile fraction is 0.2 to 0.6 units.[1] When beta-glycerophosphate is the substrate for the laboratory assay, the normal range is 0.6 to 1.1 Bodansky units.[1] The total and tartrate-labile enzyme activity in normal adult males and females is not significantly different—again emphasizing the negligible prostatic contribution to normal serum activity.

The serum acid phosphatase activity in normal subjects does not appear to have a circadian fluctuation.[2] This is in contrast to the well-known and defined diurnal pattern exhibited by patients with carcinomas of the prostate gland.[2]

LABORATORY CONSIDERATIONS

Stability and Sample Preference

In the practice of clinical laboratory medicine, it is nearly axiomatic that of all the enzymes measured in the laboratory, acid phosphatase suffers the most from instability. Factors at play in the stability of serum acid phosphatase are (1) pH, (2) temperature at storage, and (3) substrate acidity of the acid phosphatase being measured. Of these three, pH is the most critical and temperature the least important.[11] As a consequence of these variables and interplay with others, we cannot give a completely standardized protocol for the presentation of test serum. When serum is separated from the clot and kept at room temperature (25° C), enzyme activity decreases considerably within one to two hours owing to the increase in pH as a result of the loss of carbon dioxide. This increase in pH, which may go from 7.6 to 8.5 in several hours, may be slowed by tightly stoppered containers. The serum activity is better preserved at room temperature when the clot and serum are *not* separated, or when the serum is buffered to pH 6.2 to 6.6 with disodium hydrogen citrate. If one compares separated serum with clot/serum samples under the same conditions, serum manifests a 14–50% (mean of 33%) greater loss of activity. Countering this recommendation, however, is the possibility of erythrocytic acid phosphatase contaminating a serum measured by a substrate that is attacked by both red cell and prostatic acid phosphatase.

Because the serum acid phosphatase activity is influenced by factors such as inactivation and an unpredictable contribution of enzyme from platelets during clotting, it is likely that the most appropriate sample for determining the acid phosphatase activity is fresh plasma, buffered with citrate to a pH of 6.2 to 6.6.[4]

Multiple Molecular Forms

The early investigations dealing with the variable responses of acid phosphatase to different substrates and inhibitors and chromatographic and purification studies clearly suggested that the tissue acid phosphatases existed in more than one molecular form.[1,3,4] Since then, immunochemical, chromatographic, and electrophoretic evidence has substantiated the molecular heterogeneity of acid phosphatase. Compared to the well-characterized isoenzymes of lactate dehydrogenase and creatine kinase, it is also abundantly clear that much remains to be learned concerning the molecular variants of acid phosphatase.[1,3,4]

Chromatography of prostatic phosphatase with Sephadex G-200 or with DEAE-cellulose rather consistently yields two peaks of enzyme activity.[1] Isoelectric focusing of these two fractions yields at least four active peaks for each fraction. To date, there has been found no marked difference in the relative rate of hydrolysis of a number of phosphate esters, at a concentration of 2 mM, by the two purified fractions.[1]

Starch gel electrophoresis of prostatic acid phosphatase usually yields about 20 bands of activity. All bands are almost totally inhibited by 5 mM L-(+)-tartrate.[1] Experiments with neuraminidase indicate that the electrophoretic heterogeneity of the enzyme arises from a single enzyme protein, bearing a variable number of acid residues. The large number of molecular variants demonstrated by gel electrophoresis or isoelectric focusing differ from each other basically in the number of neuraminic acid residues attached to the same protein molecule. The molecular weights of the variants do not differ from each other by more than 5%. The average molecular weight is about 100,000.[1] A similar electrophoretic phenomenon is present with the molecular variants of alkaline phosphatase.[2]

The isoenzyme characterization of various tissue acid phosphatases continues. The cell-isoenzyme specificity demonstrated by the formed elements of the blood, particularly the erythrocyte and leukocyte, has already been used to shed more light on the physiology, biochemistry, cell biology, and function of these enzymes and their cells.[4] Practical and research applications of the prostatic acid phosphatases, however, lag behind. Normal *plasma* contains only a tartrate-resistant isoenzyme. Normal serum has two isoenzymes: the tartrate-resistant form found in normal plasma and a tartrate-labile isoenzyme derived from platelets during the clotting process.[1,3,4] In patients with metastatic carcinomas of the prostate gland, two different isoenzymes appear and they represent the major components of the prostatic enzyme. Both are tartrate labile and are not found in either normal plasma or serum.[1,3,4] These "prostatic isoenzymes," however, are shared by other tissues (pancreas, spleen, bone marrow, kidney, lung, bone, skin, adrenal gland, and intestine). Furthermore, all are tartrate labile and may be indistinguishable from the prostatic isoenzymes.

Methods of Assay

Because of the intimate clinical association of acid phosphatase activity and carcinoma of the prostate gland and the rather wide tissue distribution of the acid phosphatases, investigations concerning methodologic development have been devoted to distinguishing "prostatic" acid phosphatase from that of the erythrocyte and other tissues which may be found in serum/plasma. We have already seen that while there exists great clinical potential for separation of acid phosphatase isoenzymes, this potential is far from being achieved and is seriously hampered by differences in substrate specificity of the isoenzymes and a paradoxical similarity of the physicochemical properties of the isoenzymes.[1–3]

Accordingly, present investigations have followed two routes, including (1) a search for a substrate specific for the prostatic acid phosphatase, and (2) a search for differential inhibitors which will either inhibit nonprostatic acid phosphatases or specifically inhibit the prostatic enzyme.[2] To date, these efforts have been only partially successful but have spawned a large number of methods with different eponymic designations and units. Most methods have one or more unique features that prevent interchanging of test results.[1,2] King,[12] perhaps, has viewed these investigations in their proper perspective in the following statement: "It is obvious that the action of any compound (inhibitor) can, at most, apply to some of the acid phosphatases of human tissue and even with a single enzyme, that derived from the prostate, their effects also vary considerably with the substrate used."

Substrates

The substrates that have been used for the measurement of serum acid phosphatase activity have been beta-glycerophosphate or various phenolic or naphtholic phosphates.[2] Methods using the former substrate measure the inorganic phosphate released. If aromatic substrates are used, the organic moiety is usually measured. Detection systems have involved the Folin-Ciocalteu reagent, azo-coupling, or direct photometry of chromogenic substrates like p-nitrophenyl phosphate or phenolphthalein phosphate.[2] Table 6–1 lists available substrates and related information.

In normal sera the rate of action of the acid phosphatase present varies with the substrate (usually an organic phosphate) and its concentration in the reaction mixture.[1] To illustrate this variance, Bodansky[1] has indicated that normal average activities by various methods may all be converted into micromoles of substrate hydrolyzed in one hour at 37°–38° C by 100 ml of serum to yield the following comparison: beta-glycerophosphate, 6.1; phenyl phosphate, 15; phenolphthalein diphosphate, 18; p-nitrophenyl phosphate, 145; beta-naphthyl phosphate, 69; alpha-naphthyl phosphate, 14. These relative action rates on substrates are subject to even greater variation in patients whose activity is elevated.

In view of the preceding, selection of an appropriate substrate is difficult.[4] Some are insensitive to small increments of prostatic acid phosphatase activity; either the blank is large (e.g., beta-glycerophosphate) or the substrates are sensitive to nonprostatic phosphatases present in serum (e.g., phenyl phosphate and p-nitrophenyl phosphate). Other substrates are introduced prematurely and with considerable fanfare as being nearly exclusively "prostate-specific." Alpha-naphthyl phosphate is an example of this group. Clinical testing, however, has shown that it is hydrolyzed by platelet acid phosphatase and is hampered by a large number of false positives (12% of a male population without prostatic carcinoma and in a similar number of females).[13,14]

Table 6-1

Acid phosphatase methods

Substrate	Buffer	Product (Measured by)	Opt. pH	Incubation Time	Serum Quantity	Normal Adult Value Mean	Range
Beta-glycerophosphate (Bodansky)[37]	Acetate	Phosphate (Sodium molybdate)	5.0	3 hr	1.0 ml	45 Bu/dl	0.04–0.88
(Shinowara, Jones, Reinhart)[38]		Phosphate (sodium molybdate)	5.0	1 hr	0.02 ml		0.0–1.1
Phenyl phosphate[a]							
(Gutman-Gutman)[39]	Acetate	Phenyl (Folin-Ciocalteu)	4.8	3 hr	0.5 ml	2.2 KAU/dl	0.5–4.6 (upper limit)
(Herbert)[40]	Acetate	(Folin-Ciocalteu)	4.8	1 hr	0.5 ml	5.0 KAU/dl	
(Kaplan-Narahara)[41]	Acetate	(Diazo-red B salt)	5.0	1 hr	0.05 ml	$0.55 \pm .32$ mM/dl	0.15–2.8
(Hansen)[42]	Citrate	(Amino antipyrine)	4.9	1 hr	0.1 ml	$1.8 \pm .61$ KAU/dl	1.0–4.0
(Brooks-Purdy)[43]	Citrate	(Coulometric)	4.9	3 hr	0.5 ml		
Alpha-naphthyl[a]							
(Babson-Read)[44]	Citrate	α-naphthol (diazotized 5-nitro-o-anisidine)	5.2	30 min	0.2 ml	$1.4 \pm .2$ IU/l	0.9–2.5
(Campbell-Moss)[45]	Citrate	(Spectrofluorometric)	5.2	15 min	0.1 ml	5.0 mM/min/l	(upper limit)
(Fabiny-Byrd-Ertingshausen)[50]	Citrate	(Fast-analyzer)	5.2	16 min	40 µl		0.0–0.9 µ/l
Phenolphthalein diphosphate (Huggins-Talalay)[46]	Acetate	Phenolphthalein (Glycine buffer pH 11.2)	5.5	1 hr	0.5 ml	5.9 U/dl	3–10
Monophosphate (Coleman)[47]	Citrate	Phosphate ($Na_2(O_3\text{-}Na_4EDTA$)	6.0	30 min	0.1 ml		
Thymolphthalein monophosphate (Roy-Brower-Hayden)[15]	Citrate	Thymolphthalein ($NaOH + Na_2CO_3$)	6.0	30 min	0.2 ml	$0.28 \pm .09$ IU/l	0.11–0.60
Para-nitrophenol phosphate (Hudson-Brendler-Scott)[51]	Acetate	Para-nitrophenol (NAOH)	5.4	30 min	0.1 ml	$1.55 \pm .34$ mMu/l	1.00–2.30
(Andersch-Szczypinski)[52]	Citrate	Para-nitrophenol (NAOH)	4.8	30 min	0.2 ml	0.27 mMu/l	0.03–0.63
Adenosine 3'-monophosphate (Goldberg-Ellis)[48]	Acetate	Ammonia (Phenol-hypochlorite)	5.6	1 hr	0.05 ml	1.8 ± 1.0 IU/l	0.9–3.1
Naphthol AS-BI (Vaughan-Guilbault, Hackney)[49]	Citrate	Naphthol (fluorescence)	5.5	3 min			

[a]Has been automated (Klein, Auerbach, and Morgenstern).[53]

At the present time, sodium thymol-phthalein monophosphate, which yields its own chromogen on enzymatic hydrolysis, appears to be the best choice for measuring the prostatic enzyme.[15,16] Although it is not hydrolyzed as rapidly as alpha-naphthyl phosphate by prostatic acid phosphatase, it has less activity with nonprostatic acid phosphatase and therefore gives the appearance of greater specificity.

Inhibitors

The use of various antagonistic compounds (inhibitors) has met with variable success, and their use diminishes as investigations bring us closer to (1) prostatic isoenzyme definition and (2) prostate-specific substrates.

Prostatic acid phosphatase is taken to be represented by "formaldehyde-stable," "copper-resistant," and "tartrate-labile."[1] Magnesium, calcium, chromium, cobalt, manganese, nickel, and zinc all have variable inhibiting effects on both red cell and prostatic acid phosphatase.[1,2] Fluoride is a powerful inhibitor of acid phosphatase, particularly of prostatic phosphatases.[1,2] Oxalate, but not citrate or EDTA, produces a moderate inhibition on human acid phosphatase. Heparin also inhibits prostatic acid phosphatase.[1,2]

Only the L(+) form of tartrate is active as an inhibitor. It inhibits about 95% of the activity of prostatic acid phosphatase, whereas the acid phosphatase from the erythrocyte remains relatively unaffected.[2] As noted in the discussion of multiple molecular forms, acid phosphatases from the kidney, liver, and spleen are also 70 to 85% tartrate-inhibitable; hence misleading inhibition studies can be obtained if one seeks prostatic acid phosphatase.[2] It should be also noted that L(+) tartrate is not an efficient inhibitor of prostatic phosphatase when p-nitrophenyl phosphate is used as the substrate.[2]

Formaldehyde (0.5 of 1%) totally inhibits red cell acid phosphatase and does not affect the prostatic fraction. Other acid phosphatases are 10 to 60% inhibited. This form of differential inhibition has not found widespread use because hepatic, renal, and splenic sources are still capable of increasing the nonformaldehyde inhibitable fractions.[2]

Ethanol inhibits red cell acid phosphatase by 70–80% under conditions yielding a 90–100% inhibitor of the prostatic enzyme. Hence it is not useful in identifying the latter fraction.[2] Important, however, is the observation that hepatic and splenic acid phosphatases are not inhibited by ethanol and that the absence of an inhibitor may be significant when used with other methods.

Lability of the acid phosphatases at 37°C does not differentiate hepatic or prostatic acid phosphatases.[2]

SERUM ACID PHOSPHATASE IN PROSTATIC CARCINOMA

Acid phosphatase activity in the prostate gland is localized primarily in the glandular and ductal epithelia.[17] This tissue enzyme activity increases with the age of the subject, i.e., 1.5 King-Armstrong units/g of tissue in children and an activity ranging between 522–2284 King-Armstrong units/g in the adult prostate gland.[18] It has been further shown that, on the average, neoplastic prostate tissue (carcinoma) contains *less* acid phosphatase, on a gram to gram basis, than does either normal or hyperplastic prostate glands.[19]

With the foregoing data as the theoretical background, the measurement of acid phosphatase (total and "prostatic") has served as the cornerstone for the biochemical diagnosis of carcinoma of the prostate gland. As we have indicated in previous sections of this chapter, this cornerstone is an imperfect foundation with the following differences: (1) imperfect specificity even to isoenzyme fractionation, (2) overlapping of inhibition studies, and (3) interpretations highly dependent on the test reaction conditions, particularly in reference to the substrate used. Nevertheless, the measurement of acid phosphatase has withstood the test of time and within the proper clinical content (which is important in the evaluation of an enzymatic analysis) may be considered nearly diagnostic.[2,20]

Given this appropriate clinical context, it has been considered that an increase in serum acid phosphatase activity is evidence for a neoplastic extension *beyond* the capsule of the prostate gland. While this may be true for the mean average of several hundred cases, this correlation is not perfect.[2]

In patients with prostatic carcinoma metastatic to bone, 80% will manifest abnormal serum acid phosphatase activity. Twenty percent of the patients with neoplastic extension into the periprostatic soft tissue will also have abnormal serum activity.[2] Woodard[21] claims that nearly 5% of the patients with neoplasm confined to the gland will also manifest an increased serum activity.

There does not appear to be a consistent correlation between the level of acid phosphatase and amount or location of metastases, although we—and others—using repeated or serial determinations, have shown an increasing level of activity with progression of the disease.[22]

On occasion, serum activity remains relatively low or, more rarely, normal, despite active metastatic growth. No completely satisfactory answer has been offered but several have been proposed, including (1) low or dedifferentiation of the neoplasm, (2) insufficient invasion of vascular or lymphatic channels, (3) some "barrier" to egress from metastatic sites, (4) inhibition by serum components, (5) termal denaturation, and (6) rate of production of the acid phosphatase or modification by prior treatment.

A *persistently* elevated total acid phosphatase activity (regardless of substrate) requires a thorough clinical and biochem-

ical evaluation. An elevated activity, particularly of the tartrate-inhibitable type as obtained by the use of substrates more nearly reflecting prostatic acid phosphatase in patients with presumably localized and operable carcinoma of the prostate gland, is strong evidence of metastases.[2]

Circadian variation in serum activity, which persists in the patient with carcinoma of the prostate gland despite removal of the testes, often makes serial enzyme interpretation difficult.[2] Since peak circadian variation is not reached at the same time each day, apparent increases or decreases of activity may occur if only *isolated* serum samples are relied on.[2] In this respect it should go without saying that an exclusion of carcinoma of the prostate gland *cannot* be made on a single measurement of a suspect's acid phosphatase activity (total or prostatic, or both).[2]

While there is some unpredictability of serum activity in prostatic cancer, estimations of activity may be useful in following the effectiveness of therapy for carcinoma of the prostate gland. In some patients a complete normalization of activity may ensue; in others it may remain at slightly increased levels. Approximately 10% of patients with carcinoma of the prostate gland do not respond clinically to hormonal therapy and this is manifested by a failure of the acid phosphatase activity to fall.

The responses to different modes of therapy are variable. Huggins et al., in a series of three reports,[23-25] demonstrated the effects of castration, estrogens, androgens, and desoxycorticosterone in patients with elevated acid phosphate. Castration and estrogen therapy in responsive patients produced a rapid fall in serum acid phosphatase levels. Serum alkaline phosphatase activity, concomitantly measured, manifested a rise over the first two to three weeks, followed by a gradual decline (Figure 6–1). Desoxycortico-

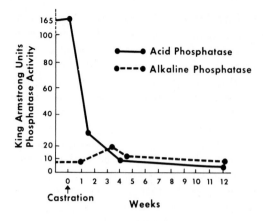

Figure 6–1. Following castration there is an immediate fall in serum acid phosphatase; the final level achieved depends upon pretherapy levels. Alkaline phosphatase usually demonstrates a posttherapy elevation.

sterone prompted a rise in the acid phosphatase. Since these pioneering studies, there has been ample reaffirmation of the effects of castration on acid phosphatasemia, i.e., a precipitous drop in activity within 24 hours of the orchidectomy. With respect to the alkaline phosphatase, if this enzyme is normal prior to therapy, there is an immediate postoperative increase. If the alkaline phosphatase is increased at the onset of treatment, a small decline in alkaline phosphatase activity occurs during the first week, and this is followed by a gradual elevation to levels exceeding the pretherapy base line activity.[26]

If one uses the decline in acid phosphatase activity as a guide to effective and/or modality of treatment, the cumulative data (again irrespective of substrate and inhibitors) clearly demonstrate that castration produces a significantly greater number of patients responding by a declining acid phosphatasemia.[27]

We can also conclude that alternative test media such as urine and prostatic secretions are not satisfactory substitutes for either the diagnosis or followup of patients with carcinoma of the prostate

gland. Urinary output of the enzyme is not only highly variable, but the kidney itself is probably the source of most of the tartrate-inhibitable fractions in urine. The same criticism of variability of secretion applies to the use of prostatic secretions as a test medium. Additionally, *normal* secretions manifest much higher levels than secretions from neoplastic glands.[28,29]

Effect of Prostatic Massage

Claims that massage of prostate glands suspected of harboring carcinoma can be used as a provocative test by showing enhancement of serum acid phosphatase activity have been poorly documented. In truth, the converse is true (Table 6–2). Prostatic massage is as likely to cause an increased level of serum acid phosphatase in patients with benign hyperplasia as with carcinoma. When the baseline acid phosphatase is within normal limits, the increment due to massage usually dissipates within 24 hours after the manipulation of the gland. A longer persistence follows massage of patients with above normal baseline activity.[30]

Effect of Prostatic Infarction and Operative Manipulation

As may be expected, infarcts of the prostate gland may be accompanied by an increased acid phosphatase activity in

Table 6–2

Effect of prostatic massage on acid phosphatase[a]

		Patients	
	Normal	Prostatic carcinoma	Prostatic hypertrophy
Total	98	25	173
No change	54%	48%	70%
Elevated	46%	48%	30%
Decreased	——	4%	——

[a]Summary of review of literature.

serum.[31] The available data, however, suggest that this is not constant and of relatively low frequency (8–30% of reported cases).

Transurethral resection is also accompanied by an increased acid phosphatasemia. In this instance, there is a strong correlation between the magnitude of rise and the amount of prostatic tissue removed. If more than 30 g are resected, nearly all subjects manifest a rise in serum activity that persists beyond 24 hours. Lesser amounts of tissue have a lower incidence of accompanying acid phosphatasemia (less than 15 grams, 65% of patients; 15–30 g, 85% of patients). In these groups, normalization of serum activity is achieved within 24 hours.[32]

Miscellaneous Stimuli

Psychic-sexual stimulation is capable of increasing urinary acid phosphatase but has no effect on serum levels.[33] Urinary retention has also been associated with an acid phosphatasemia.[26] This occurrence, however, is not common.

PHOSPHOHEXOSEISOMERASE (PHI) AND ALDOLASE IN PATIENTS WITH PROSTATIC CARCINOMA

In our opinion, both of these "ubiquitous enzymes" play an important role in the evaluation of a patient with known carcinoma of the prostate gland. This statement especially pertains to PHI studies.

Many authors share our opinion that the total acid phosphatase is not an accurate indicator of relapse; others suggest that prostatic acid phosphatase is a better parameter to follow the effectiveness of treatment.[34]

Bodansky[35] has demonstrated an excellent correlation between serum PHI levels and the growth and activity of metastatic prostatic carcinoma; this, often in the face of a nonresponsive acid phosphatase. Schwartz et al.[36] have confirmed these observations and regard PHI activity as superior to acid or alkaline phosphatase

for the followup of patients undergoing treatment for prostatic carcinoma.

NONPROSTATIC DISORDERS AND HYPERACIDPHOSPHATASEMIA

In this chapter we have emphasized that the clinical laboratory confirmation of carcinoma of the prostate gland is one built largely on empiric grounds and therefore to be considered in the light of the clinical context. The following list, after Batsakis et al.,[2] is a partial tabulation of nonprostatic causes of elevated serum/plasma acid phosphatase: *primary diseases of bone* (Paget's disease, osteogenesis imperfecta, osteogenic sarcoma, osteopetrosis, and osteoporosis); *secondary disorders of bone* (hyperparathyroidism, multiple myeloma, and metastatic carcinomas); *hepatobiliary disease* (viral hepatitis, chlorpromazine hepatitis, extrahepatic obstruction, and cirrhosis); *diseases of the kidney* (chronic glomerulonephritis and gouty nephropathy); *diseases of the reticuloendothelial system with hepatic or osseous manifestations, or both* (Gaucher's disease, Niemann-Pick disease, eosinophilic granuloma, reticulum cell sarcoma, and Hodgkin's disease); and *carcinomas with hepatitis or osseous metastases, or both* (breast, stomach, colon, kidney, and adrenal cortex).

The incidence of these causes varies, but Bodansky[1] has presented statistics on a large number of subjects with diseases other than that of the prostate gland. He relates the following: 19% in patients with skeletal metastases; 2% in patients with liver metastases; 6% in those patients with neoplasms but without either bone or liver involvement; and 10% in patients with primary bone tumors. In the category of nonneoplastic diseases of bone, elevations were present in 21% of 96 patients with Paget's disease, in 33% of nine patients with hyperparathyroidism and in 4% of patients with miscellaneous diseases of bone. These figures, again, are substrate dependent.

References

1. Bodansky, O.: Acid phosphatase. Adv. Clin. Chem., 15:43, 1972.
2. Batsakis, J. G., et al.: Diagnostic Enzymology. Amer. Soc. Clin. Path., Chicago., Ill., 1970.
3. Lam, K. W., et al.: Biochemical properties of human prostatic acid phosphatase. Clin. Chem., 19:483, 1973.
4. Yam, L. T.: Clinical significance of the human acid phosphatases. A review. Am. J. Med., 56:604, 1974.,
5. Kirchheim, D., et al.: Histochemistry of the normal, hyperplastic and neoplastic human prostate gland. Invest. Urol., 1:403, 1964.
6. DeDuve, C., et al.: Tissue fractionation studies. 6. Intracellular distribution patterns of enzymes in rat-liver tissue. Biochem. J., 60:604, 1955.
7. Goldfischer, S., et al.: The localization of phosphatase activities at the level of ultrastructure. J. Histochem. Cytochem., 12:72, 1964.
8. Zucker, M. B., and Borrelli, J.: A survey of some platelet enzymes and functions: The platelets as the source of normal serum acid glycerophosphatase. Ann. N.Y. Acad. Sci., 75:203, 1958.
9. Zucker, M. B., and Borrelli, J.: Platelets as a source of serum acid nitrophenylphosphatase. J. Clin. Invest., 38:148, 1959.
10. Zucker, M. B., and Woodard, H. Q.: Elevation of serum acid glycerophosphatase activity in thrombocytosis. J. Lab. Clin. Med., 59:760, 1962.
11. Daniel, O.: The stability of acid phosphatase in blood and other fluids. Br. J. Urol., 26:152, 1954.
12. King, J.: Practical Clinical Enzymology. London and New York, D. Van Nostrand, 1965.
13. Amador, E., et al.: Serum acid α-naphthyl phosphatase activity. Am. J. Clin. Pathol., 51:202, 1969.
14. Bruhn, H. D., and Keller, H.: A comparison of methods for the estimation of "prostatic acid phosphatase." Ger. Med. Mon., 12:109, 1967.
15. Roy, A. V., et al.: Sodium thymolphthalein monophosphate: A new acid phosphatase substrate with greater specificity for the prostatic enzyme in serum. Clin. Chem., 17:1093, 1971.
16. Demetriou, J. A., et al.: Acid Phosphatase. In Clinical Chemistry: Principles and Technics, Edited by R. J. Henry, D. C. Cannon, and J. W. Winkelman (2d Ed.). Harper and Row, 1974.
17. Györkey, F.: The appearance of acid phosphatase in human prostate gland. Lab. Invest., 13:105, 1964.
18. Gutman, A. B., and Gutman, E. B.: "Acid" phosphatase and functional activity of the prostate (man) and preputial glands (rat). Proc. Soc. Exp. Biol. Med., 39:529, 1938.
19. Woodard, H. Q.: Quantitative studies of beta-glycerophosphatase activity in normal and neoplastic tissues. Cancer, 9:352, 1956.
20. Batsakis, J. G., and Briere, R. O.: Interpretive Enzymology, Springfield, Ill., C C Thomas, 1967.
21. Woodard, H. Q.: The clinical significance of serum acid phosphatase. Am. J. Med., 27:902, 1959.
22. Herger, C. C., and Sauer, H. R.: Serum acid phosphatase determination in carcinoma of prostate. Urol. Cutan. Rev., 45:283, 1941.
23. Huggins, C., and Hodges, C. V.: Studies on prostatic cancer. I. The effect of castration, of estrogen and of androgen injection on serum phosphatases in metastatic carcinoma of the prostate. Cancer Res., 1:293, 1941.
24. Huggins, C., et al.: Studies on prostatic cancer; The effect of castration on advanced carcinoma of the prostate gland. Arch. Surg., 43:209, 1941.
25. Huggins, C., et al.: Studies on prostatic cancer. III. The effects of fever, of desoxycorticosterone and of estrogen on clinical patients with metastatic carcinoma of the prostate. J. Urol., 46:997, 1941.
26. Wray, S.: The significance of the blood acid and alkaline phosphatase values in cancer of the prostate. J. Clin. Pathol., 9:341, 1956.
27. Woodard, H. Q., and Dean, A. L.: The significance of phosphatase findings in carcinoma of the prostate. J. Urol., 57:158, 1947.
28. Muhsen, J.: Possible significance of the prostatic secretion acid phosphatase as a diagnostic and a prognostic index in carcinoma of the prostate. J. Urol., 72:928, 1954.
29. Kent, J. R., and Bischoff, A.: Acid phosphatase content of prostatic exprimate from patients with advanced prostatic carcinoma. A potential prognostic and therapeutic index. Cancer, 25:858, 1970.
30. Dybkaer, R., and Jensen, G.: Acid serum-phosphatase levels following massage of the prostate. Scand. J. Clin. Lab. Invest., 10:349, 1958.
31. Silber, I., et al.: The incidence of elevated acid phosphatase in prostatic infarction. J. Urol., 103:765, 1970.
32. Marberger, H., et al.: Changes in serum acid phosphatase levels consequent to prostatic manipulation or surgery. J. Urol., 78:287, 1957.
33. Gustafson, J. E., et al.: The effect of psychic-sexual stimulation on urinary and serum acid phosphatase and plasma nonesterified fatty acids. Psychosom. Med., 25:101, 1963.
34. Fishman, W. H., et al.: Serum "prostatic" acid phosphatase and cancer of the prostate. N. Engl. J. Med., 255:925, 1956.
35. Bodansky, O.: Serum phosphohexose isomerase in cancer. III. As an index of tumor growth in metastatic carcinoma of the prostate. Cancer, 8:1087, 1955.
36. Schwartz, M. K., et al.: Comparative values of phosphatases and other serum enzymes in following patients with prostatic carcinoma. Consideration of phosphohexose isomerase, glutamic oxalacetic transaminase, isocitric dehydrogenase and acid and alkaline phosphatases. Cancer, 16:583, 1963.
37. Bodansky, A.: Phosphatase studies. II. Determination of serum phosphatase. Factors influencing the accuracy of the determination. J. Biol. Chem., 101:93, 1933.
38. Shinowara, G. Y., et al.: The estimation of serum inorganic phosphate and "acid" and "alkaline" phosphatase activity. J. Biol. Chem., 142:921, 1942.

39. Gutman, E. B., and Gutman, A. B.: Estimation of "acid" phosphatase activity of blood serum. J. Biol. Chem., 136:201, 1940.

40. Herbert, F. K.: The estimation of prostatic phosphatase in serum and its use in the diagnosis of prostatic carcinoma. Q. J. Med. N.S., XV:221, 1946.

41. Kaplan, A., and Narahara, A.: The determination of serum acid phosphatase activity. J. Lab. Clin. Med., 41:825, 1953.

42. Hansen, P. W.: A simplification of Kind and King's method for determination of serum phosphatase. Scand. J. Clin. Lab. Invest., 18:353, 1966.

43. Brooks, M. A., and Purdy, W. C.: Coulometric determination of activity of acid or alkaline phosphatases in serum. Clin. Chem., 18:503, 1972.

44. Babson, A. L., and Read, P. A.: A new assay for prostatic acid phosphatase in serum. Tech. Bull. Regist. Med. Technol., 29:82, 1959.

45. Campbell, D. M., and Moss, D. W.: Spectrofluorimetric determinaton of acid phosphatase activity. Clin. Chim. Acta, 6:307, 1961.

46. Huggins, C., and Talalay, P.: Sodium phenolphthalein phosphate as a substrate for phosphatase tests. J. Biol. Chem., 159:399, 1945.

47. Coleman, C. M.: Chromogenic acid phosphatase substrates. Clin. Chem., 12:529, 1966.

48. Goldberg, D. M., and Ellis, G.: An assessment of serum acid and alkaline phosphatase determinations in prostatic cancer with a clinical validation of an acid phosphatase assay utilizing adenosine-3'-monophosphate as substrate. J. Clin. Pathol., 27:140, 1974.

49. Vaughan, A., et al.: Fluorometric methods for analysis of acid and alkaline phosphatase. Anal. Chem., 43:721, 1971.

50. Fabiny-Byrd, D. L., and Ertingshausen, G.: Kinetic method for determining acid phosphatase activity in serum with use of the "centrifichem." Clin. Chem., 18:841, 1972.

51. Hudson, P. B., et al.: A simple method for the determination of serum acid phosphatase. J. Urol., 58:89, 1957.

52. Andersch, M. A., and Szczypinski, A. J.: Use of p-nitrophenylphosphate as the substrate in determination of serum acid phosphatase. Am. J. Clin. Pathol., 17:571, 1947.

53. Klein, B., et al.: Automated determination of acid phosphatase. Clin. Chem., 11:998, 1965.

Chapter 7

Isoenzymes in Prostatic Carcinoma

C. W. MONCURE

The use of isoenzymes in the diagnosis and management of prostatic disease is relatively new in the clinical laboratory. However, advances in basic research in this area promise to expand the clinical application of this technique in urology and diagnostic pathology. Anticipating this expansion, this chapter has three objectives, including: (1) to define and briefly review the nature of isoenzymes; (2) to discuss current studies on the isoenzymes which relate to the prostate; and (3) to point out new methodologies which appear likely to play a role in future urologic diagnostic procedures.

The human prostate is a rich source of hydrolytic enzymes that appear in secreted seminal plasma and of intracellular enzymes that regulate metabolism of the glandular epithelium. Although many intracellular and secretory enzymes are altered by hormonal manipulation and by neoplastic changes, clinical enzymology in prostatic disease has, in most hospitals, been limited to serum acid phosphatase determinations. Even this classic diagnostic aid has been the subject of much controversy.

The problems inherent in interpreting alterations in enzyme levels in various body fluids stem from the multiple tissue sources within the body that can potentially contribute to abnormal accumulation of *extracellular enzymes*. The identification of multiple molecular forms of individual enzymes (isoenzymes) provides one approach to achieving a degree of tissue specificity in laboratory diagnosis.

In a given species, isoenzymes are enzymatically active proteins which catalyze the same reaction but differ in certain physicochemical properties. In the strict sense of this definition, the reaction in question should be the physiologic reaction which occurs in vivo. In vitro analysis should employ the natural substrate reacting in as near to physiologic conditions as possible. In the laboratory, however, many enzymes are detected only through the use of artificial substrates reacting under somewhat empiric conditions.

Indeed, little is known about the physiologic function of many enzymes which can be detected in serum and tissues. This is particularly true of "nonspecific" esterases and phosphatases and is a major source of difficulty in evaluating prostatic isoenzymes.

A broad definition of isoenzymes based on in vitro reactions would then include both "true" physiologic isoenzymes, such as those of lactate dehydrogenase and groups of enzymes which catalyze a common in vitro reaction, but are involved in different physiologic processes. The alkaline phosphatase isoenzymes of bone, liver, small bowel, and placenta may fall in this latter category.

It is important to establish this concept and to keep this difference in mind because the limits of physicochemical variations which permit separation of isoenzymes differ in these two groups.

Separation of isoenzymes is most commonly accomplished by electrophoresis; however, other physicochemical separation techniques based on molecular weight or antigenicity may also be applied. The molecular charge (and therefore electrophoretic mobility) on an enzyme at a given pH may vary as a result of either amino acid substitution or variation in charged side groups (such as sialic acid) which are not an integral part of the polypeptide chain. Alterations of this type may occur in a molecule without changing the enzyme's catalytic function (substrate receptor site) or its antigenicity (major antigenic determinant). However, in groups of enzymes classified together only on the basis of one common in vitro reaction, major differences in molecular structure may occur.

These differences may be reflected in variations in substrate selectivity, susceptibility to inhibitors, and antigenicity. Major variations such as inhibitor sensitivity may be used to subclassify enzymes into categories which may be further resolved on the basis of minor variations in charged side chains. In enzymology, it becomes important to determine the significance and nature of physicochemical variation in order to distinguish isoenzyme alterations of diagnostic value from alterations due to genetic drift within the population.

ISOENZYMES OF ACID PHOSPHATASE

The early studies of Kutscher and his co-workers[1] and the classic work of Huggins and Hodges[2] have firmly bound the clinical evaluation of acid phosphatase to the diagnosis of prostatic carcinoma. However, the heterogeneous and ubiquitous nature of this enzyme has complicated the interpretation of serum levels and has given rise to numerous variations in methodology in an attempt to achieve specificity. Differential inhibition and substrate selectivity are widely employed in the clinical laboratory. Electrophoretic separation of acid phosphatase has been extensively investigated, but no standard method has been accepted for diagnostic purposes. More recently immunologic techniques have been employed to identify tissue specific acid phosphatase.

Separation by Inhibitors

Acid phosphatase was demonstrated in man in 1942 as an erythrocytic enzyme, and the majority of modifications of clinical assays have been directed toward differentiating the erythrocytic and prostatic components. Gutman et al.[3] first demonstrated that the red cell enzyme was resistant to fluoride in concentrations which inhibited the prostatic enzyme. Herbert[4] subsequently reported inhibition of prostatic acid phosphatase by ethanol and negligible inhibition of "normal serum." These observations were confirmed and extended by Abul-Fadl and King,[5] who investigated the effect of various ions and organic compounds. The major differential inhibitors are summarized in Table 7–1.

Of the various inhibitors of prostatic acid phosphatase only L(+) tartrate has achieved widespread clinical application. The popularity of this inhibitor has unfortunately given rise to a misconception that tartrate inhibition is "specific" for prostatic acid phosphatase.

Whereas the prostatic enzyme is highly

Table 7–1

% Inhibition or Activation (Phenyl Phosphate in pH-5.0 Acetate Buffer)[a]

Substance	Prostate in Saline	Red Cells in Water
Arsenate, 0.001 M	− 66	− 80
Citrate, 0.001 M	+ 8	+ 5
Cyanide, 0.001 M	+ 12	+ 8
Fluoride, 0.001 M	− 96	− 8
Formate, 0.001 M	0	0
Oralate, 0.001 M	− 22	− 27
Salicylate, 0.001 M	0	0
Tartrate (L), 0.001 M	− 94	0
Tartrate (D), 0.001 M	0	0
Tauroglycocholate, 0.01 M	− 76	− 77
Ethanol preincubation, 40%	− 80	− 75
Formaldehyde, 0.5%	0	−100
Stilbestrol	0	0
Acetone preincubation, 40%	−100	− 70
Copper,[b] 0.0002 M	− 8	− 96
Iron,[b] 0.0005 M	− 80	− 9

[a]Selectively compiled from Abul-Fadl and King.[5]
[b]No effect in citrate buffer.

sensitive to L(+) tartrate, and prostatic disease is the most likely cause of serum elevations of tartrate-sensitive acid phosphatase, it is now clear that many other tissues also contain a form of this enzyme which is inhibited by L(+) tartrate.[6]

Separation by Substrate Selectivity

As the natural substrate of prostatic acid phosphatase is unknown, all in vitro assays and histochemical stains employ synthetic phosphate esters. The rates of hydrolysis of these esters differ with enzymes from various tissues. Again, because of the clinical importance of the prostatic enzyme and the danger of falsely elevated results from the red cell enzyme (hemolysis), most diagnostic assays have been formulated to differentiate these two forms of acid phosphatase.

Commonly employed substrates include phenyl phosphate,[7] para-nitrophenyl phosphate,[8] beta-glycerophosphate,[9] phenolphthalein phosphate,[10] beta-naphthyl phosphate,[11] alpha-naphthyl phosphate,[12] Naphthol AS-BI phosphate,[13] and thymolphthalein phosphate.[14]

Tsuboi and Hudson[15] and later Babson and Read[12] evaluated relative activity of erythrocytic and prostatic acid phosphatase on various substrates. Beta-glycerophosphate and alpha-naphthyl phosphate were shown to be preferentially hydrolyzed by prostatic acid phosphatase.

Sodium thymolphthalein phosphate was introduced in 1971 by Roy et al. and was demonstrated to have an even greater selectivity for prostatic acid phosphatase; however, electrophoretic studies combined with the evaluation of preferred substrates[16] suggest that none of the currently employed substrates is truly prostate specific.

An important potential application of preferred substrate hydrolysis suggested by Seligman,[17] is the development of synthetic substrate analogs with chemotherapeutic effects which would not be activated until the substrate moiety had been hydrolyzed. Such agents would potentially become active chemotherapeutic agents at the site of prostatic cancer metastasis but remain inactive in other sites.

Separation by Electrophoresis

Electrophoretic separation of acid phosphatase isoenzyme has been accomplished with serum and numerous tissue extracts. The methodology employed has varied considerably, and consequently no standard diagnostic technique or isoenzyme pattern has gained widespread acceptance. While not a comprehensive review, Table 7–2 summarizes the methodology and results obtained in 26 papers on acid phosphatase isoenzymes. Clearly the techniques of electrophoresis and enzyme staining are an important source of variation in results. Furthermore, many of the tabulated results show further variation when the enzyme preparation is fractionated with and without a detergent (Triton X-100), suggesting that one or more forms of the enzyme are membrane bound.

While the data are subject to various interpretations, this author suggests that they warrant the following tentative conclusions:

1. At least three, and probably four enzyme populations exist, which may have little physiologic relationship with each other.
2. Each major acid phosphatase population may be further subdivided into isoenzymes which may share common physiologic functions.
3. The major groups of acid phosphatases include: (a) intracellular red cell acid phosphatases, (b) intracellular acid phosphatases associated with lysosomes, and (c) acid phosphatases which are formed as secretory products with extracellular function.

Intracellular membrane-bound acid phosphatases not involved in lysosomal function may constitute another major group.

Hopkinson[23,24] has shown that red cell acid phosphatases are reproducibly separable into three isoenzymes forming five phenotypic isoenzyme patterns (A, BA, B, CA, and CB). It is believed that these are under the control of three genes.

It is not clear whether any of these acid phosphatase isoenzymes may exist in the prostate or tissues other than red cells. Kaye et al. have demonstrated an isoenzyme in skin fibroblasts which resembles the red cell enzymes in its electrophoretic mobility and inability to hydrolyze alpha-naphthyl phosphate.[42] Beckman and Beckman also point out that isoenzyme patterns of tissue extracts may vary from patient to patient as well as with technique.[29,33] At pH 5.2, they could resolve up to 17 bands of activity on starch gel. At pH 8.6, only four major zones were detected, which they designate A, B, C, and D. Kidney usually showed A, B, and D, but in one patient only B and D were detected. Heart, skeletal muscle, liver, and intestine usually showed only B and D, but individual cases also contained A. A genetic variation of the placental C band was also described. Regrettably no prostatic specimens were included in this study.

The greatest variability in acid phosphatase occurs in the intracellular forms which can be found in tissues other than red cells and which, at least in part, are associated with the lysosomes. These enzymes are especially prominent in the reticuloendothelial system and may become valuable diagnostic aids in hematology. The numeric designations 0, 1, 2, 3, 3B, 4, and 5 employed by Li et al.[16] and by Yam et al.[37] are convenient for discussing this group of isoenzymes and will be used herein unless otherwise designated.

Since bone marrow acid phosphatase

Table 7–2

Summary of Methodology of Substrate Selectivity

Enzyme Source	Number Isoenzymes	Electrophoresis Media	pH	Year	Reference
1. Semen	1	SG	10	1959	18
2. Serum	3	SG	9.0	1960	19
3. Serum	2	SG	8.6	1960	20
4. Prostate	13	SG	6.2	1962	21
5. Brain	2	AG	8.4	1963	22
6. Red cells	3	SG	6.0	1963	23
7. Red cells	3	SG	6.0	1964	24
8. Liver	4	DEAE	7.0–6.0	1964	25
9. Plasma					26
Normal	3	SG	8.5	1965	
Hyperparathyroid	3	SG	8.5	1965	
Osteopetrosis	3	SG	8.5	1965	
Gaucher's	5	SG	8.5	1965	
Prostatic carcinoma	4	SG	8.5	1965	
10. Serum					27
Normal	1	PA	*	1966	
Multiple myeloma	1	PA	*	1966	
Carcinoma prostate	1	PA	*	1966	
Gaucher's	5	PA	*	1966	
11. Prostate, liver, kidneys	Up to 17 total	SG	6.0	1966	28
Leukocytes	3 Major	PA	5.8	1966	
12. Various tissues	3 to 4	SG	8.6	1967	29
	Up to 17	SG	5.2	1967	
Heart, muscle, kidney, skin, liver, pancreas, intestine, placenta					
13. Kidney (rat)	3 cortex	AG	8.4	1958	30
	2 medulla	AG	8.4	1958	30
14. Various tissues	6	SG	8.6 and 7.5	1967	31
15. Various tissues	1 to 5	PA	*	1968	32
16. Placenta	4	SG	7.5	1970	33
Polys	4	SG	7.5	1970	
Lymphocytes and platelets	3	SG	7.5		
17. Leukocytes	5	PA	4.0	1970	34
18. Leukocytes	7	PA	4.0	1970	35
19. Red cells	5 to 7	SG	5.9	1971	36
20. Leukemic reticulo-endotheliosis	6	PA	4.0	1971	37
21. Subretinal fluid	1	PA	4.5	1972	38
22. Endometrium	3	PA	9.5	1972	39
23. Plasma and various tissues	5	PA	4.0	1973	16
24. Eosinophilic	2	PA	8.5 and 4.5	1973	40
Leukemia	3	PA	8.5 and 4.5	1973	40
25. Prostatic	3	PA	4.3	1973	41
26. Fibroblasts	5	SG and PA	4.0	1974	42

Key: SG, starch gel; AG, agar gel; PA, polyacrylamide gel; and DEAE, DEAE cellulose chromatography.

levels have been proposed as diagnostic aids in prostatic cancer,[43,44] it is important to recognize that numerous constituents of bone marrow aspirates other than red cells and prostatic cancer may contribute to total marrow acid phosphatase.

Osteoclasts are rich in acid phosphatase which is tartrate resistant and probably migrates in position 5. Osteoclastic acid phosphatase is probably responsible for minor serum enzyme elevation in Paget's disease, osteoporosis, nonprostatic malignancies with bone metastases, and other conditions in which there is increased bone resorption.

Platelets and megakaryocytes contain an isoenzyme which is inhibited by tartrate and migrates in zone 3. According to Li,[16] normal plasma contains only tartrate-resistant isoenzyme 5, while normal serum contains 5 and tartrate-inhibited 3, which is released from platelets during clotting. It would appear, therefore, that platelets and osteoclasts may be the primary source of normal serum acid phosphatase.

The platelet isoenzyme may contribute to circulating enzyme levels during intravascular coagulation, but increased serum levels associated with thromboembolic disorders[45] probably reflect red cell lysis as well as platelet release.

Granulocytes, monocytes, histiocytes, and plasma cells exhibit strong acid phosphatase activity, whereas lymphocytes, lymphoblasts, myeloblasts, and erythroblasts have relatively weak activity as judged by histochemical staining.[46-48] In these cell lines, the acid phosphatases appear to be predominantly of lysosomal origin. However, clear differences in substrate hydrolysis and inhibition exist. Granulocytes and monocytes have isoenzymes which migrate in zones 2 and 4 and hydrolyze alpha-naphthyl phosphate, whereas the lymphocytic enzyme migrates in zone 3 and has little activity against this substrate.[6] The storage cells of Gaucher's disease are rich in acid phos-

phatase, which is only slightly inhibited by tartrate, if at all.[49] In some cases[27] this enzyme is present in five bands on acrylamide electrophoresis. Other investigators[16] report 3 bands, and in one case the activity did not migrate into the gel.[35] This variation remains unexplained. Yam et al. have also reported a fast (zone 5) isoenzyme which is tartrate resistant in the "hairy cells" of leukemic reticuloendotheliosis.[37]

When prostatic extracts are evaluated by this acrylamide technique, two bands of activity in zones 2 and 4 are detected.[6] Both of these are tartrate sensitive. Thus by this method, granulocytic acid phosphatase and prostatic acid phosphatase are quite similar.

While studying acid phosphatase in neoplasia, one must consider the possible appearance of an oncofetal isoenzyme such as the Regan isoenzyme of alkaline phosphatase.[50] Although this is an intriguing prospect, little data are available to support the existence of such an isoenzyme. Beckman and Beckman[29,33] have reported four acid phosphatase isoenzymes (starch gel) in human placentas, one of which could only be detected in placental or fetal tissue. However, the appearance of this isoenzyme in prostatic cancer or other neoplasms has not been observed.

Primitive blast cells have been reported to contain a tartrate-inhibited isoenzyme which hydrolyzes alpha-naphthyl phosphate and exhibits a unique electrophoretic mobility, 3b.[35] This blast isoenzyme may represent a "fetal" form; however, variations in methodology make it impossible to relate this enzyme to the placental enzyme.

Prostatic acid phosphatase appears to be primarily a secretory product, although lysosomal forms of this enzyme may also occur in prostatic cells. Extreme heterogeneity of prostatic acid phosphatase is revealed by starch gel electrophoresis when prostatic tissue is used as the source of the enzyme. Sur et al.[21] have demonstrated up to 13 bands of activity. These authors also noted that only a single fast band of activity was observed when seminal plasma was studied.

These observations suggest that the heterogeneity of the tissue enzyme may represent variation in side groups on a single molecular form of the enzyme. The cells may contain numerous incomplete forms of the final secretory product. This view is supported by the work of Smith and Whitby,[51] Ostrowski et al.,[52] and Chu et al.[53] These investigators have demonstrated that apparently multiple molecular forms of acid phosphatase can be reduced to a single protein enzyme by neuraminidase digestion. Variation in isoelectric point appears to depend on the number of sialic acid groups bound to the peptide chain. It is possible that prostatic neoplasms may produce "incomplete" variants of acid phosphatase by failing to incorporate the usual number of sialic acid molecules into the enzyme; however, such variants have not been recognized.

By acrylamide electrophoresis, prostatic acid phosphatase shows activity primarily in zone 2 with weak activity in zone 4.[16] As tartrate-inhibitable forms of acid phosphates with this electrophoretic mobility are present in granulocytes and other tissues,[16,35] this isoenzyme pattern cannot be used to specifically identify prostatic acid phosphatase.

Immunologic Separation

Prostate-specific antigens in dogs were suggested by the in vivo studies of Flocks et al.[54] and by Macalalag and Prout.[55] Shulman et al.[56] subsequently demonstrated antibodies which reacted with human prostatic acid phosphatase. Subsequent studies in this laboratory[44,57–60] and others[61,62] attest to the apparent antigenic specificity of prostatic acid phosphatase.

By Ouchterlony immunodiffusion, Shulman and Ferber[63] have demonstrated up to five precipitin bands with acid phosphatase activity when selected antiprostate antisera were reacted with prostate. The exact nature of this apparent antigenic heterogeneity is not clear but warrants further investigation.

Prostatic acid phosphatase is not inactivated when precipitated by specific antibody, and therefore simple gel immunodiffusion studies coupled with histochemical staining of the enzyme can be employed to immunochemically identify prostatic acid phosphatase. We have employed radial immunodiffusion to compare prostatic acid phosphatase levels in serum and bone marrow (Figure 7–1).[44,59] In our experience, levels of prostatic acid phosphatase in a patient's marrow which are greater than concurrent serum levels indicate stage IV disease and usually correlate with the demonstration of tumor cells in the marrow. Normal marrow components, Gaucher's cells, and nonprostatic tumor cells have not led to any erroneous diagnosis or staging in 150 patients evaluated by this technique. In only one patient has a cross reaction with nonprostatic acid phosphatase been observed. The patient was a female with chronic myelogenous leukemia with "storage cells" resembling Gaucher's cells.[64] A questionable positive marrow reaction was obtained by radial immunodiffusion, using antiserum raised against partially purified (DEAE fractionation) prostatic acid phosphatase.[44]

Further studies are in progress. However, this antiserum appears to contain antibodies which react with prostatic acid phosphatase and a minor antibody component which cross-reacts with the leukemic marrow. Antiserum against Gaucher's spleen has been developed which produces two precipitin bands with acid phosphatase activity when reacted with Gaucher's spleen, but which shows no reactivity with prostate or the

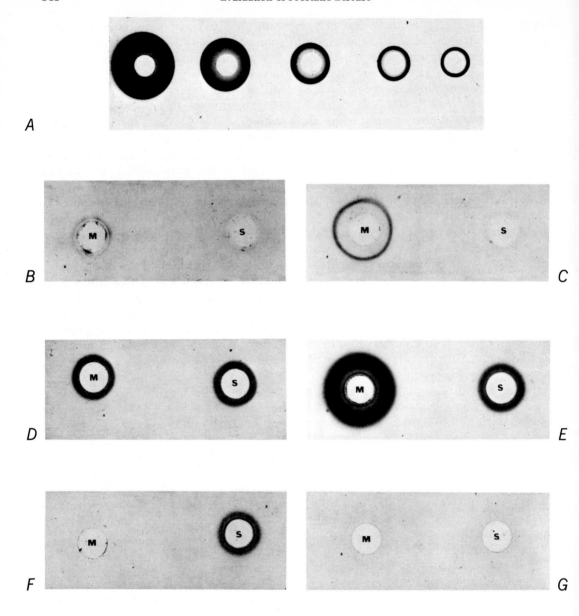

Figure 7–1. Serial dilution of prostatic acid phosphatase. A, Reduction of precipitative ring with decreasing enzyme concentration. B, Comparative immunodiffusion results. *Key:* M, marrow well; S, serum well; negative reaction in control patient with hematological disorder. C, Positive reaction in metastatic prostatic cancer and slightly elevated serum acid phosphatase; no precipitative ring has formed around serum wall. D, Negative reaction in patient with metastatic prostatic cancer and marked elevation in serum acid phosphatase. Rings are of equal size and do not prove presence of tumor in marrow. E, Positive reaction in patient with metastatic prostatic cancer and very high serum acid phosphatase; the much larger marrow ring proves tumor in marrow. F, Negative reaction in patient with benign prostatic hyperplasia and elevated serum acid phosphatase following transurethral resection; no precipitative ring around marrow well. G, Negative reaction in patient with Gaucher's disease, elevated serum acid phosphatase and Gaucher's cells in marrow sample; antiserum does not precipitate nonprostatic acid phosphatase.

marrow of the patient with chronic myelogenous leukemia with "storage cells." Other patients with myelogenous leukemia have shown no reaction with either anti-Gaucher or antiprostate antisera.

ISOENZYMES OF ALKALINE PHOSPHATASE

The characteristic bony metastases of prostatic carcinoma are reflected in an elevation of bone alkaline phosphatase. The detection of this isoenzyme should be a valuable parameter for following the course of the disease and the efficiency of therapy. Unfortunately, no large scale prospective studies on bone alkaline phosphatase in prostatic cancer patients have been conducted.

Isoenzyme separation is essential if alkaline phosphatase is to be used for this purpose, since normal adult serum contains very little alkaline phosphatase of bone origin. Metastatic or other mass lesions of the liver will cause disproportionate elevations of total serum alkaline phosphatase.[65] Several electrophoretic separation methodologies have been developed that satisfactorily resolve alkaline phosphatase isoenzymes. Starch block,[66,67] starch gel,[18,68] and acrylamide gel electrophoresis[69,70] provide high resolution but are inconvenient for routine clinical application.

Agar-gel electrophoresis as employed by Haije and DeJong[71] or cellulose acetate electrophoresis[72] are more readily applicable and generally satisfactory for resolving at least bone, liver, and intestinal alkaline phosphatase. Although these three isoenzymes plus placental alkaline phosphatase are the only forms of the enzyme commonly reported in clinical studies, it is clear that far greater heterogeneity exists and additional tissue specific forms of the enzyme may be identified in the future. Boyer[73] has reported 16 bands in human serum although not all in the same individual. As

with acid phosphatase, the precise nature of the enzyme heterogeneity is not clear but may be a combination of variables including different physiologic enzyme populations, minor structural alterations within a given population, and genetic variability.

As with prostatic acid phosphatase, part of the electrophoretic heterogeneity of alkaline phosphatase is a reflection of the sialic acid groups on the molecules. Posen[74] has shown that the bone isoenzyme which normally appears in the alpha-2 region remains in the gamma-globulins following treatment with neuraminidase. Alterations in mobility following neuraminidase have also been reported by Robinson and Pierce[75] and by Moss et al.[76] Intestinal alkaline phosphatase does not appear to be altered by neuraminidase.

In routine clinical chemistry laboratories, selective inhibition by heat[77,78] and 0.005 M L-phenylalanine[79,80] can readily identify intestinal and placental alkaline phosphatase and differentiate them from other tissue isoenzymes, including liver and bone. Liver, bone, and intestinal alkaline phosphatase are inactivated by heating at 56°C for 30 minutes. The placental enzyme is stable under these conditions. Placental and intestinal isoenzymes are inhibited by 0.005 M L-phenylalanine, while liver and bone are not.

The differentiation of liver and bone is less clear-cut but is possible through selective heat denaturation. At 56°C, bone alkaline phosphatase is almost completely inactivated in 15 minutes, whereas the liver enzyme is only partially inactivated in this time. An automated assay with a carefully regulated inactivation phase should provide a practical approach to this problem.

The immunologic specificity of alkaline phosphatase has not been fully evaluated, but several studies suggest at least three major antigenic forms exist in man.

Schlamowitz and Bodansky[81] developed antisera against human intestinal and bone alkaline phosphatase using an osteogenic sarcoma as a source of bone isoenzyme. These antisera exhibited strong reactivity with the homologous antigens and no cross reactivity with each other; however, the antibone alkaline phosphatase did cross react with liver and kidney alkaline phosphatase. On the other hand, Sussman et al.[82] have shown that antisera prepared against human liver and placenta react with homologous antigens, but show no cross reactivity with bone, intestine, kidney, or neutrophils.

Of special interest in the immunology of alkaline phosphatase is the demonstration by Fishman et al. that the Regan isoenzyme,[50] which is occasionally produced by a variety of neoplasms, is biochemically and immunologically identical to placental alkaline phosphatase,[83] and this may be considered an oncofetal antigen. The occurrence of the Regan isoenzyme in patients with prostatic carcinoma is probably rare, but no firm data on the subject are available.

ISOENZYMES OF LACTATE DEHYDROGENASE

The value of lactate dehydrogenase (LDH) isoenzymes in the diagnosis of cardiac, liver, and muscle disorders has led to widespread clinical application of this test. In malignant diseases very high total serum LDH levels may occur, or isoenzyme patterns may show abnormalities, whereas total levels remain within normal limits. Wieme et al.[84] have reported marked elevation of LDH-3 in 38 of 76 patients with bronchogenic carcinoma and normal total LDH. Small but significant elevations were seen in 22 other patients.

Numerous investigators[85–87] have demonstrated increases in cationic LDH isoenzymes in malignant tissues compared to normal tissue from the same organ. This presumably is a reflection of increased anaerobic glycolysis in the neoplastic tissue. Patients with prostatic carcinoma[88] have elevations in LDH-4 and LDH-5, which may return to normal during remission.

While of great value in following patients with an established diagnosis of prostatic cancer, elevations in LDH-5 or LDH-4 are not specific for prostatic malignancy. Similar elevations have been reported in malignancy of stomach,[89] colon,[90] lung,[91] brain,[22] cervix,[92] and breast.[93]

To increase the diagnostic value of LDH isoenzymes in patients with prostatic carcinoma, it is necessary to select specimens in some manner which imposes a degree of "prostate specificity" on the test. The most direct approach is the evaluation of LDH isoenzymes in prostatic tissue. Oliver et al.[94] have studied over 600 surgical specimens by LDH electrophoresis and assigned an index to each derived from the ratio of LDH-5 to LDH-1. In their series a 5/1 index of greater than 1 was found in 78% of those cases diagnosed as malignant and less than one in 86% of those with benign disease. Flocks and Schmidt[95] report comparable results on 200 patients and describe two patients with LDH ratios (these authors use LDH 1/LDH 5 rather than LDH 5/LDH 1) suggestive of cancer but benign by histology who were proven to have cancer on repeat biopsy.

Elhilali et al.[96] have observed similar differences in LDH isoenzymes in benign and malignant prostatic tissue and suggest that evaluation of LDH isoenzymes in prostatic fluid may provide a nonsurgical approach to the diagnostic procedure. They indicate however that the LDH 5/1 index of prostatic fluid from patients with benign disease is greater than 2, and further evaluation of this approach is necessary.

In evaluating prostatic fluid isoenzymes, one must keep in mind that if the vasa deferentia are patent and even slight spermatogenesis persists a sixth isoenzyme of LDH (LDH-X) is likely to be detected between LDH-3 and LDH-4.[97]

Another possible nonsurgical approach to selective prostatic LDH evaluation has been proposed by Belitsky et al.[98] These investigators have compared LDH 5/1 ratios in patient's serum before and after prostatic manipulation. Their data from 36 patients with prostatic cancer suggest an increase in the 5/1 index following prostatic massage. It is likely to occur if prostatic cancer is present even though the premanipulation index is low. Elevations following massage are occasionally observed in patients with benign disease, however, and again the test cannot be considered specific.

A major limitation to the clinical application of LDH 5/1 ratios on serum, prostatic fluid or even tissue may be the effect of active infection. Granulocytes have been reported to be high in LDH-5,[99] and acute inflammatory processes may contribute to high LDH 5/1 indices. Although promising in concept, the diagnostic accuracy of the currently available LDH studies is relatively low and increased LDH 5/1 ratios in tissues, prostatic fluid, or postmassage serum serve best to raise the index of suspicion of malignancy and prompt further evaluation of the patient. As pointed out by Flocks, a tissue LDH index suggestive of carcinoma but histologically benign warrants a repeat biopsy especially if no inflammatory disease is present.

Immunochemical studies of LDH[100] do not demonstrate tissue specificity but illustrate an important form of antigenic heterogeneity which may be encountered in other enzymes. LDH contains two types of subunits, A and B. LDH-1 contains four type A subunits, whereas LDH-5 contains four type B subunits. The intermediate isoenzymes are hybrids of A and B. Neutralizing antibodies of three types can be demonstrated against subunit pairs AA, AB, and BB. These have been termed alpha alpha, alpha beta, and beta beta respectively. Alpha alpha antibodies react only with LDH isoenzymes containing at least two A subunits, beta beta with isoenzymes containing at least two B subunits, and alpha beta with isoenzymes containing both A and B subunits in any combination.

ISOENZYMES OF LEUCINE AMINOPEPTIDASE

The enzyme commonly referred to as leucine aminopeptidase (LAP) is an acrylamidase which hydrolyzes L-leucyl-beta naphthylamide. It was first shown to have electrophoretic heterogeneity by Lawrence et al. in 1960[20]; however, no standard isoenzyme nomenclature has been established for LAP. Normal serum contains a single zone of activity which varies in its location somewhat with the electrophoretic technique. On starch gel, most investigators report LAP in the fast alpha 2 region[101]; paper or cellulose acetate electrophoresis, however, show activity in the alpha 1 region. Human liver extracts show a similar pattern,[102] suggesting that liver may be the primary source of normal serum LAP. An additional band appears in the serum of pregnant women which appears to be placental in origin.[101]

Beckman et al.[103] have described multiple forms of LAP in numerous human tissues, including four bands in placenta, three in kidney, two in liver, lung, spleen, and heart, a major slow band in intestine, and single fast bands in erythrocytes and brain. Treatment with neuraminidase suggested that the slower components contain sialic acid groups. The fast (anodal) bands were not altered by neuraminidase.

Serum LAP has been proposed as a diagnostic aid in pancreatic and liver disease but has not gained widespread application, and little is known about serum levels or isoenzyme patterns in patients with prostatic carcinoma. The prostate is rich in LAP, and Mattila[104] has reported detecting two antigenically distinct forms of LAP in human prostate. By immunizing rabbits with prostate, this investigator developed antisera which produced two precipitin bands against prostate with LAP activity in Ouchterlony immunodiffusion. When reacted with kidney, only one LAP band was formed. The author suggests that two antigenic forms be considered—renal LAP and prostate LAP. However, the tissue specificity of LAP has not been thoroughly investigated. In our laboratory, we have developed antiprostate antisera which give results identical to those reported by Mattila et al. with prostate and kidney; however, our antibody against renal LAP reacts with lines of identity by Ouchterlony diffusion with other tissues including liver and small bowel. The prostate LAP band does not occur when the antisera is reacted with these tissues, but absorption with tissue homogenates removes antibody activity. This suggests that "prostatic LAP" may be present in very low concentrations in other tissues but may, nonetheless, be of diagnostic value owing to its high concentration in the prostate.

In conclusion, we may say that the variety of enzymes and isoenzymes which occur in the prostate offers a valuable set of parameters which can guide us in the diagnosis of prostatic cancer and may provide a means of evaluating the disease both in grade and stage. The occurrence of similar or closely related enzymes in other tissues introduces a complex problem of distinguishing prostatic enzymes from nonprostatic enzymes.

It appears that conventional inhibition and electrophoretic separation techniques have much to offer in some specific situations, but they do not fully resolve the heterogeneity of such enzymes as acid and alkaline phosphatase or leucine aminopeptidase.

The introduction of immunologic techniques for the identification of specific enzymes opens a new dimension of clinical enzymology which may unveil an entire new population of immunoisoenzymes with diagnostic tissue specificity. While promising in many respects, antigenic typing of enzymes must be undertaken with caution. The evolution of different but related proteins regularly results in molecules which are structurally identical in some regions but different in others. This gives rise to the possibility of multiple antigenic sites on a single enzyme molecule, some specific, some shared by other enzymes. We have excellent examples of this in the various antigenic determinants on immunoglobulin molecules and in the antigenic similarity of glycopeptide hormones. To fully resolve the heterogeneity of prostatic and nonprostatic isoenzymes, we must attain a thorough understanding of their biochemical structure and selectively identify their antigenic determinants. With this information, truly monospecific antisera can be developed which would be of great value not only in diagnostic enzymology but also in studying prostatic physiology and the pathophysiology of prostatic carcinoma.

References

1. Kutscher, W., and Wolbergs, H.: Prostataphosphatase. Hoppe-Seyler's ztschr. f. physiol. Chem., 236:237, 1935.
2. Huggins, C., and Hodges, C. V.: Studies on prostatic cancer. I. The effect of castration, of estrogen and of androgen injection on serum phosphatases in metastatic carcinoma of the prostate. Cancer Res., 1:293, 1941.
3. Gutman, E. B., and Gutman, A. B.: Erythrocyte phosphatase activity in hemolyzed sera and estimation of serum acid phosphatases. Proc. Soc. Exp. Biol. Med., 47:513, 1941.
4. Herbert, F. K.: The differentiation between prostatic phosphatase and other acid phosphatases in pathological human sera. Biochem. J., 39:iv, 1945.
5. Abul-Fadl, M. A. M., and King, E. J.: Properties of the acid phosphatases of erythrocytes and of the human prostate gland. Biochem. J., 45:51, 1949.
6. Yam, L. T.: Clinical significance of the human acid phosphatases. A review. Am. J. Med., 56:604, 1974.

7. Gutman, E. B., and Gutman, A. B.: Estimation of "acid" phosphatase activity of blood serum. J. Biol. Chem., *136*:201, 1940.

8. Modder, C. P.: Investigations on acid phosphatase activity in human plasma and serum. Clin. Chim. Acta, 43:205, 1973.

9. Woodard, H. Q.: The clinical significance of serum acid phosphatase. Am. J. Med., *27*:902, 1959.

10. Huggins, C, and Talalay, P.: Sodium phenolphthalein phosphate as a substrate for phosphatase tests. J. Biol. Chem., *159*:399, 1945.

11. Seligman, A. M., et al.: The colorimetric determination of phosphatases in human serum. J. Biol. Chem., *190*:7, 1951.

12. Babson, A. L., and Read, P. A.: A new assay for prostatic acid phosphatase in serum. Am. J. Clin. Pathol., *32*:88, 1959.

13. Vaughan, A., et al.: Fluorometric methods for analysis of acid and alkaline phosphatase. Anal. Chem., *43*:721, 1971.

14. Roy, A. V., et al.: Sodium thymolphthalein monophosphate: A new acid phosphatase substrate with greater specificity for the prostatic enzyme in serum. Clin. Chem., *17*:1093, 1971.

15. Tsuboi, K. K., and Hudson, P. B.: Acid phosphatase. III. Specific kinetic properties of highly purified prostatic phosphomonoesterase. Arch. Biochem. Biophys., *55*:191, 1955.

16. Li, C. Y., et al.: Acid phosphatases in human plasma. J. Lab. Clin. Med., *82*:446, 1973.

17. Seligman, A. M.: Proceedings of the National Prostatic Cancer Project Workshop, 1974, in Cancer Chemother. Rep., *59*(1):233, 1975.

18. Estborn, B.: Visualization of acid and alkaline phosphatase after starch-gel electrophoresis of seminal plasma, serum and bile. Nature, *184*:1636, 1959.

19. Dubbs, C. A., et al.: Subfractionation of human serum enzymes. Science, *131*:1529, 1960.

20. Lawrence, S. H., et al.: A species comparison of serum proteins and enzymes by starch gel electrophoresis. Proc. Soc. Exp. Biol. Med., *105*:572, 1960.

21. Sur, B. K., et al.: Apparent heterogeneity of prostatic acid phosphatase. Biochem. J., *84*:55P, 1962.

22. Gerhardt, W., et al.: Changes in LDH-isozymes, esterases, acid phosphatases and proteins in malignant and benign human brain tumors. Acta Neurol. Scand., *39*: 85, 1963.

23. Hopkinson, D. A., et al.: Red cell acid phosphatase variants: A new human polymorphism. Nature, *199*:969, 1963.

24. Hopkinson, D. A., et al.: Genetical studies on human red cell acid phosphatase. Am. J. Hum. Genet., *16*:141, 1964.

25. Reith, A., et al.: Über die isozyme der sauren phosphatase und ihre intracellulärelokalisation in der menschlichen und der ratten leber. XV. Mitteilung über fermentaktivitätsbestimungen in der menschlichen leber. Klin. Wochenschr., *42*:915, 1964.

26. Grundig, E., et al.: Vergleichende unter-suchungen von "sauren" plasma phosphatasen bei verschiedenen knochenerkrankungen. Clin. Chim. Acta, *12*:157, 1965.

27. Goldberg, A. F., et al.: Electrophoretic separation of serum acid phosphatase isoenzymes in Gaucher's disease, prostatic carcinoma and multiple myeloma. Nature, *211*:41, 1966.

28. Lundin, L. G., and Allison, A. C.: Acid phosphatase from different organs and animal forms compared by starch-gel electrophoresis. Biochim. Biophys. Acta, *127*:527, 1966.

29. Beckman, L., and Beckman, G.: Individual and organ-specific variations of human acid phosphatase. Biochem. Genet., *1*:145, 1967.

30. Pla, G. W., et al.: Renal acid phosphatase isoenzymes. Enzymologia, *34*:40, 1958.

31. Ramot, B., and Streifler, C.: Serum and tissue acid α-naphthylphosphatase isozymes in various diseases. Isr. J. Med. Sci., *3*:505, 1967.

32. Rozenszajn, L., et al.: The acid phosphatase isoenzymes in normal and pathological sera and tissue homogenates. J. Lab. Clin. Med., *72*:786, 1968.

33. Beckman, G., et al.: A rare subunit variant shared by five acid phosphatase isozymes from human leukocytes and placentae. Hum. Hered., *20*:81, 1970.

34. Li, C. Y., et al.: Acid phosphatase isoenzyme in human leukocytes in normal and pathologic conditions. J. Histochem. Cytochem., *18*:473, 1970.

35. Li, C. Y., et al.: Studies of acid phosphatase isoenzymes in human leukocytes. Demonstration of isoenzyme cell specificity. J. Histochem. Cytochem., *18*:901, 1970.

36. White, I. N. H., and Butterworth, P. J.: Isoenzymes of human erythrocyte acid phosphatase. Biochim. Biophys Acta, *229*:193, 1971.

37. Yam, L. T., et al.: Tartrate-resistant acid phosphatase isoenzyme in the reticulum cells of leukemic reticuloendotheliosis. N. Engl. J. Med., *284*:357, 1971.

38. Lam, K. W., et al.: Subretinal fluid: Isoenzymes and cytologic studies. Invest. Ophthalmol., *11*:1037, 1972.

39. Sumner, N. A., and Brush, M. G.: Isoenzymes of acid phosphatase in human endometrium. Biochem. J., *128*:103p, 1972.

40. Pajdak, W., and Lisiewicz, J.: Heterogeneity of enzymes in leukaemic eosinophils. Scand. J. Haematol., *11*:325, 1973.

41. Reif, A. E., et al.: Acid phosphatase isoenzymes in cancer of the prostate. Cancer *31*:689, 1973.

42. Kaye, C. I., and Nadler, H. L.: Acid phosphatase isoenzymes in human skin fibroblasts. Proc. Soc. Exp. Biol. Med., *145*:157, 1974.

43. Chua, D. T., et al.: Acid phosphatase levels in bone marrow: Value in detecting early bone metastasis from carcinoma of the prostate. J. Urol., *103*:462, 1970.

44. Moncure, C. W., et al.: Immunological and histochemical evaluation of marrow aspirates in patients with prostatic carcinoma. J. Urol., *108*:609, 1972.

45. Schoenfeld, M. R.: Increased serum acid phosphatase after arterial embolism. Am. Heart J., 67:92, 1964.

46. Rabinovitch, M., and Andreucci, D.: A histochemical study of "acid" and "alkaline" phosphatase distribution in normal human bone marrow smears. Blood, 4:580, 1949.

47. Rozenszajn, L., et al.: Acid phosphatase activity in normal human blood and bone marrow cells as demonstrated by the azo dye method. Acta Haematol., 30:310, 1963.

48. Kaplow, L. S., and Burstone, M. S.: Cytochemical demonstration of acid phosphatase in hematopoietic cells in health and in various hematological disorders using azo dye techniques. J. Histochem Cytochem., 12:805, 1964.

49. Tuchman, L. R, et al.: Studies on the nature of the increased serum acid phosphatase in Gaucher's disease. Am. J. Med., 27:959, 1959.

50. Fishman, W. H., et al.: A serum alkaline phosphatase isoenzyme of human neoplastic cell origin. Cancer Res., 28:150, 1968.

51. Smith, J. K., and Whitby, L. G.: The heterogeneity of prostatic acid phosphatase. Biochim. Biophys. Acta, 151:607, 1968.

52. Ostrowski, W., et al.: The role of neuraminic acid in the heterogeneity of acid phosphomonoesterase from the human prostate gland. Biochim. Biophys. Acta, 221:297, 1970.

53. Chu, T. M., et al.: The tumor antigen and acid phosphatase isoenzymes in prostatic cancer. National Prostatic Cancer Project Workshop, 1974. Cancer Chemother. Rep., 59(1):97, 1975.

54. Flocks, R. H., et al.: Studies on the antigenic properties of prostatic tissues. J. Urol., 84:134, 1960.

55. Macalalag, E. V., Jr., and Prout, G. R., Jr.: Anti-canine prostatic fluid serum and prostatic degeneration. Invest. Urol., 4:321, 1967.

56. Shulman, S., et al.: The detection of prostatic acid phosphatase by antibody reactions in gel diffusion, J. Immunol., 93:474, 1964.

57. Moncure, C. W., et al.: Prostatic acid phosphatase antisera. Invest. Urol., 5:331, 1968.

58. Moncure, C. W., and Prout, G. R., Jr.: Antigenicity of human prostatic acid phosphatase. Cancer, 25:463, 1970.

59. Moncure, C. W.: Prostatic acid phosphatase: A Potpourri. MCV Q Med Coll. Va. Q, 9:235, 1973.

60. Moncure, C. W.: Investigation of specific antigens in prostatic cancer. National Prostatic Cancer Project Workshop, 1975. Cancer Chemother. Rep., 59(1):105, 1975.

61. Milisauskas, V., and Rose, N. R.: Immunochemical quantitation of prostatic phosphatase. Clin. Chem., 18:1529, 1972.

62. Ablin, R. J.: Immunochemical identification of prostatic tissue-specific acid phosphatase. Clin. Chem., 19:786, 1973.

63. Shulman, S., and Ferber, J. M.: Multiple forms of prostatic acid phosphatase. J. Reprod. Fertil., 11:295, 1966.

64. Lee, R. E., and Ellis, L. D.: The storage cells of chronic myelogenous leukemia. Lab. Invest., 24:261, 1971.

65. Ewen, L. M.: Separation of alkaline phosphatase isoenzymes and evaluation of the clinical usefulness of this determination. Am. J. Clin. Pathol., 61:142, 1974.

66. Keiding, N. R.: Differentiation into three fractions of the serum alkaline phosphatase and the behavior of the fractions in diseases of bone and liver. Scand. J. Clin. Lab. Invest., 11:106, 1959.

67. Keiding, N. R.: The alkaline phosphatase fractions of human lymph. Clin. Sci., 26:291, 1964.

68. Markert, C. L., and Moller, F.: Multiple forms of enzymes: Tissue, ontogenetic, and species specific patterns. Proc. Nat. Acad. Sci. U.S.A., 45:753, 1959.

69. Epstein, E., et al.: An indigogenic reaction for alkaline phosphatase in disk electrophoresis. Am. J. Clin. Pathol., 48:530, 1967.

70. Sussman, H. H., et al.: Human alkaline phosphatase. Immunochemical identification of organ-specific isoenzymes. J. Biol. Chem., 243:160, 1968.

71. Haije, W. G., and DeJong, M.: Iso-enzyme patterns of serum alkaline phosphatase in agar-gel electrophoresis and their clinical significance. Clin. Chim. Acta, 8:620, 1963.

72. Romel, W. C., et al.: Detection of serum alkaline phosphatase isoenzymes with phenolphthalein monophosphate following cellulose acetate electrophoresis. Clin. Chem., 14:47, 1968.

73. Boyer, S. H.: Alkaline phosphatase in human sera and placentae. Science, 134:1002, 1961.

74. Posen, S.: Alkaline phosphatase. Ann. Intern. Med., 67:183, 1967.

75. Robinson, J. C., and Pierce, J. E.: Differential action of neuraminidase on human serum alkaline phosphatases. Nature, 204:472, 1964.

76. Moss, D. W., et al.: Alteration in the electrophoretic mobility of alkaline phosphatases after treatment with neuraminidase. Biochem. J., 98:32c, 1966.

77. Posen, S., et al.: Heat inactivation in the study of human alkaline phosphatases. Ann. Intern. Med., 62:1234, 1965.

78. McMaster, Y., et al.: The mechanism of the elevation of serum alkaline phosphatase in pregnancy. J. Obstet. Gynaecol. Br. Commonw., 71:735, 1964.

79. Fishman, W. H., et al.: Organ-specific behavior exhibited by rat intestine and liver alkaline phosphatase. Biochim. Biophys. Acta, 62:363, 1962.

80. Fishman, W. H., et al.: Distinguishing characteristics of serum alkaline phosphatase isoenzymes. Fed. Proc., 25:748, 3158 abs, 1966.

81. Schlamowitz, M., and Bodansky, O.: Tissue sources of human serum alkaline phosphatase as determined by immunochemical procedures. J. Biol. Chem., 234:1433, 1959.

82. Sussman, H. H., et al.: Placental alkaline

phosphatase in maternal serum during normal and abnormal pregnancy. Nature, 218:359, 1968.

83. Fishman, W. H., et al.: Immunology and biochemistry of Regan isoenzyme of alkaline phosphatase in human cancer. Nature, 219:697, 1968.

84. Wieme, R. J., et al.: The influence of cytostatic treatment on serum LDH patterns of patients with bronchial carcinoma and its relation to tumor regression. Ann. N.Y. Acad. Sci., 151:213, 1968.

85. Pfleiderer, G., and Wachsmuth, E. D.: Alters- und funktionsabhängige differenzierung der lactatdehydrogenase menschlicher organe. Biochem. Z., 334:185, 1961.

86. Nissen, N. I., and Bohn, L.: Patterns of lactic acid dehydrogenase isoenzymes in normal and malignant human tissues. Eur. J. Cancer, 1:217, 1965.

87. Güttler, F.: The metabolic activity acquired by the media of cultivated malignant and non-malignant cells compared to that of human effusions. Enzyme, 8:228, 1967.

88. Denis, L. J., and Prout, G. R., Jr.: Lactic dehydrogenase in prostatic cancer. Invest. Urol., 1:101, 1963.

89. Baume, P. E., et al.: Isoenzymes of lactate dehydrogenase in human gastric mucosa and gastric carcinoma tissue. Gastroenterology, 50:781, 1966.

90. Langvad, E.: Lactate dehydrogenase isoenzyme patterns in the tumour-bearing colon. Int. J. Cancer, 3:17, 1968.

91. Langvad, E.: Lactate dehydrogenase isoenzyme patterns in bronchogenic carcinama. Eur. J. Cancer, 4:107, 1968.

92. Latner, A. L., et al.: Enzyme and isoenzyme studies in preinvasive carcinoma of the cervix. Lancet, 2:814, 1966.

93. Barnett, H., and Gibson, A.: Lactate dehydrogenase (L.D.H.) isoenzyme patterns in carcinomas of the breast. J. Clin. Pathol., 17:201, 1964.

94. Oliver, J. A., et al.: LDH isoenzymes in benign and malignant prostate tissue. The LDH V/I ratio as an index of malignancy. Cancer, 25:863, 1970.

95. Flocks, R. H., and Schmidt, J. D.: Lactate dehydrogenase isoenzyme patterns of prostatic cancer and hyperplasia. J. Surg. Oncol., 4:161, 1972.

96. Elhilali, M. M., et al.: Lactate dehydrogenase isoenzymes in hyperplasia and carcinoma of the prostate: A clinical study. J. Urol., 98:686, 1968.

97. Moncure, C. W., et al.: The ontogeny of the isozyme of lactate dehydrogenase in human testes. Surg. Forum, 17:513, 1966.

98. Belitsky, P., et al.: The effect of stilbestrol on the isoenzymes of lactic dehydrogenase in benign and malignant prostatic tissue. J. Urol., 104:453, 1970.

99. Malasková, V., and Holeyšovská, H.: Lactic dehydrogenase isoenzymes of human leuko-cytes. Clin. Chim. Acta, 24:39, 1969.

100. Markert, C. L., and Appella, E.: Immunochemical properties of lactate dehydrogenase isozymes. Ann. N.Y. Acad. Sci., 103:915, 1963.

101. Kowlessar, O. D., et al.: Localization of serum leucine aminopeptidase, 5-nucleotidase and nonspecific alkaline phosphatase by starch-gel electrophoresis: Clinical and biochemical significance in disease states. Ann. N.Y. Acad. Sci., 94:836, 1961.

102. Pineda, E. P., et al.: Serum leucine aminopeptidase in pancreatic and hepatobiliary diseases. Gastroenterology, 38:698, 1960.

103. Beckman, L., et al.: Multiple molecular forms of leucine aminopeptidase in man. Acta Genet. Stat. Med., 16:223, 1966.

104. Mattila, S.: Further studies on the prostatic tissue antigens. Separation of two molecular forms of aminopeptidase. Invest. Urol., 7:1, 1969.

Chapter 8

Prostatitis

GEORGE W. DRACH and PAUL W. KOHNEN

Prostatitis remains one of the most controversial diseases diagnosed and treated by physicians. Multiple problems contribute to the confusion generated by pathophysiology of this disease. Patients with prostatitis may or may not have symptoms,[1-4] may or may not have polymorphonuclear leukocytes or round cells in their prostatic fluid,[1,2,5,6] may or may not have "pathogens" cultured from their prostatic fluid,[2,4,7,8] may or may not have "pathogens" cultured from prostatic tissues,[7,9,10] may or may not show evidence of tissue inflammation.[7,9,11,12] and may or may not have tenderness and edema of the gland upon rectal examination with the finger.[1,4,7,13] To further complicate our concepts of prostatitis, some authors feel that a significant number of patients with prostatic symptoms have psychogenic or neurotic syndromes which cause the disease.[3,14] Perhaps the only agreement that we find, as we review the literature on prostatitis, indicates that cure is difficult no matter what methods of therapy are used.[1,14]

Perhaps it is presumptuous to assume that we can gain some order out of this confusion but, nevertheless, we will attempt to present, at least, a cogent theory

of etiology and diagnosis of prostatitis in this chapter. We will first cover some special aspects of prostatic anatomy which contribute to prostatitis. Next, we will review recent advances in diagnostic methods which have increased our ability to define the microorganisms which cause prostatitis. Then we will review prevailing theories about routes of prostatic infection and will then define types of microorganisms that cause prostatitis which we are certain exist. Some comments will follow regarding the antibacterial nature of prostatic fluid as well as the ability of the prostate to participate in both local and systemic antibody response to prostatic infection. Lastly, we will review our criteria for the histological diagnosis of prostatitis.

ANATOMY OF PROSTATE AS RELATED TO PROSTATITIS

Specific aspects of prostatic anatomy are presented elsewhere in this text. In order to standardize our discussion of prostatitis however, we will briefly discuss the terminology generated by McNeal,[15] Cameron,[16] and Blacklock,[17] namely that prostatic tissue is comprised of two major segments of multiple glandular structures which surround the urethra as it exits from the male bladder neck.

Surgically we recognize lobular divisions which surround the urethra so that, looking from within the urethra, five divisions can be discerned. These are the anterior, middle or median, posterior, and two lateral lobes. These surgeon's divisions are most obvious in those prostate glands that have undergone significant hypertrophy. Anatomically, however, some authors point out the confusion in precise terminology for the prostate.[15,16] McNeal divides the prostate into two segments, or more precisely "two separate and distinct organs."

The preprostatic segment is associated with the bladder neck, proximal sphincteric muscles, urethral glands, and that area of nodular hyperplasia which causes urinary obstruction. Since he believes that these hyperplastic glands arise from periurethral glands, he prefers the term, benign periurethral hyperplasia, instead of BPH, applied to the prostatic adenoma enucleated by the surgeon. Its inferior boundary exists at the point where the verumontanum arises from the posterior wall of the urethra.

His anatomic true prostate consists of two zones of tissue that surround the previously noted urethral tissue, partly posteriorly and laterally and extend also distally around the verumontanum. Ducts from these true prostatic glands open into the sulci beside the verumontanum, while most of the periurethral glands exit above, or superior to the verumontanum. Based on 371 autopsy studies, McNeal believes that the true prostate zones can be defined as central (a smaller wedge of tissue with its apex at the verumontanum and its base at the bladder neck) and peripheral (a larger mass of tissue which surrounds most of the central zone posteriorly, and extends further laterally and inferiorly, Figure 8–1).

Most significant was the fact that

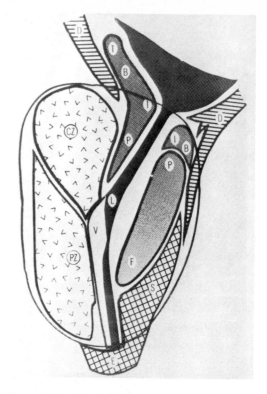

Figure 8–1. Composite of prostate. Sagittal section shows anatomic subdivisions as defined by McNeal.[15] *Key:* CZ, central zone; PZ, peripheral zone; V, verumontanum; L, urethral lumen; U, urethral stroma with longitudinal muscle; D, detrusor; T, interureteric ridge; I, internal sphincter; P, preprostatic sphincter; F, fibrous preprostatic sphincter, S, prostatic sphincter, and E, external sphincter. (From NcNeal.[15])

McNeal noted the peripheral zone "was observed to have a much greater susceptibility than the central to inflammation and carcinoma." This finding would correlate with our clinical observation that prostatitis appears to arise either in the periprostatic urethral glands or in those glands whose ducts empty into the sulci beside the verumontanum,[7] or both. More than 64 glands probably exit into these sulci.[17]

Because of this complex anatomy, clinical differentiation of the exact location of infection remains difficult: only one or two of the multiple prostatic glands, or periurethral glands, may be infected but, when prostatic fluid is collected by mas-

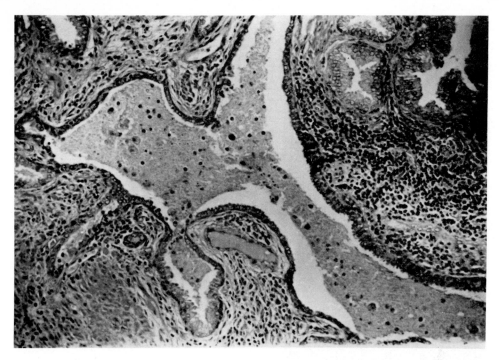

Figure 8–2. Localized inflammation. A duct in area of hyperplasia is distended with inspissated secretion. Within lumen the dark nuclei, which cannot be resolved in this illustration, are those of neutrophils and macrophages. Focal dense infiltrate of chronic inflammatory cells (right) lies adjacent to duct. Elsewhere, along periphery of duct, chronic inflammatory cells are scattered in stroma. (×120.)

sage, one collects random mixtures of normal and infected fluid from which the diagnosis is made. Fluid collection under direct vision aids diagnosis. Urethroscopic visualization of the prostatic urethra demonstrates glandular origins of thick, purulent secretions which can be aspirated directly for culture.[7] In addition, a small cup-forceps biopsy of the same area will often show inflammation (Figure 8–2), and culture of the tissue will result in growth of organisms (Figure 8–3).

In essence then, one can define some anatomic misconceptions which have led to confusion in diagnosis of prostatitis. It is no wonder that random biopsies of the prostate have often failed to demonstrate inflammation or bacteria,[9,10] since the areas sampled may have been centimeters away from the involved glands. To add to the confusion, variations in bacterial culture from prostatic fluid may depend on whether or not the infected glands were really emptied by massage. Lastly, few investigators agree on exactly which bacteria cultured from prostatic fluid or tissue are pathogens and which are not.

PROSTATITIS AND MICROORGANISMS

Bacteria and other microorganisms most often arrive at the prostate via the urethra, either by retrograde entry through the urethral meatus or antegrade entry via contaminated urine. Elite experiments and observations by Furness et al. point clearly to retrograde entry of bacteria from the fossa navicularis of the glans penis to the prostatic urethra.[18] Hematogenous dissemination may be possible, but little proof for this route of dissemination exists. Lymphatic spread from the colon or other contaminated source to the prostate seems very unlikely, since it is doubtful that the prostate has any lymphatics.[19]

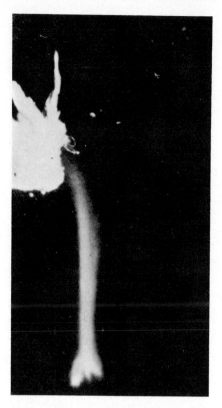

Figure 8–3. Biopsy of prostatic tissue obtained adjacent to verumontanum. Tissue (left) has column of bacteria growing downward into broth. (From Drach.[7])

Many authors have commented on the apparent relationship between prostatitis and sexual activities. Some a priori observations are appropriate. Prostatitis occurs mostly in sexually active populations.[1,3] Microorganisms obtained from the prostate resemble those cultured from the female vagina.[3,4] Certain infestations of the vagina, such as gonorrhea and trichomonas, easily invade the male urethra and occasionally the prostate, during the act of intercourse. Whether too much sexual activity, or too little, or aberrant sexual practices contribute to prostatitis, we cannot say.[5,14] Adequate data are not available.

Prostatitis may occur because of allergic responses or neurotic conditions, but it is our premise that most patients with prostatitis have a disease created by microor-

ganisms (a term which we define to include bacteria, mycotic organisms, viruses, and those organisms intermediate between bacteria and viruses). Diagnosis of prostatitis requires careful progression of studies, from history, through culture of prostatic fluid or tissues, and occasionally requires confirmatory study of tissue histology.

Symptoms and Signs

Patients with prostatitis most often complain of urinary frequency and urgency, often with nocturia and terminal dysuria. Perhaps 25% of the patients will be asymptomatic.[1,4] Less frequent complaints include lower abdominal aching, backache, testicular aching, or perineal pain.[1,7]

Urethral discharge occurs frequently and seems to be especially common upon arising in the morning. Prostatic tenderness, nodularity, or edema (bogginess) occur occasionally, but absence of these signs does not eliminate diagnosis of prostatitis. An acutely inflamed prostate is exquisitely tender, and a prostate which contains an abscess may be tender and asymmetrical.[16,20]

Bacteriologic Diagnosis

Whenever one suspects prostatitis, it is imperative to collect divided urinary specimens and prostatic fluid in order to locate the source of lower genitourinary infection. This methodology has been described extensively and will be reviewed here only briefly.[3,4,7,31]

Patients cleanse themselves, retract the foreskin if it is present, and then void the first 10–15 ml of urine into a small container. They collect the next 50–75 ml urine in a second container, without interrupting the urinary stream. These two specimens represent the urethral and bladder urines, respectively. Immediately thereafter, the physician performs prostatic examination and massage. Any prostatic fluid which is expressed flows by gravity into a wide-mouthed cup. This collection should be performed carefully to avoid contamination of the cup by the glans penis or surrounding skin or hair. This prostatic fluid specimen completes the usual collection.[7] For various reasons however, it may not be possible to collect prostatic fluid. If so, the patient should void a small quantity of urine after massage to wash any retained prostatic fluid from the urethra. This postprostatic specimen represents a close approximation of those bacteria present in prostatic fluid.[4,7]

Culture of these specimens by quantitative techniques results in a pattern of species and numbers of microorganisms on which diagnosis can be based. Meares and Stamey have emphasized that recovery of small numbers of bacteria from prostatic fluid can be evidence of disease.[4] We cannot, therefore, rely on the usual criterion of "greater than 10^5 bacteria" when we are attempting to diagnose prostatic infection.[7]

Separation of prostatitis from urethritis can be accomplished by recognizing different patterns created by the numbers of bacteria grown from divided urinary and prostatic specimens. Figures 8–4 to 8–7 illustrate the quantitative differences noted between normal men and patients

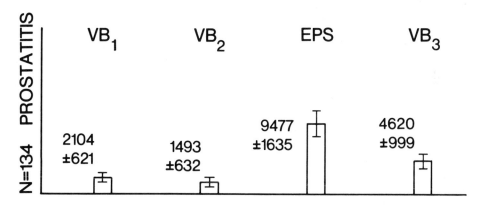

Figure 8–4. Quantitative bacterial counts of gram-positive and gram-negative bacteria grown from divided urinary specimens and EPS of patients with prostatitis. Numbers represent mean bacteria/ml ± 1 standard error. Histogram gives visual perspective of numbers of bacteria in various specimens. *Key:* VB_1 = urethral urine; VB_2 = bladder urine; EPS = prostatic fluid specimen; and VB_3 = postprostatic specimen in this and following figures. (From Drach.[7])

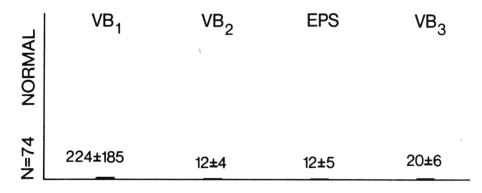

Figure 8–5. Histograms for normal males. Comparison with Figures 8–4, 6, and 7 aids differential diagnosis. (From Drach.[7])

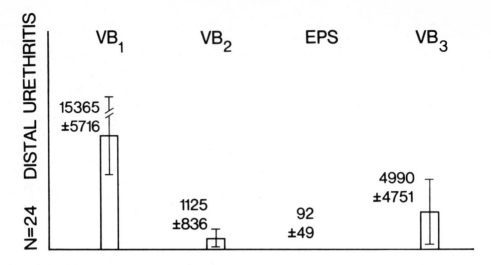

Figure 8–6. Histograms for patients with urethritis. VB_1 (urethral urine) contains significantly larger numbers of bacteria than all other specimens. (From Drach.[7])

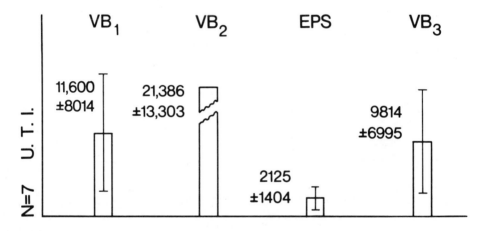

Figure 8–7. Histograms for patients with urinary tract infection. VB_2 (bladder urine) has largest number of bacteria and addition of normal prostatic fluid to VB_3 (postprostatic specimen) decreases urinary bacterial count. (From Drach.[7])

with urethritis, prostatitis, or urinary infections. Practically speaking, one may make the diagnosis of prostatitis if urethral urine and bladder urine specimens contain fewer than 3000 bacteria/ml and prostatic fluid specimen contains more than 5000 bacteria/ml. Values of 200–5000 bacteria/ml for prostatic fluid specimen should suggest prostatitis, and repeat studies should be performed after five days. If no prostatic fluid specimen is recovered,

postprostatic specimens containing over 3500 bacteria are still diagnostic when urethral urine and bladder urine have many fewer bacteria.[7]

No aspect of prostatitis generates as much controversy as does discussion of those organisms which may cause prostatitis. Part of this controversy arises from lack of precise criteria by which we can define prostatitis. Our definition of prostatitis includes:

1. One or more of the symptoms of frequency, urgency, nocturia, terminal dysuria, lower abdominal or perineal pain in the absence of other genital disease or urinary infection (optional).
2. Abnormal prostate by rectal examination (tender, boggy, calculi) (optional).
3. Prostatic fluid which shows more than 15 inflammatory cells/high-power (2 mm) field, often with clumps of cells and absence of lecithin bodies.[5,6] Gram's stain is performed to show extracellular or intracellular microorganisms, and a wet saline drop preparation is examined for possible *Trichomonas vaginalis*.
4. Microorganisms capable of creating inflammation grow in significant numbers from prostatic fluid and in significantly fewer numbers from other specimens (Figures 8–4 and 7).
5. When questions of diagnosis arise, anatomical correlation is obtained by culture of microorganisms directly from a biopsy specimen of prostatic tissue, in which the same specimen demonstrates inflammation on histologic examination.[7] This biopsy must be obtained under direct vision from that portion of the prostate observed to be the origin of purulent prostatic fluid.

PROSTATITIS AND CAUSATIVE MICROORGANISM

Gram-positive bacteria are cultured more frequently from purulent prostatic fluid than any other microorganism.[7,22,23] Exclusion of these organisms from pathogenicity because they may be found on skin or in the urethra,[1,4] does not seem valid in the face of their obvious creation of inflammatory disease of the prostate.[7,22,23] In our series of patients with prostatitis, *Staphylococcus epidermidis* was the bacterial strain recovered most frequently from prostatic fluid (Table 8–1). Streptococci (other than the beta-hemolytic strains), diphtheroids, and enterococci were found less frequently. Prostatic biopsies from some patients with gram-positive prostatitis revealed inflammation of glands in the area near the verumontanum (Figure 8–2). We find it difficult to reconcile the concept that pure or mixed prostatic infections due to gram-positive organisms are insignificant when the very same organisms (S. *epidermidis*, diphtheroids, and streptococci) are considered to be significant pathogens in the creation of acne.[24] We consider it possible that gram-positive prostatitis is truly acne of the prostate.

Gram-negative bacteria cause prostatitis in a smaller proportion of our patients than in some other reported series (Table 8–2).[4] These patients represent the major group with relapsing

Table 8–1

Gram-positive bacteria isolated from prostatic fluid of 122 patients with prostatitis

Organism	Number of Patients	% Gram-Positive	% of All Patients
S. epidermidis	57	48	37
Alpha streptococcus	32	26	21
Diphtheroids	18	15	12
Enterococci	8	7	5
S. aureus	6	5	4
Beta streptococcus	1	1	0.6
	122	102	79.6

Table 8–2

Gram-negative bacteria isolated from prostatic fluid of 26 patients with prostatitis

Organism	Number of Patients	% Gram-Negative	% of All Patients
E. coli	13	50	8
Klebsiella	5	19	3
Proteus species	4	15	2
Bacillus	2	8	1
Providencia	1	4	0.6
Pseudomonas	1	4	0.6
	26	100	15.2

urinary infections due to reinfection of urine from the infected prostate.[4,7] Patients with gram-positive prostatitis seldom develop urinary infection.[7] Only enterococci of gram-positive bacteria seem capable of creating significant urinary infection.[4]

Symptoms and signs of prostatitis among patients with gram-negative infection often indicated more severe disease than that seen in patients with gram-positive prostatitis. Gram-negative prostatitis patients were more susceptible to episodes of acute pain, dysuria, fever, and chills even when overt urinary infection did not exist.

Gonorrheal, Trichomonal, and Tubercular Prostatitis

Gonorrheal prostatitis occurs less often than it has in the past, but occasionally one finds an unsuspected prostatitis due to N. gonorrhea in a patient who has been inadequately treated or who has received penicillin therapy for a penicillin-resistant organism. Gram stain of the prostatic fluid has been very helpful to us in discovering this occasional cause of prostatitis. Confirmation must be obtained by anaerobic culture of prostatic fluid.

Similarly, prostatitis caused by trichomonas may be the cause of purulent prostatic secretions from which no organisms are cultured. Diagnosis rests on direct examination of the wet smear of prostatic fluid mixed with a drop of saline.

After all the diagnostic studies just mentioned, we are often left with patients who have an apparent prostatitis but from whom we cannot isolate, by routine microbiologic methods, any causative microorganism. When this occurs, we should first search for those rare prostatic infections caused by mycotic organisms: tuberculosis, blastomycosis, coccidioidomycosis, histoplasmosis, and related fungal infections.

Tuberculosis most often afflicts the prostate only after the upper urinary tract has also been involved. Evidence of urinary tuberculosis then leads one to suspect that the prostate is also involved. Culture of tuberculous organisms from prostatic fluid or demonstration of acid fast bacilli in prostatic tissue confirm this diagnosis.[25]

Patients with fungal infections may have the fungi isolated only in the prostate or in the prostate, vasa, and epididymis, without involvement of the bladder or upper urinary tract. Diagnosis becomes more difficult and requires direct observation of fungi in the prostatic fluid and culture of the fluid for fungal growth by special techniques.[26]

Coccidioidomycosis (Valley fever) serves as an example of a fungal disease

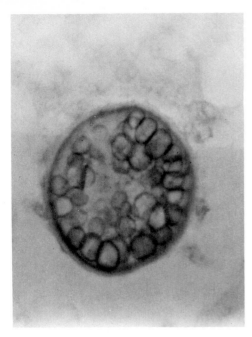

Figure 8–8. Endospore of *Coccidioides immitis* found in urine of patient with genitourinary coccidioidomycosis. (From Conner and Drach.[27])

which causes isolated prostatic involvement if the disease disseminates from its preferred location in the lungs.[27] Fungal endospores of *C. immitis* may be observed in the prostatic fluid or postprostatic specimen (Figure 8–8), and prostatic biopsy may show typical granulomatous prostatitis (Figure 8–9).

There remains still another group of patients with evidence of prostatitis from whom no bacteria, tuberculous, or fungal organisms can be isolated. Some of these patients probably have prostatitis owing to unusual pathogens whose existence depends on well-defined conditions of life and growth. Included in this group are the mycoplasma,[6] TRIC-agent (chlamydia),[28] and viruses.[29,30] Diagnosis of prostatitis caused by these unusual microorganisms requires special techniques beyond the scope of this discussion. The fact that they have been demonstrated as probable causative

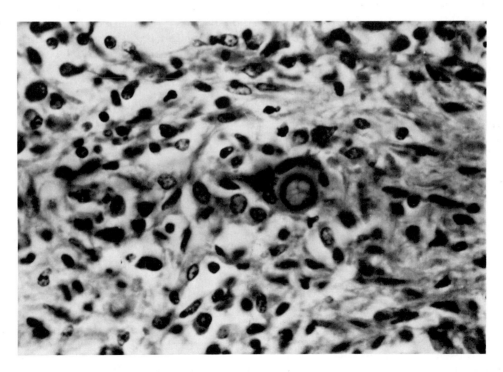

Figure 8–9. Granulomatous prostatitis. Field shows part of a granuloma. Etiologic agent in this case, a spherule of *Coccidioides immitis,* lies near center, engulfed by multinucleated giant cell. Other inflammatory cells include histiocytes, lymphocytes, and plasma cells. (×480.)

agents in some patients with prostatitis indicates that our lack of understanding of the etiology of all cases of prostatitis may be partly due to our inability, at this time, to demonstrate or grow from prostatic fluid, all of the microorganisms that can invade the prostate and create prostatitis.

What about "granulomatous prostatitis"?[16,31,32] An entity of this type probably exists. On the other hand, we may be observing prostatic response to chronic infection created by one of the agents mentioned in the previous paragraph. Hence, without a proven etiologic agent, our description remains incomplete, even though we can describe a histologic appearance which is characterized by granulomatous inflammation in the absence of those organisms known to cause granulomatous disease. Autoimmune or allergic phenomena have been implicated in causation of granulomatous prostatitis.[16] Perhaps the most important aspect of this entity is the fact that on rectal examination of the prostate, one feels nodular firm lesions that can mimic carcinoma of the prostate. Biopsy provides the only accurate means of differentiating the two conditions.

Host Responses to Prostatitis

Prostatic fluid contains nonprotein components which kill gram-positive and gram-negative organisms.[33,34] Activity against these two groups of bacteria appears to reside in two separate parts of the prostatic fluid. In addition, prostatic fluid and tissue contain proteins which participate in resistance to invasion of the posterior urethra and prostate by microorganisms.[35,36] Obviously, if microorganisms multiply in prostatic glands, these resistance mechanisms have been overwhelmed and are no longer effective.

If prostatitis is truly an infection of tissues created by bacteria or other microorganisms, we would expect some local and systemic antibody response to these microorganisms. Investigation into this aspect of prostatitis has been meager, but some information is available.

Bacteria isolated from the prostatic fluid of patients with prostatitis are coated with antibody, usually of the IgA and IgG classes.[37] In our laboratory we have done immunoelectrophoresis studies on prostatic fluid from 22 patients with proven bacterial prostatitis. Table 8–3 illustrates the types of immunoglobulins found in these patients, confirming the immunofluorescent labeling methods reported by earlier investigators.[36,37]

In addition we have performed direct bacterial agglutinations, using sera obtained from hosts with prostatitis from gram-positive or gram-negative bacteria. Mean reciprocal agglutination titers for nine patients with gram-negative bacterial prostatitis was 5.11, while the mean titer for eight patients with prostatitis caused by gram-positive organisms was 5.14. This difference between groups is insignificant and implies that both types of prostatitis create some systemic immune response.[23] Unfortunately, sera for serial titration were not available from this group of patients.

We can summarize our discussion to this point by stating that inflammatory disease of the prostate may arise from a variety of causes: gram-positive or gram-negative bacteria, tuberculosis, fungi, parasites, mycoplasma, TRIC agent, viruses, and autoimmune or allergic phenomena. Anatomic studies of prostates indicate that the major areas of prostatic inflammation lie near the ver-

Table 8–3

Classes of immunoglobulin detected in prostatic fluid from 22 patients with prostatitis

Parameter	IgA	IgG	IgM	IgE
Number	16	22	4	1
Percent	72.7	100	18.2	4.5

umontanum, and may be related to the periurethral glandular tissue or to true prostatic tissue. Because we have emphasized biopsy of observed areas of prostatic inflammation as one method of enhancing diagnosis of prostatitis,[7] we will now present our method for histologic diagnosis and classification of prostatitis.

HISTOPATHOLOGY

In histologic sections of the prostate, the most common pattern of inflammation is a localized process involving a duct, an acinus, or a group of acini. The lumen of the duct or gland is dilated and filled with inspissated secretion, together with neutrophils and macrophages. Neutrophils may be found between epithelial cells. Scattered neutrophils and aggregates of chronic inflammatory cells—lymphocytes and plasma cells—lie in the surrounding stroma (Figure 8–10). This lesion, then, is a localized response to infection and includes both acute and chronic inflammatory cells.

In contrast, acute infection may spread throughout the prostate. A dense infiltrate of neutrophils may involve many glands and large areas of stroma. Necrosis and localization of this process may ultimately lead to abscess formation (Figure 8–11).

Small foci of lymphocytes and plasma cells in the prostatic stroma are exceedingly common. Serial sections indicate that many such lymphoid aggregates are not related to ductal or glandular inflammation (Figure 8–12). They cannot be correlated with clinical prostatitis and their significance is not known. The diagnosis of chronic prostatitis remains a clinical rather than a histopathologic diagnosis.

Mycotic prostatitis, typified by coccidioidomycosis in Figure 8–9, is similar to the chronic granulomatous prostatitis seen in tuberculosis of the prostate. Iden-

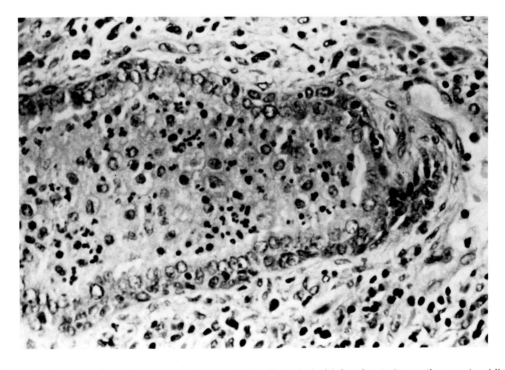

Figure 8–10. Localized inflammation. Part of duct is distended with inspissated secretion, neutrophils, macrophages, and cell debris. Chronic inflammatory cells infiltrate surrounding stroma. (×300.)

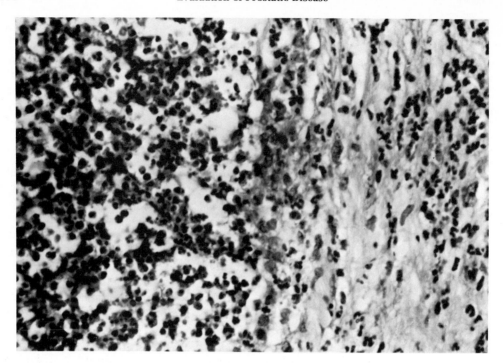

Figure 8–11.   Acute *spreading* inflammation. Part of distended acinus (left) is filled with neutrophils and nuclear debris. Lining epithelium is undergoing degeneration and necrosis. Neutrophils infiltrate stroma (right). This prostate contained one grossly visible abscess and several microabscesses. (×300.)

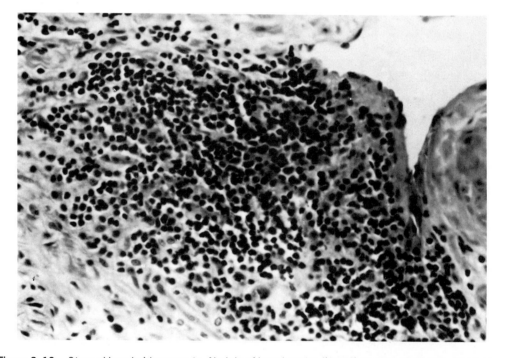

Figure 8–12.   Stromal lymphoid aggregate. Nodule of lymphocytes lies adjacent to small vein. There is no ductal or acinar inflammation in section. Significance of such lymphoid aggregates is not known. They should not be used as criterion for histopathologic diagnosis of "chronic prostatitis." (×300.)

tification of the organisms in tissue sections or differential cultures of prostatic fluid or tissue provides a specific diagnosis.

Prostatic calculi may be found within lumens of glands or within prostatic tissue stroma. Apatite seems to be the major component of these endogenous calculi, although carbonate-apatite and whitlockite are also found in some prostatic calculi. If the calculus lies exposed to urinary flow, elements of urine may be found in the calculus. Hence, uric acid, calcium oxalate, cystine, or struvite may be found in prostatic calculi which are exposed to the urinary stream.[38,39]

Limited observations imply that prostatic calculi may harbor bacteria just as urinary calculi do. Bacteria buried deep within the calculus persist in spite of antibiotic therapy. When therapy ceases, infection can be recreated by these protected bacteria.[4]

Granulomatous prostatitis without infectious origin has already been mentioned. Clinically it is difficult to differentiate this hard, painless, prostatic nodule or induration from carcinoma. Biopsy reveals a chronic inflammatory process with destruction of normal glandular architecture by eosinophilic infiltration, and central fibrinoid necrosis with nearby histiocytes, giant cells, and active fibroblasts. Small blood vessels show intimal swelling.

In summary, diagnosis of prostatitis requires careful attention to localization of infection to the prostate by careful differential collection and microbiologic examination of urine and prostatic fluid. Microorganisms that cause prostatitis include gram-positive and gram-negative bacteria, mycotic organisms, trichomonas, mycoplasma, TRIC agent (chlamydia), viruses, and probably other undefined microorganisms. Abacterial prostatitis occurs less often than previously suspected. One postulated reason for excessive diagnosis of abacterial prostatitis (sometimes called prostatosis) is the unwillingness of some investigators to accept many strains of gram-positive organisms as pathogenic in prostatic infections. In addition, highly specialized detection and culture techniques are required to identify some of the unusual organisms, such as chlamydia, which may cause prostatitis.

Random needle biopsies of prostatic tissue via perineal or rectal routes often fail to demonstrate inflammation or organisms in tissues of patients with prostatitis because of sampling error. Direct vision transurethral biopsies of areas which exude pus from which organisms are cultured result in demonstration of inflammation of periurethral or prostatic glands and surrounding tissue. Only a few of the multiple prostatic glands may be involved in prostatitis. Those glands which discharge into the prostatic urethra near the sulci lateral to the verumontanum seem to be most often involved in prostatitis. Humoral immune responses, local and systemic, are generated by patients with prostatitis, but this response does not appear to be effective in curing infection. Multiple methods of therapy of prostatitis result in depressingly poor cure rate. Study of factors which contribute to this poor cure rate remains our major challenge.[40]

References

1. Blacklock, N. J., and Reeves, D. S.: Chronic prostatitis. Br.: Med. J., 3:351, 1972.
2. Mobley, D. F.: Chronic prostatitis. South Med. J., 67:219, 1974.
3. Meares, E. M., Jr.: Bacterial prostatitis vs. "prostatosis." A clinical and bacteriological study. J.A.M.A., 224:1372, 1973.
4. Meares, E. M., Jr., and Stamey, T. A.: The diagnosis and management of bacterial prostatitis. Br. J. Urol., 44:175, 1972.
5. Jameson, R. M.: Sexual activity and the variations of the white cell content of the prostatic secretion. Invest. Urol., 5:297, 1967.
6. Messent, J. J.: Association of threads in the urine with non-gonococcal urethritis and prostatitis. Br. J. Vener. Dis., 46:469, 1970.
7. Drach, G. W.: Problems in diagnosis of bacterial prostatitis: Gram-negative, gram-positive and mixed infections. J. Urol., 111:630, 1974.

8. Murnaghan, G. F., et al.: Chronic prostatitis—an Australian view. Br. J. Urol., 46:55, 1974.

9. Schmidt, J. D., and Patterson, M. C.: Needle biopsy study of chronic prostatitis. J. Urol., 96:519, 1966.

10. Landes, R. R., and French T. N.: Bacterial prostatitis: Incidence in the obstructive prostate. J. Urol., 110:427, 1973.

11. Nielsen, M L., et al.: Inflammatory changes in the noninfected prostate gland. A clinical, microbiological and histological investigation. J. Urol., 110:423, 1973.

12. Boström, K.: Chronic inflammation of human male accessory sex glands and its effect on the morphology of the spermatozoa. Scand. J. Urol. Nephrol., 5:133, 1971.

13. Austen, G., Jr.: The test of time. IX. Prostatitis: Acute and chronic. Bost. Med. Q., 17:27, 1966.

14. Mendlewicz, J., et al.: Chronic prostatitis: Psychosomatic incidence. Psychother. Psychosom., 19:118, 1971.

15. McNeal, J. E.: The prostate and prostatic urethra: A morphologic synthesis. J. Urol., 107:1008, 1972.

16. Cameron, K. M.: Pathology of the prostate. Br. J. Hosp. Med., 11:348, 1974.

17. Blacklock, N. J.: Anatomical factors in prostatitis. Br. J. Urol., 46:47, 1974.

18. Furness, G., et al.: Epididymitis after the luminal spread of NSU corynebacteria and gram negative bacteria from the fossa navicularis. Invest. Urol., 11:486, 1974.

19. Smith, M. J. V.: The lymphatics of the prostate. Invest. Urol., 3:439, 1966.

20. Trapnell, J., and Roberts, M.: Prostatic abscess. Br. J. Surg., 57:565, 1970.

21. Meares, E. M., Jr., and Stamey, T. A.: Bacteriologic localization patterns in bacterial prostatitis and urethritis. Invest. Urol., 5:492, 1968.

22. Nickel, A. C.: The bacteriology of chronic prostatitis and seminal vesiculitis and elective localization of the bacteria as isolated. J. Urol., 24:343, 1930.

23. Maged, Z., and Khafaga, H.: Bacteriological and serological study of chronic prostatitis patients. Br. J. Vener. Dis., 41:202, 1965.

24. Marples, R. R., et al.: Microbiology of comedones in acne vulgaris. J. Invest. Dermatol., 60:80, 1973.

25. Borthwick, W. M.: Present position of urinary tuberculosis. Br. J. Urol., 42:642, 1970.

26. Orr, W. A., et al.: Genitourinary tract involvement with systemic mycosis. J. Urol., 107:1047, 1972.

27. Conner, W. T., and Drach, G. W.: Genitourinary aspects of disseminated coccidioidomycosis. J. Urol. (In press).

28. Mardh, P.-A., et al.: Chlamydia in chronic prostatitis. Br. Med. J., 4:361, 1972.

29. Nielsen, M. L., and Vestergaard, B. F.: Virological investigations in chronic prostatitis. J. Urol., 109:1023, 1973.

30. Morrisseau, P. M., et al.: Viral prostatitis. J. Urol., 103:767, 1970.

31. Brown, H. E.: Granulomatous prostatitis: Its clinical significance. J. Urol., 105:549, 1971.

32. Towfighi, J., et al.: Granulomatous prostatitis with emphasis on the eosinophilic variety. Am. J. Clin. Pathol., 58:630, 1972.

33. Stamey, T. A., et al.: Antibacterial nature of prostatic fluid. Nature, 218:444, 1968.

34. Fair, W. R., and Wehner, N.: Antibacterial action of spermine: Effect on urinary tract pathogens. Appl. Microbiol., 21:6, 1971.

35. Rusk, J., et al.: The antibacterial activity of semen and its relation to semen proteins. Scand. J. Urol. Nephrol., 7:23, 1973.

36. Ablin, R. J., et al.: Localization of immunoglobulins in human prostatic tissue. J. Immunol. 107:603, 1971.

37. Jones, S. R.: Prostatitis as cause of antibody-coated bacteria in urine. New Engl. J. Med., 291:365, 1974.

38. Sutor, D. J., and Wooley, S. E.: The crystalline composition of prostatic calculi. Br. J. Urol., 46:533, 1974.

39. Eykyn, S., et al.: Prostatic calculi as a source of recurrent bacteriuria in the male. Br. J. Urol., 46:527, 1974.

40. Drach, G. W.: Trimethoprim/sulfamethoxazole therapy of chronic bacterial prostatitis. J. Urol., 111:637, 1974.

Chapter 9

Histologic Grading and Clinical Staging of Prostatic Carcinoma

DONALD F. GLEASON and The Veterans Administration Cooperative Urological Research Group

Careful autopsy studies reveal many small, well-differentiated "latent" adenocarcinomas of the prostate. The incidence increases steadily with advancing age and has been reported to be present in more than 80% of U.S. males in the tenth decade of life.[1] The incidence of clinically diagnosed carcinoma of the prostate is much lower but is second only to cancer of the lung in U.S. males. Yet cancer of the prostate ranks only third as a cause of death, following cancer of the lung and cancer of the colon and rectum.

This disparity between incidence and mortality rates is a clear expression of the unusually wide range of biologic malignancy of prostate cancer. Some patients with prostatic cancer suffer rapid progression of their cancers leading to early death. Others show a much slower progression. Some patients appear to live out a normal life span in spite of a histologic diagnosis of cancer. Only about 30% of the patients in the Veterans Administration Cooperative Urological Research Group (VACURG) studies of cancer of the prostate actually die of their cancer. From Whitmore's estimates, there may be several hundred small latent carcinomas for every fatal prostatic cancer.[2]

Cancer of the prostate also has a wide spectrum of histologic appearances, ranging from small foci of well-differentiated but abnormal glands to anaplastic undifferentiated tumors, with a spectrum of intermediate appearances.

Many workers have reported correlations between the apparent histologic differentiation and the eventually expressed biologic malignancy of the tumors. At least 12 well-documented reports have appeared since 1942, describing various correlations with mortality rates, size of prostate, extent of tumor within the prostate, clinical stage of the tumor when first diagnosed, and the presence or absence of metastases.[3-14]

It is disturbing that this information is not widely applied. One might conclude that histologic grading has no value in the management of prostatic cancer. Most clinical studies group their patients according to the clinical stage of the tumor, which does of course, correlate well with the eventual course.

Some urologists do work more closely with their pathologists, at least in separating out the small, well-differentiated tumors found unexpectedly in prostatic tissue resected for obstruction or in biopsies of suspicious prostatic nodules. Paradoxically, identification of these low-grade tumors may determine that the patient is eligible for a radical prostatectomy or that the patient requires only minimal treatment, depending on other factors.

It is more common to accept the diagnosis of cancer and begin treatment immediately, ranging from estrogenic hormone therapy to orchiectomy, radical prostatectomy, chemotherapy, cryosurgery, or radiotherapy. Most physicians feel, with the best of motives, that some possibly beneficial treatment should be instituted as soon as possible for the patient with an established diagnosis of carcinoma of the prostate.

Probably the real reason that histologic grading is not widely practiced is that it is difficult for pathologists to be confident that they can apply the published grading systems exactly as their authors intended. Descriptions and representative photomicrographs convey neither a clear impression of the ranges covered by the various grades nor the boundaries between them. Many tumors have more than one histologic pattern.

The author devised a histologic classification of prostatic cancer which showed close correlation with mortality rates.[15-17] The accumulated experience with almost 3000 tumors from the VACURG studies confirms that the histologic grade of the tumors is strongly correlated with the behavior of the tumors. The VACURG data also indicate that histologic grading provides predictive information *in addition* to that provided by clinical staging, i.e., *within* the clinical stages. Grading and staging can be combined to provide a powerful tool which can identify a substantial proportion of patients who are at very low risk from their prostatic cancers. The potential hazards of some forms of treatment are probably greater than the risk that the cancer will progress in these patients.

VETERANS ADMINISTRATION COOPERATIVE UROLOGICAL RESEARCH GROUP (VACURG)

The VACURG studies were begun in 1960 as controlled, randomized, prospective comparisons of the various treatments available for cancer of the prostate.[18] These studies are described in more detail in Chapter 13.

Study I (1960–1967) compared placebo with 5 mg of diethylstilbestrol (DES)/day following radical prostatectomy in stage I

Table 9–1

VACURG staging system and incidence of cases

Stage	Rectal Examination	Serum Prostatic Acid Phosphatase	Distant Metastases (X-ray or Biopsy)	Number of Cases
I	No palpable tumor	Normal[a]	None	296
II	Palpable nodule	Normal	None	243
III	Local extension outside prostate	Normal	None	1328
IV	Any findings	Elevated and/or present		1044
				2911

[a]Normal ≤ 1.0 King-Armstrong units/100 ml.

and II patients. (The VACURG staging system is shown in Table 9–1.) Stage III and IV patients were randomized into four treatment groups: placebo, 5 mg DES/day, orchiectomy alone, and orchiectomy plus 5 mg DES/day. Early analyses revealed no significant differences between the survival rates of the placebo and DES groups. Further analyses revealed that 5 mg DES/day reduced cancer mortality rates significantly but were also associated with a significant increase in cardiovascular deaths (including myocardial infarction, congestive heart failure, pulmonary embolism, and cerebrovascular accidents) which more than offset the reduced cancer mortality.[19–21] Of the 2313 patients admitted to Study I, 1294 cases had been graded histologically for the most recent analysis in September 1974.

In Study II (1967–1969) stage I and II patients were randomized between radical prostatectomy and no radical prostatectomy. No significant difference in survival between these two groups has appeared (September 1974), but the groups are small and the periods of follow-up are relatively short. In Study II the effects of placebo were compared with 0.2 mg DES, 1 mg DES, and 5 mg DES/day in the stage III and IV patients. The 1 mg dose of DES was as effective as the 5 mg dose in controlling the cancers, but the 1 mg dose of DES did not cause increased cardiovascular deaths in comparison with the placebo group. The 0.2 mg DES treatment did not cause increased cardiovascular deaths but was ineffective in reducing cancer mortality. The adverse cardiovascular effects of 5 mg DES/day were confirmed.[22] Of the 561 patients admitted to Study II, 540 patients had histologic grading of their tumors available for this analysis.

Study III was begun in 1969 and patients are still being admitted (February 1975). Stage I and II patients were randomized as in Study II if they were judged

able to tolerate radical prostatectomy but were randomized between placebo and 1 mg DES/day if they were judged unable (too old or too ill) to tolerate the operation or refused to consider surgical intervention. Stage III and IV patients were randomized into four treatment groups: 1 mg DES/day, 2.5 mg of conjugated equine estrogens (Premarin)/day, 30 mg of medroxyprogesterone acetate (Provera)/day, or 30 mg of Provera plus 1 mg DES/day. No significant differences in survival have been noted between these groups (September 1974). Histologic grading was available for 1077 patients from this on-going study.

Thus 2911 cases with histologic grading were available for correlation with the follow-up data in September 1974. The cause of death in each case was determined by a rotating Evaluation Committee of three of the participating physicians (of which the author was not a member). In all cases the original diagnosis was made by the local pathologist of the participating hospital and confirmed by the author. The histologic grading was performed on the original microscopic sections. Subsequent biopsy or resection material obtained within three months of the initial positive biopsy was also incorporated into the histologic grading, but tissue obtained more than three months after the initial biopsy is being studied separately for changes in the tumor histology.

HISTOLOGIC GRADING

The histologic grading system considers only the degree of glandular differentiation and the growth pattern of the tumor in relation to the prostatic stroma. The grading is performed under low magnifications (40–100×) and can be performed almost as rapidly as one can examine all the tissue available. Very little time is added to that required to make the diagnosis. The grading can be performed on small biopsies. Approxi-

Table 9-2

Histologic patterns of adenocarcinoma of the prostate

Pattern	Margins of Tumor Areas	Gland Pattern	Gland Size	Gland Distribution	Stromal Invasion
1	Well defined	Single, separate, round	Medium	Closely packed	Minimal, expansile
2	Less definite	Single, separate, rounded, but more variable	Medium	Spaced up to one gland diameter, average	Mild, in larger stromal planes
3	Poorly defined	Single, separate, more irregular	Small, medium, or large	Spaced more than one gland diameter, rarely packed	Moderate, in larger or smaller stromal planes
or 3	Poorly defined	Rounded masses of cribriform or papillary epithelium	Medium or large	Rounded masses with smooth sharp edges	Expansile masses
4	Ragged infiltrating	Fused glandular masses or "hypernephroid"	Small	Fused in ragged masses	Marked, through smaller planes
5	Ragged, infiltrating	Almost absent, few tiny glands or signet ring cells	Small	Ragged anaplastic masses of epithelium	Severe, between stromal fibers or destructive
or 5	Poorly defined	Few small lumina in rounded masses of solid epithelium central necrosis?	Small	Rounded masses and cords with smooth, sharp edges	Expansile masses

mately 60% of the cases were graded on the basis of a needle biopsy only.

A deliberate attempt was made to subdivide the two ends of the spectrum of apparent histologic malignancy, leading to five grades rather than to the usual three or four grades.

The following description of the five patterns is also presented in tabular form in Table 9–2.

Pattern 1. Very well-differentiated (Figure 9–1). The tumor consists of single, separate, round to oval glands, which are quite uniform in size. They grow abnormally in closely packed, roughly rounded masses with definitely limited edges relative to the uninvolved tissue. Pattern 1 was seen in 102 cases (3.5%).

Pattern 2. Well-differentiated (Figure 9–2). The tumor consists of single, separate, round to oval glands, which are similar in size and shape but vary more than those of pattern 1. They also show more stromal spacing between the glands (up to one gland diameter, average). The tumor masses are less well circumscribed and not as definitely rounded as in pattern 1. Pattern 2 was seen in 709 cases (24.4%).

Pattern 3. Moderately differentiated. This is the most common pattern and includes two distinctive appearances. One is an extension of patterns 1 and 2, with single, separate glands which may be much smaller (Figure 9–3) or much larger (Figure 9–4), or about the same size (Figure 9–5) as those in patterns 1 and 2. The individual glands are more irregular in size and shape than in patterns 1 and 2, many being more elongated or angular. They may be closely packed together (Figure 9–4) but are much more commonly quite widely separated by stroma (one or more gland diameters, average), as in Figures 9–3 and 5.

The areas of tumor are usually quite irregular in outline, without a clearly definable boundary. Larger glands may have some papillary infoldings or a thick epithelium containing additional tiny glandular lumina (Figure 9–4). These latter appearances provide the

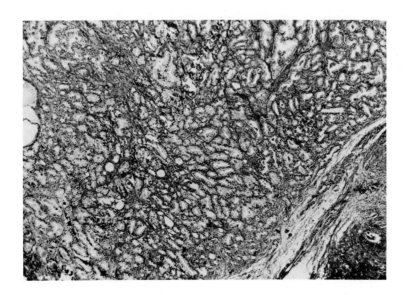

Figure 9–1. Pattern 1. Very well-differentiated. Single, separate, uniform, well-differentiated glands, closely packed together. Area of tumor has definite edge. (All photomicrographs 70× before reduction).

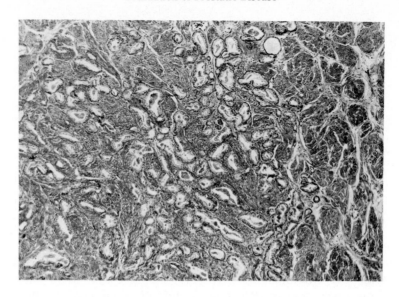

Figure 9–2. Pattern 2. Well-differentiated. Single, separate glands, slightly more variable in size and shape than pattern 1, separated up to one gland diameter (average). Boundary of tumor less definite than pattern 1.

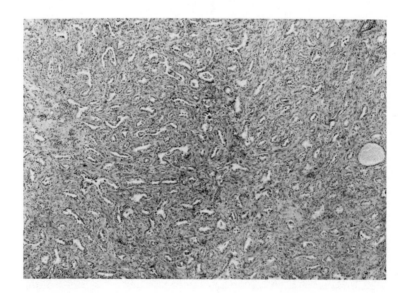

Figure 9–3. Pattern 3. Moderately differentiated. (Small gland variety.) Single, separate glands with moderate to marked variation in size and shape, usually separated more than one gland diameter (average). Boundary of tumor usually poorly defined.

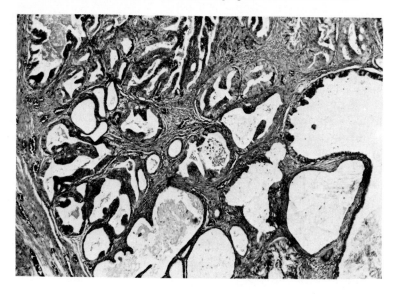

Figure 9–4. Pattern 3. Moderately differentiated (large gland variety). Single, separate glands with moderate to marked variation in size and shape, usually separated more than one gland diameter (average). Boundary of tumor usually poorly defined.

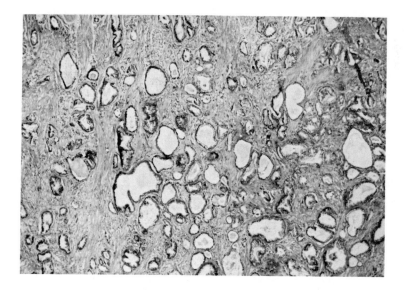

Figure 9–5. Pattern 3. Moderately differentiated (medium size glands). Single, separate glands with moderate to marked variation in size and shape.

transition to the second distinctive appearance in pattern 3, namely, the occurrence of sharply circumscribed masses of papillary or cribriform tumor, or both. These vary in size and may be quite large, but the essential feature is the smooth and usually rounded edge around all the sharply circumscribed masses of tumor (Figure 9–6). Any or all of these patterns may appear in one case. There may be tiny glands, large irregular glands and sharply circumscribed papillary and cribriform masses, all included under the designation of pattern 3 (Figure 9–7). Pattern 3 was seen in 2554 cases (87.7%).

Pattern 4. Poorly differentiated. The tumor consists of irregular masses of *fused* glands (Figure 9–8). That is, the glands are not single and separate but coalesce and branch. The fusion may be so extreme that the appearance is that of solid masses of epithelium containing multiple glandular lumina lined by poorly oriented layers of polygonal cells. Some cells may have two surfaces facing separate rounded gland spaces.

The multiple glandular lumina are usually of small or medium size. In contrast to the sharply circumscribed and smoothly rounded masses in pattern 3, the pattern 4 tumors grow in very raggedly outlined masses, appearing to infiltrate the stroma very aggressively. Also included are essentially similar tumors composed of large cells with very pale cytoplasm, sometimes resembling the clear cell adenocarcinoma of the renal cortex or "hypernephroma" (Figure 9–9). Pattern 4 was seen in 353 cases (12.1%).

Pattern 5. Very poorly differentiated. The tumor shows minimal glandular differentiation and consists of raggedly infiltrating masses of epithelial cells with only a few poorly formed glandular lumina or signet ring cells to confirm that it is an adenocarcinoma (Figure 9–10). A second rare pattern is also included in pattern 5. This consists of sharply circumscribed broad cords and masses of compactly arranged epithelial cells with only occasional poorly formed tiny glandular lumina,

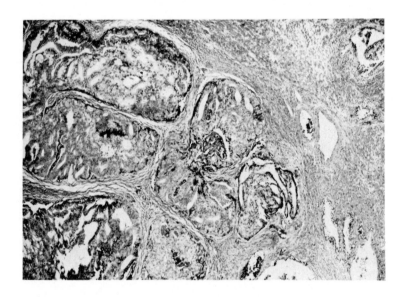

Figure 9–6. Pattern 3. Moderately differentiated (papillary/cribriform variety). Masses of papillary or cribriform tumor in smoothly and sharply limited rounded masses.

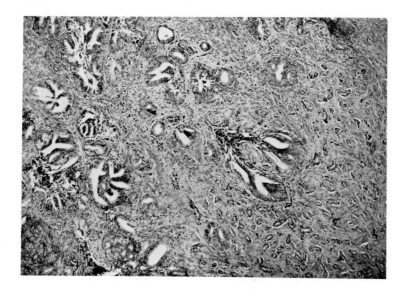

Figure 9–7. Pattern 3. Moderately differentiated. Frequently observed mixture of small, medium and large single separate glands plus papillary masses with smooth, sharp edges.

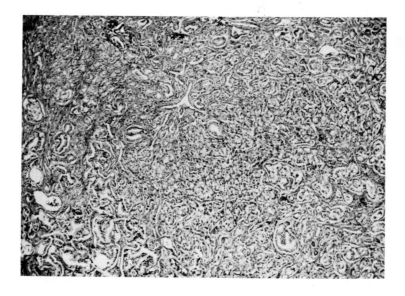

Figure 9–8. Pattern 4. Poorly differentiated. Ragged, infiltrating masses of fused-glandular epitheliuum.

Figure 9–9. Pattern 4. Poorly differentiated. Large clear cells infiltrating diffusely in cords and nests. Few well-formed glands but vacuoles common.

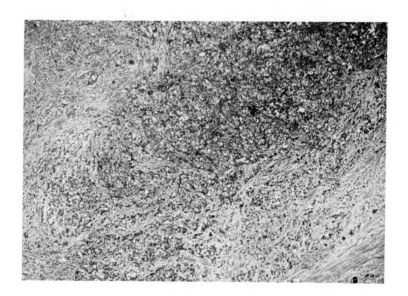

Figure 9–10. Pattern 5. Very poorly differentiated. Diffusely infiltrating anaplastic cells.

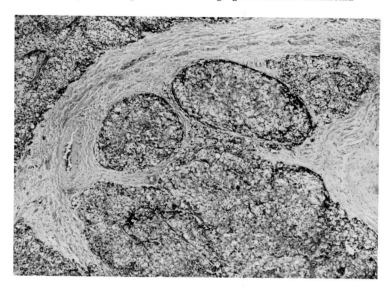

Figure 9–11. Pattern 5. Very poorly differentiated. Sharply circumscribed cords and masses of solid epithelium. Occasional tiny gland lumina are usually present in the masses. Central necrosis may yield a "comedocarcinoma" appearance.

sometimes with central necrosis of the masses like the "comedocarcinoma" of the breast (Figure 9–11). Pattern 5 was seen in 657 cases (22.6%).

The percentages add up to about 150% since 50% of the tumors showed at least two different patterns.

These patterns can be represented schematically in a simplified drawing (Figure 9–12) since the classification does not consider cytological details. It is based entirely on the microscopic outline of the tumor tissue and its relation to the uninvolved prostate. All of the black in the drawing represents tumor glands and tumor tissue with all cellular detail obscured (except in the right side of the pattern 4 area, in which the tiny open structures are intended to depict the large cells of the clear cell carcinoma).

The classification avoids any preconceived ideas of histogenetic origin such as resemblance to fetal or adult glands or ducts. It attempts to avoid terms which may be subject to differences in interpretation. Perhaps pattern 1 includes the "back-to-back glands" favored by some

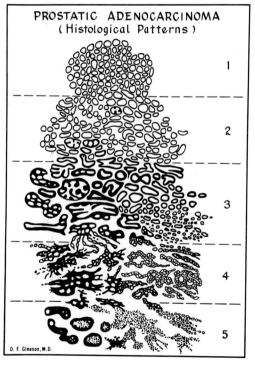

Figure 9–12. Simplified drawing of histologic patterns, emphasizing degree of glandular differentiation and relation to stroma. All black in the drawing represents tumor tissue and glands with all cytologic detail obscured except in right side of pattern 4 where tiny open structures are intended to suggest the "hypernephroid" pattern.

pathologists, but others seem to include under that description the fused glands assigned to pattern 4. The term "cribriform" is useful to describe masses of epithelium containing multiple glandular lumina and can perhaps be applied to some of the ragged masses of epithelium containing multiple glandular lumina in pattern 4. To avoid confusion, this classification restricts "cribriform" to those sharply circumscribed masses seen in pattern 3.

MULTIPLE HISTOLOGIC PATTERNS IN ONE TUMOR

A strong effort was made to limit the histologic grade to a single pattern in each case. A few large glands or a few tiny squeezed glands at the center or the periphery of a mass in pattern 1 tumor did not change it to patterns 2 or 3. A few elongated glands or a few small cribriform masses did not change a pattern 2 tumor to pattern 3. An occasional small area of fused glands did not change a pattern 3 tumor to pattern 4. A small focus of disorganized cells did not change a pattern 3 or 4 tumor to pattern 5.

Nevertheless, many cases clearly showed more than one pattern of growth. These usually seemed to be separate foci but were sometimes contiguous and less commonly seemed to show transition from one pattern to another.

Two different patterns were recorded when definitely present. The pattern most extensive in area was identified as the "primary" pattern and the less extensive pattern as the "secondary" pattern. This decision eventually revealed several significant characteristics of the tumors.

The two patterns were simply recorded as two digits for each case. For example, 2–3 indicated a tumor with more than 50% pattern 2 and less than 50% pattern 3; a tumor designated 5–4 contained more than 50% pattern 5 and less than 50% pattern 4. For uniformity in the statistical treatment, two digits were also recorded for tumors with only one histologic pattern. Thus 3–3 indicated a tumor with only pattern 3 present.

Occasionally small areas of a third pattern were observed. They were also recorded but are not considered in this report. They were rare and the number of possible combinations is large. Many more cases will be needed to obtain enough observations in the various triplet combinations to yield significant data.

The presence or absence of perineural space invasion was also recorded. Beginning in Study II, a rough measure of the percent area of the tissue occupied by tumor was recorded (in TUR and prostatectomy specimens). The occasionally observed extension of tumor outside the prostatic capsule in needle biopsies, TUR specimens, and prostatectomy specimens was also recorded.

Follow-up Data

For a measure of biologic malignancy, the death rate (deaths/patient-year of follow-up) was employed. This statistic was calculated by dividing the number of deaths in the group under consideration by the sum of the follow-up times for all the patients (both living and dead) in that group. Follow-up time was measured from the date of admission to the study, to the date of death or, from the date of admission to the study, to the date of the last follow-up visit for those patients still alive. Time was actually recorded in months but is expressed in years for this report. The total follow-up time for the 2911 patients was 9730.4 years, ranging from 0 to 14 years/patient.

This statistic is a single numeric measure of the mortality rate experienced by a group of patients. For example, a value of 0.05 deaths/patient-year indicates five deaths/100 patient-years of follow-up. These five deaths might have occurred among 100 patients followed for one year or 10 patients followed for 10 years, or any combination of follow-up periods

Table 9–3

Incidence and coincidence of primary and secondary histologic patterns

Secondary Patterns	Primary Patterns					Totals
	1	2	3	4	5	
1	14	52				66
2	32	65	306		1	404
3	3	251	1239	76	153	1722
4	1	1	178	36	29	245
5		1	348	32	93	474
	50	370	2071	144	276	2911

totaling 100 years. As a reference of magnitude, the preceding value (0.05 deaths/patient-year) is approximately that to which "normal" 70-year-old U.S. males are subject.[23]

This statistic includes all the available survival information from a group of patients, regardless of how long each patient has been followed. It has a powerful smoothing effect on erratic random variations, even in small groups, and it is simple to calculate.

Deaths/patient-year can also be calculated in the same manner for cause-specific deaths such as "deaths due to cancer of the prostate" or "deaths due to cardiovascular disease," using only deaths due to the specific cause in the numerator, but continuing to use the total follow-up time for all the patients in the group in the denominator.

RESULTS

The observed incidence of the primary and secondary histologic patterns revealed an encouraging relationship (Table 9–3). Cases with single pattern tumors are found on the diagonal (1–1, 2–2, and so on); 1464 cases (50.3%) had two different patterns which were not randomly distributed but were strongly correlated. That is, low-grade primary patterns tended to be associated with low-grade secondary patterns and high-grade pat-

terns with high-grade patterns. The opposite corners of the matrix contained few cases or were empty.

Mortality Rates and Histologic Patterns

Mortality rates (deaths/patient-year) were calculated for patient groups according to their primary histologic patterns and then calculated according to their secondary histologic patterns. Strong correlation was found between the mortality rates and the primary pattern. There was a very similar although somewhat weaker correlation with the secondary pattern (Table 9–4; Figure 9–13). Both correlations were stronger, of course, when only deaths due to cancer were included in the numerators.

Mortality Rates and Multiple Patterns

Faced with more than one histologic pattern in one tumor, pathologists have customarily categorized the tumor by its most malignant component: "A tumor is as bad as its worst part." The present data afforded an opportunity to test this "aphorism." The patients were therefore grouped according to the highest ("worst") pattern in each case and then regrouped according to the lowest ("best") pattern.

The cancer mortality rates did correlate closely with the "worst" pattern, but surprisingly the correlation with the

Table 9–4

Death rates—all deaths, cancer deaths—by histologic patterns

	Histologic Patterns					
	1	2	3	4	5	Totals
Primary Pattern						
No. Patients	50	370	2071	144	276	2911
Total Yrs Followup	264.1	1507.4	7013.2	368.3	577.4	9730.4
No. Dead	25	168	1238	89	213	1733
No. Dead—CA	1	22	350	41	124	538
Dead/total yrs	0.095	0.111	0.177	0.242	0.369	0.178
Dead—CA/total yrs	0.004	0.015	0.050	0.111	0.215	0.055
Secondary Pattern						
No. Patients	66	404	1722	245	474	2911
Total Yrs Followup	242.5	1786.0	5690.5	687.3	1324.1	9730.4
No. Dead	25	206	1013	152	337	1733
No. Dead—CA	3	26	282	49	178	538
Dead/total yrs	0.103	0.115	0.178	0.221	0.255	0.178
Dead—CA/total yrs	0.012	0.015	0.050	0.071	0.134	0.055

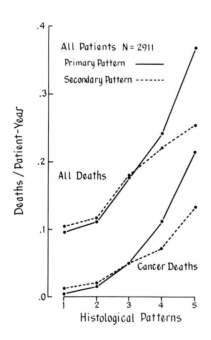

Figure 9–13. Cancer and total mortality rates calculated separately according to the primary (predominant) and the secondary histologic pattern for each case.

"best" pattern appeared stronger (identified patients with higher cancer death rates) than either the "worst" pattern or the primary (predominant) pattern (Figure 9–14).

However, the "worst" pattern isolated a group with *no* cancer deaths—the pure pattern 1 cases, while the "best" pattern isolated a group with very high cancer mortality—the pure pattern 5 group. At the other end of each spectrum, the "worst" pattern 5 group included cases with secondary pattern 3 and 4 tumors with lower mortality, while the "best" pattern 1 group included cases with secondary pattern 2 and 3 tumors with appreciable cancer mortality.

It appeared that, at least for cancer of the prostate, the biologic malignancy of the tumor was more closely related to its average histologic pattern than to its "worst" or "best" pattern. Averaging the primary and secondary patterns would gain the advantages of both the "worst" and "best" groupings. That is, averaging would assign the lowest scale value to the pure pattern 1 tumors and the highest

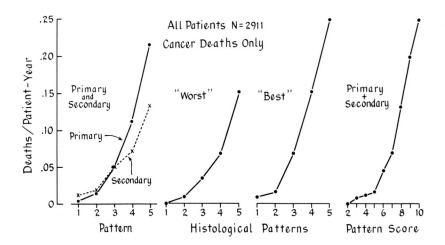

Figure 9–14. Cancer mortality rates by histologic patterns, calculated separately for primary and secondary patterns (same as Figure 9–13), "worst" pattern, "best" pattern, and sum of primary and secondary patterns. See text.

scale value to the pure pattern 5 tumors. The primary and secondary pattern numbers were added together for each case thus achieving the scaling effect of averaging. Division by two was omitted avoiding fractional grades.

A new scale was created which ranged from 2 to 10 and was designated the *pattern score*. Stronger and more regular correlation was found between mortality rates and this averaging pattern score (Table 9–5; Figures 9–14 and 15) than with any other histologic scale.

Simple histologic grading can separate patients into groups which experience markedly different mortality rates. For example, from Table 9–5 one can calculate that 724 patients (24.9%) with a pattern score from 2 to 5 had a cancer death rate of only 0.012, or 1.2 cancer deaths/100 patient-years. The remaining 2187 patients with pattern scores from 6 to 10 had a cancer death rate of 0.124 deaths/patient-year, or 10 times as high.

Histologic Grading and Initial Clinical Findings

In addition to the eventually observed death rate correlations, there were strong correlations between the tumor grades and various tumor-related clinical findings in the initial pretreatment examinations of the patients. For example, there were strong correlations between the histologic pattern scores and the presence of identifiable metastases, pain due to the cancer, dilatation of the upper urinary tract, and abnormal elevation of the serum prostatic acid phosphatase level (Figure 9–16). There were similar but weaker correlations between the tumor grades, the initial body weight and the hemoglobin level.

Histologic Grading and Clinical Staging

There was strong correlation between the formally defined clinical stage of the tumor, the histologic patterns and the pattern scores. There was a striking shift

Table 9–5

Death rates—all deaths, cancer deaths—by histologic pattern score

| | Histologic Pattern Score (primary + secondary patterns) | | | | | | | | | |
	2	3	4	5	6	7	8	9	10	Totals
No. Patients	14	84	68	558	1240	256	537	61	93	2911
Total Yrs. Followup	46.3	381.0	272.4	2423.8	4057.7	718.5	1527.6	137.3	165.8	9730.4
No. Dead	7	34	31	279	726	158	384	44	70	1733
No. Dead–CA	0	3	3	37	179	49	199	27	41	538
Dead/total years	0.151	0.089	0.114	0.115	0.179	0.220	0.251	0.320	0.422	0.178
Dead–CA/total yrs.	0	0.008	0.011	0.015	0.044	0.068	0.130	0.197	0.247	0.055

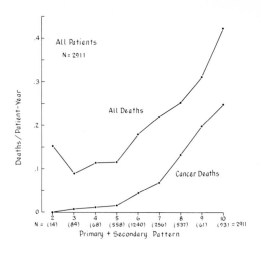

Figure 9–15. Cancer and total mortality rates by histologic pattern score (sum of primary and secondary patterns). Cancer mortality rates same as in Figure 9–14.

from lower to higher clinical stages with increasing tumor grades (Table 9–6). It was also noteworthy that in each of the clinical stages, each of the histologic patterns was actually observed with appropriately varying incidence.

The follow-up data for the clinical stages themselves revealed mortality rates similar to those of other published series (Table 9–7). The breakdown of the VAC-URG stage IV cases, as shown in Table 9–7, confirms that patients with elevated prostatic acid phosphatase levels, but with no demonstrable metastases, are definitely at higher risk than stage III patients with normal acid phosphatase levels. A useful separation of patients into six groups can be made, using only the clinical stage and the serum prostatic acid phosphatase level.

When the patients were grouped according to their clinical stages, histologic grading still showed strong correlations with mortality rates *within* the clinical stages (Figure 9–17). The death rates associated with the histologic pattern scores showed overlapping of death rates between the clinical stages. For example,

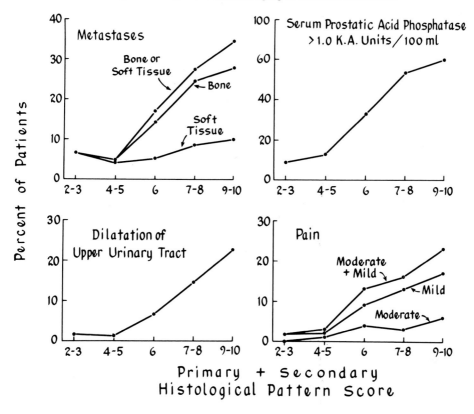

Figure 9–16.   Correlation of histologic pattern scores with the incidence of some clinical findings in the pretreatment examinations.

Table 9–6

Percent distribution of clinical stages by histologic pattern scores

Pattern Score	Stage				Total (%)
	I	II	III	IV	
2–3	40.8	12.3	34.6	12.3	100
4–5	22.2	11.0	52.6	14.2	100
6	6.9	9.8	50.4	32.9	100
7–8	3.2	4.9	37.1	54.8	100
9–10	3.9	1.3	29.9	64.9	100

Table 9–7

Mortality data by clinical stages

Stage	N	Serum Prostatic Acid Phosphatase[a]	Distant Metastases	Five-Year Survival[b]	Deaths/ Patient-year	CA Deaths/ Patient-year
I	296	N	0	61%	0.10	0.008
II	243	N	0	68	0.08	0.007
III	1328	N	0	45	0.16	0.028
IV	1044	± or[c]	±	25	0.28	0.144
	578[d]	+	0	32	0.23	0.095
	78[d]	N	+	23	0.30	0.148
	374[d]	+	+	14	0.39	0.252
	2911			41%	0.18	0.055

[a]N = 1.0 or less, + = more than 1.0 King-Armstrong units/100 ml.
[b]Five-year survival rate calculated from death rates.
[c]Either phosphatase elevated, or metastases present, or both.
[d]In 14 cases the reason for assignment to Stage IV was not available.

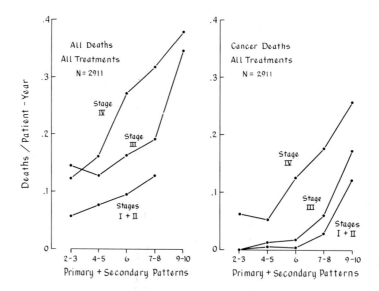

Figure 9–17. Cancer and total mortality rates by histologic pattern scores, calculated separately by clinical stages. Stage I and II combined, and histologic pattern scores grouped to attain at least 12 cases for each point, except that the stage I–II, pattern score 9–10 group contained only eight cases with a total mortality rate of 0.73 deaths/patient-year but only one cancer death.

stage I and II patients with high histologic scores had higher cancer death rates than stage III patients with low histologic scores. Stage III patients with high histologic scores had higher cancer death rates than stage IV patients with low histologic scores.

These results indicated that histologic grading had predictive power, in addition to that provided by clinical staging, and suggested that grading and staging could be combined for stronger predictive discrimination.

Combined Histologic Grading and Clinical Staging

Rather than calculate a complex multiple regression equation, a simpler method was used to combine grade and stage. It was noted that the clinical stage and the primary and secondary histologic grades were associated with mortality rates which were fortuitously quite similar for each item with the same numerical "name" (Table 9–8). That is, the rates for stage I and pattern 1 were similar. The stage III rate was similar to the pattern 3

Table 9–8

Deaths/patient-year for clinical stage, primary and secondary histologic patterns

Stage	Death Rate	Histologic Patterns	Death Rates	
			Primary	Secondary
I	0.10	1	0.10	0.10
II	0.08	2	0.11	0.12
III	0.16	3	0.18	0.18
		4	0.24	0.22
IV	0.28	5	0.37	0.26

Table 9–9

Death rates—all deaths, cancer deaths by combined grading and staging categories

Category	N	Total Years	Dead	Dead–CA	Dead Total Years	Dead–CA Total Years
3	5	12.1	0	0	0.000	0.000
4	36	156.4	11	0	0.070	0.000
5	37	136.9	11	0	0.080	0.000
6	156	623.8	55	2	0.088	0.003
7	180	730.6	75	5	0.103	0.007
8	438	1865.5	219	24	0.117	0.013
9	662	2407.4	390	46	0.162	0.019
10	229	781.3	129	32	0.165	0.041
11	586	1692.7	410	181	0.242	0.107
12	134	314.8	91	39	0.289	0.124
13	348	818.3	270	160	0.330	0.196
14	35	82.0	26	21	0.317	0.256
15	65	108.6	46	28	0.424	0.258
	2911	9730.4	1733	538	0.178	0.055

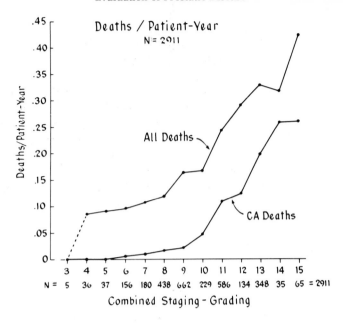

Figure 9–18. Cancer and total mortality rates by combined grading and stage. See text for explanation.

rates and so on. These observations suggested again that the three variables could be averaged for each patient, and more sophisticated mathematical analysis confirmed that the three items had roughly equal predictive weights. Therefore the numerical values of the primary and secondary patterns and the clinical stage were simply added together, achieving the effect of averaging without dividing by three. It was noted, however, that stage IV required a weighting value of 5 rather than 4, as suggested in Table 9–8.

This combined grading and staging score was designated the *category*, which could range from 3 to 15. (Stage I + primary pattern 1 + secondary pattern 1 = 3. Stage IV [= 5] + primary pattern 5 + secondary pattern 5 = 15.) Calculation of the mortality rates for each of these categories yielded very strong correlations for all deaths, and particularly for cancer deaths (Table 9–9; Figure 9–18). It was noteworthy that there were no cancer deaths in categories 3, 4, and 5, and that the cancer death rates were very low in

categories 6 and 7 (0.003 and 0.007 deaths/patient-year, respectively).

Treatment Results with Combined Grading and Staging

Combined grading and staging revealed differences in response to DES therapy (Figure 9–19). Patients in categories 8 and lower showed no significant differences in cancer death rates related to therapy.

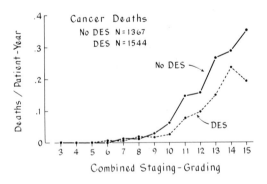

Figure 9–19. Cancer mortality rates with and without diethylstilbestrol (DES) therapy. (DES = 1 or 5 mg DES/day. No DES = placebo or 0.2 mg DES/day.) See text.

Patients in categories 9 and higher showed a definite reduction in cancer death rates if they had received 1 mg or 5 mg of DES/day, compared with patients who received placebo or 0.2 mg DES/day. Contrary to our previous report on 1032 patients from Study I,[17] patients in category 15 did show a decreased cancer death rate on DES therapy in the present analysis. In the previous report there were only eight patients on placebo and nine patients on 5 mg DES and no difference in cancer death rates was observed. In the present report there are 29 patients on placebo or 0.2 mg DES and 36 patients on 1 or 5 mg DES.

Combined Grading and Staging and Treatment Decisions

The total death rates and the cancer death rates for patients on placebo or 0.2 mg of DES provide some information on the natural history of "untreated" adenocarcinoma of the prostate. The low death rates and absence of any response to treatment in the lower categories suggest that some patients should not be subjected to any hazardous treatment. Certainly patients in categories 3, 4, and

5, who experienced no cancer deaths, fall into such a group. The data suggest that the limits of that group can be extended.

The cancer death rates and the total death rates show a definite upward inflection in the region of categories 8, 9, and 10 (Figure 9–18). For category 9 the cancer death rate was 0.019, or about one cancer death/53 patients/year. For category 8, the cancer death rate was 0.013, or about one cancer death/77 patients/year. A value judgment is involved as to when to treat carcinoma of the prostate, but these death rates are quite low. For all patients in categories 8 and lower, the cancer death rate was 0.009, or one cancer death/111 patients/year and there was no detectable effect from DES therapy in that group (Figure 9–19). There were 852 patients in that group (29.2% of the total 2911).

For all patients in categories 9 and higher, the cancer death rate was nine times as high, at 0.082, or about one cancer death/12 patients/year.

A tentative separation of the patients into the two suggested groups emphasizes the low cancer death rates and the absence of any response to therapy in the lower category group (Figure 9–20). The

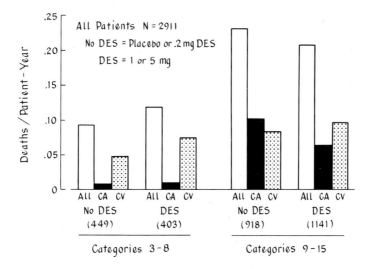

Figure 9–20. Tentative separation of patients by combined grading-staging categories. Note low cancer death rates and absence of effect of DES therapy in categories 3–8. Note high cancer death rates and significant difference in cancer death rates with DES therapy in categories 9–15.

increased cardiovascular mortality (and total mortality) in the treated group would probably be avoided by treating with only 1 mg of DES, or none at all.

In the higher category group (Figure 9–20), the cancer death rate of the patients on placebo or 0.2 mg of DES is nine times as high as that of the comparable lower category group. It is significantly reduced in the higher category group receiving 1 mg or 5 mg of DES (p = 0.025 for the ratio of the death rates tested by the F-distribution).

Importance of Other Histologic Findings

There was strong correlation between the histologic pattern scores and the extent of the tumor (percent area involved) in the prostatectomy and TUR specimens (Table 9–10). The higher grade tumors tended to involve a larger proportion of the resected tissue than the lower grade tumors. There was also definite correlation between cancer death rates and the extent of the tumor (data not presented), but this was much weaker than the correlation of the extent of the tumor with the tumor grades.

The presence or absence of perineural space invasion showed no significant correlation with cancer mortality rates, the survival curves being virtually identical. This was somewhat surprising since perineural space invasion was rarely seen in pattern 1 and 2 tumors and this might have been expected to correlate with their low mortality rates. This may have been negated by the fact that perineural invasion was also rarely seen in highly malignant tumors perhaps, because nerves were destroyed. Many of the needle biopsies and TUR biopsies contained very few nerves.

In a small number of needle biopsies and TUR specimens, it could be seen that the tumor had extended outside the prostatic capsule. There was some increase in the cancer death rates associated with this phenomenon in comparison with cases of comparable grade tumors in which that observation was not made. However, one could not assume that all the latter patients did not have similar extension.

CORRELATION OF HISTOLOGIC AND BIOLOGIC MALIGNANCY

The data presented confirm conclusively that the spectrum of histologic patterns of adenocarcinoma of the prostate is strongly correlated with its spectrum of biologic malignancy. This association has been reported by many authors for over thirty years and for various measures of clinical malignancy including mortality rates, size of prostate, extent of tumor within the prostate, the clinical stage of the tumor and the presence of metastases.[3–14]

The data presented here show that the histologic grades of the tumors are strongly correlated with the incidence of identifiable metastases, elevated serum

Table 9–10

Extent of tumor by histologic pattern score (TUR and prostatectomy specimens, only)

Pattern Score	Percent Area Involved by Tumor					
	<5%	5–9%	10–19%	20–49%	≥50%	Total (%)
2–3	40%	40%	17%	3%	0%	100
4–5	17	25	22	23	13	100
6	7	12	11	27	43	100
7–8	4	5	5	20	66	100
9–10	4	3	4	19	70	100

prostatic acid phosphatase, the formally defined clinical stage of the tumor, ureteral obstruction, and pain due to the cancer. In addition to these direct manifestations of prostatic cancer, the tumor grades also showed weaker correlations with secondarily affected variables, such as the initial body weight and hemoglobin level.

All of these clinical features might be regarded as measures of the extent to which the cancer has already progressed when it is first diagnosed. Byar et al. have shown that these clinical features (and others) can be combined into a multivariate factor exponential model which relates these variables to the subsequent mortality experience and permits identification of groups of patients at various levels of mortality risk.[24] This mathematical model also allows evaluation of the relative importance of each variable.

The data presented here also show conclusively that the histologic grades correlate very strongly with the subsequently observed death rates.

Corriere and associates,[12] using the present author's grading system, showed correlation of tumor grades with clinical stages and mortality rates. They were also able to show some correlations between histology and mortality rates within clinical stages.

In the present study, based on a large number of patients from the VACURG studies, it was possible to show strong correlations between tumor grades and death rates within the clinical stages. Further, it could be shown that histologic grading provided significant information in addition to the well-known predictive value of the clinical stages. Grading and staging can be combined into predictive categories which provide more useful information than either grade or stage. Thus, essential pretreatment information separates patients into groups which have a very wide range of mortality risks, ranging from a group with no cancer deaths and a mildly elevated total death rate, to a group with approximately 25% cancer deaths/year and a total death rate of over 40%/year. A spectrum of groups with intermediate death rates is also delineated.

It must be emphasized that these are groups of patients, and it is no consolation for a patient to be assigned to a favorable group if his cancer progresses more rapidly than that of another patient assigned to a less favorable group. Nevertheless, the differences between the death rates of these groups are large and they appear strong enough to support decision points based on observed death rates for the management of this disease.

It must also be pointed out that the Veterans Administration patient population consists of groups of men of clustered ages (corresponding to the major wars) moving through time together. There was some increase in total death rates in Studies II and III compared with Study I which was apparently related to the increasing mean age of the patient groups. This may reverse when the veterans of World War II become a larger fraction of our patients. Our statistics involving age-related variables may not correspond exactly to those observed in the general population but the essential between-group comparisons such as those between grades, stages and treatments, should not be distorted by these considerations.

Death Rate Statistics

The death rate—deaths/patient-year—was very helpful for comparing the various groups. In comparison with the common fixed-interval analysis of three, or five, or 10-year survival data, the death rate is capable of finer discrimination because it incorporates all the available mortality information. The fixed-interval comparison must discard all the patients who could not, or have not, been followed for the chosen interval and also loses the information as to how long the patient survived within that interval. Fixed-interval rates must vary according to the interval selected and the total mortality rate must eventually become 100%.

In contrast with the visual comparison of survival curves, the death rates, calculated from the same data, provide quantitative values which are suitable for statistical tests. Specifically, the ratio of two death rates is distributed as Snedecor's F-distribution when the rates are obtained from independent populations with exponential survival distributions.

The death rate, calculated from actual data, is quite stable with the passage of time, even for relatively small groups of patients. This simply calculated statistic actually yields what statisticians call the maximum likelihood estimate of the rate constant, or hazard, for the exponential survival distribution. If death rates were truly exponential, the fraction of the remaining patients dying each year (and cumulatively per total patient-years) would remain constant until the last patient died. It would not be necessary to wait 10 years, or 20 years, or until all the patients were dead, to be confident that

some characteristic or some treatment had significant value. Statistically significant differences might be demonstrated in shorter intervals.

Indeed, it has been noted that survival curves for malignancy and other chronic diseases do suggest exponential processes. Survival curves are often presented on semilogarithmic scale, usually without explanation, and often do appear linear on that scale for much of their course. The exponential distribution has been shown to fit patients with prostate cancer quite well.[24]

In fact, however, it is known that the survival curve of a group of "normal" individuals is not an exponential curve but rather a steadily increasing fraction of deaths/year, the fraction doubling about every eight years for U.S. males from 50 to 90 years old.[23,25] This must yield survival curves which accelerate downward on a semilogarithmic scale, even for specific chronic diseases, as the accelerating "normal" force of mortality becomes larger in proportion to a (possibly) constant force of mortality for the specific disease under consideration.

If the *increase* over the "normal" mor-

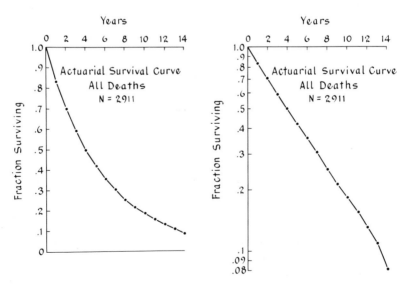

Figure 9–21. Actuarial survival curve for all 2911 patients on linear and semilogarithmic scales. Survival curve suggests exponential death rate.

tality rate due to the disease being studied is large and exponential, it might dominate the shape of the curve. The overall survival curve for the 2911 patients in this study does suggest an exponential function (Figure 9–21).

It would, of course, be essential to plot the survival curves and examine their shape, since the death rate calculation will always yield a single averaging value and may average out significant changes in the death rate occurring with the passage of time. For example, the adverse cardiovascular effects associated with DES therapy noted in the VACURG studies appear to be dissipated within a very few years.[21] The data of Nefzger and Mostofi[26] indicate that many testicular malignancies are fatal within three years, but most of the remaining patients appear to have been cured by the surgery and subsequently suffer only slightly reduced survival rates. Zumoff, Hart, and Hellman[25] have documented similar changes in death rates with passing time in several different categories of chronic disease.

In relatively small groups, the number of remaining patients rapidly becomes so small that a single death has a marked effect on the death rate for that year and the curves tend to become randomly erratic after the first few years. However, total deaths/total patient-years is not strongly affected by the small number of deaths in the later years, and the death rate is a powerful tool for comparing matched or randomized groups of patients.

Additional Histologic Correlations

It is commonly felt that the finding of small amounts of tumor in an adequate biopsy ought to be associated with a better prognosis than the finding of large amounts of tumor. The present material supports that idea but the correlation appears to be secondary to the correlation between the extent of the tumor and the histologic grade, which is much stronger than the correlation between the extent of the tumor and the death rates.

There is no indication in the data as to which tumors will respond to estrogenic hormone therapy. However, the pattern 1 and 2 tumors are of such low malignancy that it is impossible to demonstrate any effect of DES therapy on them. It is probably useless to include patients with such low-grade tumors in treatment comparison studies.

The question as to whether the tumor histology changes with time is important to the concept of grading tumors but the question cannot be answered directly from the present data. The VACURG studies did not include systematic rebiopsy of the tumors. The small number of repeat biopsies which are available suggest that many of the tumors maintain their initial appearance for long periods of time, even though these rebiopsies are heavily biased toward patients whose cancers were progressing clinically.

The author has seen clear instances of transformation of prostatic cancer to higher grades of malignancy, but these are rare. The data suggest but do not prove that the majority of prostatic cancers have a definite pattern of histology and a definite degree of malignancy and that these are maintained for long periods. The long survivals and rare cancer deaths observed among the low-grade tumors could not be obtained if there was frequent and inexorable progression to higher grades of malignancy.

Other considerations support the same conclusion. The increasing incidence of small "latent" carcinomas with advancing age at autopsy indicates not only that such tumors continue to arise throughout later life but also that many of those tumors have been present for several decades. For example, if the approximate incidence of small "latent" carcinomas is 10% at age 55, 20% at age 65, and 30% at age 75, then two-thirds of the tumors in the 75-year-old men must have been present for at least 10 years and one-third must have been present for at least 20 years!

One cannot exclude the possibility that higher grade tumors may have arisen from, and then obliterated, previous well-differentiated tumors. Nevertheless, as important as the question of changes in histology and malignancy may be from a conceptual standpoint, the practical question is moot—the observations, the calculations, and the interpretations *include* all the effects of such changes whatever they may have been. The correlation between tumor grade and behavior can be taken at face value.

In view of the well-documented value of grading, the general failure to apply this knowledge is distressing. A few authors have not found histologic classification useful for prostatic carcinoma,[27-29] but this only emphasizes that histologic grading is necessarily a subjective procedure. Systems based on histogenesis, identifying tumors by their resemblance to fetal or adult structures, and systems relying heavily on cytologic details do not seem to yield strong correlations.

The main problem appears to be that grading is subjective and requires some effort and experience to learn and apply confidently. Histologic classification of the hematologic malignancies, however, is practiced quite widely and successfully, even though they are less common and more complex than prostatic carcinoma.

The VACURG grading system depends entirely on the glandular differentiation of the tumor and the relation of the tumor growth to the prostatic stroma. Most successful grading systems do depend basically on these two factors, explicitly or implicitly. We have tried to facilitate adoption of the VACURG grading system by dissecting the histologic details into a tabular array, presenting a simplified drawing of the histologic details, and

providing a mechanism for dealing with multiple patterns in one tumor.

It is entirely possible that successful grading systems can be based on cytologic or histochemical details but they will be time-consuming and expensive compared with histologic grading which can be performed rapidly on standard surgical pathology material. More sophisticated discriminators may be found but a powerful measure of the malignancy of prostatic carcinoma is available in its histologic structure.

The correlation of histologic and biologic malignancy should be taken at face value and applied to the study of prostatic carcinoma. It will refine treatment comparisons by reducing variation within the groups being compared.

Histologic grading should be incorporated routinely into the diagnosis of prostatic carcinoma. Grading should be combined with staging to estimate roughly the increased risk to the patient from his cancer. This risk can then be weighed in the treatment decisions. Combined grading and staging can identify patients who are at such low risk that they probably should not be subjected to any potentially dangerous treatment unless (and until) there is real evidence that their cancer is progressing. More refined decisions may be possible in the future.

References

1. Hirst, A. E., Jr. and Bergman, R. T.: Carcinoma of the prostate in men 80 or more years old. Cancer, 7:136, 1954.
2. Whitmore, W. F., Jr.: The rationale and results of ablative surgery for prostatic cancer. Cancer, 16:1119, 1963.
3. Evans, N., et al.: Carcinoma of the prostate; Correlation between the histologic observations and the clinical course. Arch. Pathol., 34:473, 1942.
4. Thompson, G. J.: Transurethral resection of malignant lesions of the prostate gland. J.A.M.A., 120:1105, 1942.
5. Pool, T. L., and Thompson, G. J.: Conservative treatment of carcinoma of the prostate. J.A.M.A., 160:833, 1956.

6. Shelley, H. S., et al.: Carcinoma of the prostate. A new system of classification. Arch. Surg., 77:751, 1958.

7. Bauer, W. C., et al.: Unsuspected carcinoma of the prostate in suprapubic prostatectomy specimens. Cancer, 13:370, 1960.

8. Emmett, J. L., et al.: Endocrine therapy in carcinoma of the prostate gland: 10-year survival studies. J. Urol., 83:471, 1960.

9. Vickery, A. L., Jr. and Kerr, W. S., Jr.: Carcinoma of the prostate treated by radical prostatectomy. A clinicopathological survey of 187 cases followed for 5 years and 148 cases followed for 10 years. Cancer, 16:1598, 1963.

10. Wiederanders, R. E., et al.: Prognostic value of grading prostatic carcinoma. J. Urol., 89:881, 1963.

11. Mellinger, G. T., et al.: The histology and prognosis of prostatic cancer. J. Urol., 97:331, 1967.

12. Corriere, J. N., Jr., et al.: Prognosis in patients with carcinoma of the prostate. Cancer, 25:911, 1970.

13. Belt, E., and Schroeder, F. H.: Total perineal prostatectomy for carcinoma of the prostate. J. Urol., 107:91, 1972.

14. Hanash, K. A., et al.: Carcinoma of the prostate: a 15-year-followup. J. Urol., 107:450, 1972.

15. Gleason, D. F.: Classification of prostatic carcinomas. Cancer Chemother. Rep., 50:125, 1966.

16. Bailar, J. C. III, et al.: Survival rates of patients with prostatic cancer, tumor stage and differentiation—preliminary report. Cancer Chemother. Rep., 50:129, 1966.

17. Gleason, D. F., et al.: Prediction of prognosis for prostatic adenocarcinoma by combined histological grading and clinical staging. J. Urol., 111:58, 1974.

18. The Veterans Administration Co-op Urological Research Group: Carcinoma of the prostate: A continuing co-operative study. J. Urol., 91:590, 1964.

19. The Veterans Administration Cooperative Urological Research Group: Carcinoma of the prostate: Treatment comparisons. J. Urol., 98:516, 1967.

20. The Veterans Administration Co-op Urological Research Group: Treatment and survival of patients with cancer of the prostate. Surg., Gynecol. Obstet., 124:1011, 1967.

21. Blackard, C. E., et al.: Incidence of cardiovascular disease and death in patients receiving diethylstilbestrol for carcinoma of the prostate. Cancer, 26:249, 1970.

22. Byar, D. P.: The Veterans Administration Cooperative Urological Research Group's studies of cancer of the prostate. Cancer, 32:1126, 1973.

23. U.S. Center for Health Statistics—Department of Health, Education and Welfare. United States Life Tables: 1959–1961. U.S. Public Health Services Publication Number 1252, Volume 1, number 3. Washington, D.C. U.S. Government Printing Office, 1968 .

24. Byar, D. P., et al.: An exponential model relating censored survival data and concomitant information for prostatic cancer patients. J. Natl. Cancer Inst., 52:321, 1974.

25. Zumoff, B., et al.: Considerations of mortality in certain chronic diseases. Ann. Intern. Med., 64:595, 1966.

26. Nefzger, M. D., and Mostofi, F. Ķ.: Survival after surgery for germinal malignancies of the testis. I. Rates of survival in tumor groups. Cancer, 30:1225, 1972.

27. Foot, N. C., Humphreys, G. A., and Coats, E. L.: Carcinoma of the prostate. A review of 162 cases with a pathologic classification. N.Y. State J. Med., 50:84, 1950.

28. Franks, L. M., et al.: An assessment of factors influencing survival in prostate cancer: The absence of reliable prognostic features. Br. J. Cancer, 12:321, 1958.

29. Jewett, H. J., et al.: The palpable nodule of prostatic cancer. Results 15 years after radical excision. J.A.M.A., 203:403, 1968.

The Veterans Adminstration Cooperative Urological Research Group

George T. Mellinger, M.D.,
  VAH, Wichita, Kansas (Chairman)
Prince D. Beach, M. D.,
  VAH, Houston, Texas (Co-chairman)
Earl Haltiwanger, M. D.,
  VAH, Atlanta, Georgia
Paul W. Gonick, M. D.,
  VAH, Bronx, New York (retired)
Lino J. Arduino, M. D.,
  VAH, Des Moines, Iowa (retired)
Maxwell Malament, M. D.,
  VAH, East Orange, New Jersey (deceased)
Howard C. Kramer, M. D.,
  VAH, Baltimore, Maryland
Arthur J. Bischoff, M. D.,
  VAH, Long Beach, California (retired)
Henry I. Berman, M. D.,
  VAH, Louisville, Kentucky (retired)
Paul O. Madsen, M. D.,
  VAH, Madison, Wisconsin
Clyde E. Blackard, M. D.,
  VAH, Minneapolis, Minnesota
James S. Elliot, M. D.,
  VAH, Palo Alto, California
Leslie E. Becker, M. D.,
  VAC, Leavenworth, Kansas
William L. Parry, M. D.,
  VAH, Oklahoma City, Oklahoma
W. Pope Jordan, Jr., M. D.,
  VAH, Memphis, Tennessee
Francis F. Bartone, M. D.,
  VAH, Omaha, Nebraska
Winston K. Mebust, M. D.,
  VAH, Kansas City, Missouri
Maurice J. Gonder, M. D.,
  VAH, Buffalo, New York
John R. Kent, M. D.,
  VAH, Long Beach, California

David A. Parker, M. D.,
  VAH, Tucson, Arizona
R. E. H. Puntenney, M. D.,
  VAH, Des Moines, Iowa
John Ravera, M. D.,
  VAH, Long Beach, California
Andrew Sporer, M. D.,
  VAH, East Orange, New Jersey
Donald Gleason, M. D.,
  VAH, Minneapolis, Minnesota
Raymond Yesner, M. D.,
  VAH, West Haven, Connecticut
U. S. Seal, Ph. D.,
  VAH, Minneapolis, Minnesota
Joseph Jorgens, M. D.,
  VAC, Los Angeles, California
Richard P. Doe, M. D.,
  VAH, Minneapolis, Minnesota
Lyndon E. Lee, Jr., M. D.,
  VACO, Washington, D.C.
John C. Bailar, III, M. D.,
  NCI, Bethesda, Maryland
David P. Byar, M. D.,
  NCI, Bethesda, Maryland
Robert B. Higgins, M. D.,
  VAH, Portland, Oregon
F. K. Mostofi, M. D.,
  AFIP, Washington, D.C.
Lloyd S. Rogers, M. D.,
  VAH, Syracuse, New York
A. Hardy Ulm, III, M. D.,
  VAH, New York, New York (deceased)
Venancio R. Quiambo, M. D.,
  VAH, Cincinnati, Ohio
Additional Participating Hospital:
  VAH, Lake City, Florida

Chapter 10

Diagnosing and Staging of Prostatic Carcinoma

GEORGE R. PROUT, JR.

The purpose of this paper is to bring together data that relate to the use of certain tests or techniques, or both that have, or seem likely to have, value in establishing the diagnosis of prostatic carcinoma and to define the clinical stages of prostatic carcinoma, taking into account the accumulated information available concerning the biology of the disease.

A classification according to the TNM system is also proposed and outlined.

DIAGNOSIS

History

Clinically manifest prostatic carcinoma most often produces symptoms of frequency and nocturia. Frequently, they are of short duration in contrast to the patient with benign hyperplasia. While other symptoms, e.g., hematuria and dysuria, may occur, the complaint of back pain with or without associated weight loss is a

Supported in part by a grant from the National Cancer Institute, National Institutes of Health, USPHS (No. Ca 12414) and the Skerry Vore Foundation, New York.

complaint suggesting metastases in any elderly male, particularly with suspicious findings on digital rectal examination. Myriad symptomatology may be ascribed to prostatic carcinoma and for a detailed account the interested reader is referred to other sources.[1-3]

Physical Examination

The vast majority of men with prostatic carcinoma have no findings suggestive of the disease; it is those in whom it is *clinically manifest* that various significant findings are described. The earliest palpable change is conventionally considered to be a "discrete nodule of firm or stony consistency."[4] Extension of the process usually involves the capsule and the ipsilateral lobe. Thus the entire lobe may be infiltrated with an almost unique type of induration. Extension into the periprostatic tissues may not be detectable. As a consequence, underestimation of stage is quite common.

The presence of an isolated indurated nodule detected by rectal examination has the probability of being neoplastic in about 50% of the patients.[4] Inflammatory processes, active and ancient, calculi and tuberculosis are among those nonneoplastic disorders that may mimic carcinoma. As the neoplastic process establishes itself in the extraprostatic tissues, the likelihood of accurate diagnosis by palpation alone increases, but there is a finite limitation that will always exist.

Detectable carcinoma may be disseminated to peripheral lymph nodes, particularly those of the groin and the supraclavicular region, but these are usually very late events. The involved nodes are characteristically very firm and, upon excision, they may not yield an answer as to their source since there is little that is characteristic about prostatic metastases examined by conventional techniques. The problem is heightened, of course, when the prostate has none of the usual changes on digital examination. Accordingly, if a portion of every node removed were frozen and kept in that state, two studies might be performed that would allow for exclusion/inclusion of prostatic carcinoma. Histochemical techniques for the detection of acid phosphatase are now in widespread use,[5,6] and application will reveal cells rich in this enzyme. Of course, other neoplasms may have acid phosphatase present, but not usually in the same abundance. Our studies have shown that human prostatic acid phosphatase is immunologically unique, being antigenically unlike any acid phosphatase found in the human.[7-9] Antisera raised against ejaculate will precipitate human prostatic acid phosphatase in gel systems, and the origin of the acid phosphatase, whether from normal, benignly hyperplastic or neoplastic tissue, does not influence the precipitation. Figure 10–1 is an example of multiple gel diffusion with antisera in the center. Prostatic cellular origin is indicated by the stained bands. The positive well in the lower left was filled with an homogenate of a tumor-bearing node, the site of origin of which was unknown until this study was performed. Prostatic

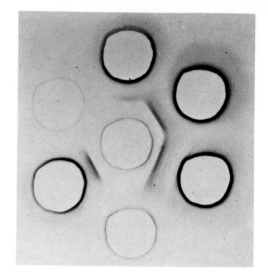

Figure 10–1. This gel diffusion study was prepared by adding homogenates of benign and malignant prostatic tissue to wells at 12, 1, and 3 o'clock. Homogenates of seminal vesicle and a lymph node in which adenocarcinoma was found were placed in wells at 6 and 8 o'clock and human serum was added to the remaining well. Absorbed goat antiserum raised against human sperm-free ejaculate was placed in center well, and preparation stained for acid phosphatase. Visible bands are precipitates of human prostatic acid phosphatase, demonstrating that node with primary tumor of unknown origin was metastatic site of prostatic carcinoma.

needle biopsy confirmed the presence of prostatic carcinoma.

Histologic Diagnosis

It has been established that transurethral resection of the prostate for neoplasms so advanced as to produce significant symptoms of obstructive uropathy will yield tissue suitable for diagnosis in excess of 90% of the patients. On the other hand, patients with clinical benign prostatic hyperplasia who undergo transurethral resection or have some enucleative type of operative procedure will have tumor gratuitously discovered in about 10% of them.[10-12] The significance of these kinds of cancer will be discussed later. It is important to note that, just as with autopsy specimens,[13] repeated sectioning of tissue at lesser intervals will produce a marked increase in the yield of positive diagnoses.[14] When the lesion is a single palpable nodule, transurethral resection is not nearly as efficient in obtaining positive tissue because of the usual deeply placed site of origin of these nodules.[15]

One of the most widely used techniques for obtaining tissue utilizes perineal or transrectal routes employing a variety of large bore needles with special cutting devices.[10,16,17] These have simplified the decision-making activities associated with the isolated nodule since the yield of positive tissue is high.[18] Information derived from needle biopsies—when of a positive nature—allows one to decide upon the treatment without electing other routes, e.g., open perineal, which may have serious consequences relating to operative trauma and sexual potency. Negative biopsies may be confirmed either immediately or after a suitable waiting period. Obviously, these procedures lack the precision of an open biopsy, but the net difference is scant and the gain to the patient is often great.

Roentgenograms

Conventional films of bone are a resource for detecting spread of tumor since changes may be present before symptoms appear. Careful examination of the roentgenograms often demonstrates that the metastatic lesions are lytic and that there are proliferative areas around these foci of lysis that produce the characteristic osteoblastic lesions of prostatic carcinoma. When clearly positive almost no other disease mimics prostatic carcinoma successfully.

The detection of bony metastases has, until recently, depended on conventional roentgenographic surveys. Skeletal films, however, often fail to detect the presence of significant metastatic deposits. Bachman and Sproul[13] examined 31 autopsy specimens of patients whose deaths

were due to advanced prostatic cancer. Bony metastases were not visualized roentgenographically in 15 patients, yet each of the 31 had tumor found in bone at autopsy. The explanation for the difference is, in a given volume of bone, nearly 50% of it must be replaced by tumor before the lesion can be detected.[19]

In recent years more sensitive means of detecting early metastatic disease have been sought and considerable interest has been directed toward the use of scintillation bone scanning following the administration of a radionuclide. The most popular nuclides have been ^{85}Sr and ^{18}Fl. These have several major drawbacks related to cost, i.e. in the case of ^{85}Sr the time delay before scanning, after administration, availability of the isotope, and scanning resolution. Our radiologic asssociates have recently used $^{99-m}$Tc coupled to a diphosphonate, a simple organophosphorus compound which has a high proclivity for actively metabolizing bone.[20] The results have been technically more satisfactory than with the use of other nuclides and there is the added advantage of both a relatively short delay (four hours following injection) before scanning, as well as the lower cost of the isotope (Figures 10–2 and 3).

Since the scanning technique is not specific for metastatic disease and the interpretation is always open to question, we have recently begun to attempt to confirm these findings by the use of selective bone biopsies. Review of our experience to date, which is still quite preliminary, suggests that bone scanning is more sensitive than conventional roentgenographic surveys in both detecting early metastatic disease and evaluating the extent of the disease. Of 21 patients' biopsies, six biopsies were taken from scan-positive regions, and four had tumor cells present. In the remaining two there were histological changes in the bone that were consistent with tumor nearby but neoplastic cells were not

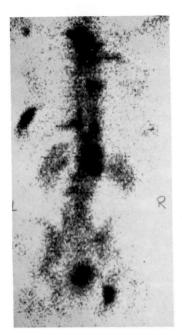 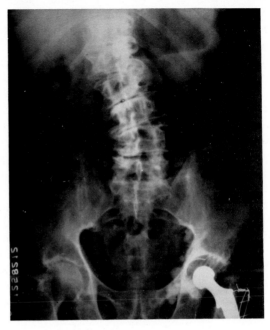

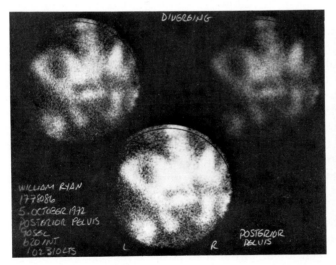 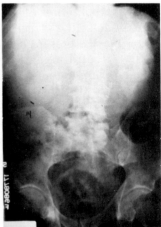

Figures 10–2 and 3. Disphosphonate scans. These $^{99\text{-m}}$Tc diphosphonate scans and associated roentgenograms demonstrate value of scans when attempting to discover presence of bony metastases. Roentgenograms are not of the highest quality but they are in no way different from many films obtained for this purpose. Time period for scanning procedure is four hours.

Table 10–1

Scans in relation to other measurements of disease[a]

	Scan	X-ray +	X-ray −	Acid P'tase +	Acid P'tase −	Alk. P'tase +	Alk. P'tase −	Biopsy +	Biopsy −	Nodes +	Nodes −
Stage B	Scan +	0	0	0	0	0	0	0	0	—	—
	Scan −	0	2	0	2	0	2	0	2	—	—
Stage C	Scan +	0	2	0	2	0	2	0	2	0	0
	Scan −	0	4	0	3	0	2	0	5	0	2
Stage D	Scan +	15	11	21	5	14	10	4/6	6/6	—	—
	Scan −	1	2	2	0	—	1	—	—	—	—

[a]37 patients scanned with prostatic carcinoma

observed. In only two of these patients, were the roentgenographic surveys positive. Three patients had positive sternal scans but negative marrow aspirates. The remainder of the patients had histologic proof of prostatic cancer and had either Stage C or Stage D disease except for two with Stage B disease (Table 10–1). The biopsies obtained from scan negative regions were all negative. There still remains a considerable problem with falsely positive scans which needs to be resolved; perhaps it will be with the use of selected open bone biopsies coupled with marrow acid phosphatase determinations. Clearly those patients with negative scans need to be followed closely for a considerable period of time before any evaluation can be made.

Biochemical Studies

This subject has been reviewed recently.[21] Because measurement of the serum acid phosphatase (SAP) is considered a semispecific test for prostatic carcinoma, it is sometimes used as a substitute for a tissue diagnosis. Actually it is a poor substitute because many disorders (prostatic infarct, multiple myeloma, osteogenic sarcoma, thromboembolic disease, and thrombocytopenia,[21–26] to mention a few) may produce elevations of the SAP and because

of the serious nature of the disease, reasonable efforts to obtain tissue by one route or another would seem essential.

Woodard[27] has separated out the various factors that are found in men with prostatic carcinoma who do have elevations of the SAP. Briefly, the higher the stage, i.e., the more tumor present, the more likely is the SAP to be elevated. She used Bodansky's method for measurement and felt that the substrate, β-glycerophosphate, was quite specific for prostatic acid phosphatase. Fishman,[28] exploiting the observation that L-tartrate inhibits prostatic acid phosphatase, has shown that this increases the specificity of the test, as well, and so this technique has gained acceptance, too. However, experience has demonstrated that that which seems so clear in the research laboratory may gain some opacity upon transfer to the general laboratory of a busy hospital.

Levels of acid phosphatase activity in the bone marrow of patients with and without prostatic carcinoma have been studied.[29] Their results suggest that otherwise undetectable prostate cancer which has metastasized to bone will be responsible for marked elevations of phosphatase activity. Similar elevations were found in patients with obvious bony metastases.

Other enzymes, such as phosphohexose

isomerase,[30] aldolase,[31] transaminase,[32] and lactic dehydrogenase (LDH) and its isozymes,[33] have been studied with regard to prostatic carcinoma; however, none seems nearly so specific for prostatic cellular activity as is SAP. It is clear that the level of the fifth isozyme of serum LDH is elevated when the disease is not in remission, and prompt decrease occurs when hormonal therapy is instituted. However, these studies seem to apply to most disseminated tumor systems, since they probably are dependent on excessive glycolysis and anaerobic glycolysis rather than on any unique characteristic of prostatic carcinoma.

Another means of detecting prostatic acid phosphatase has been developed as a result of immunologic studies. These investigations, conducted by Shulman and his associates[34-36] and by us[8,9,37] have shown that in dog and man, acid phosphatase found in the prostate is unique for that organ in those species. We found it possible to precipitate acid phosphatase of prostatic origin from the serum of patients with prostatic carcinoma[9] and we also found that metastatic prostatic carcinoma to lymph nodes would be detected by gel diffusion studies (Figure 10–1). Moncure et al. have applied these observations to studies of marrow aspirates.[7] They found a positive precipitate reaction each time tumor cells were found in the marrow and on some occasions, when no tumor cells were found, prostatic acid phosphatase was precipitated, indicating marrow involvement. Further refinement of these immunologic techniques may appreciably improve the precision of diagnosis and detection of prostatic carcinoma.

Carcinoembryonic Antigen

The evaluation of this test is currently being conducted. Only preliminary data are available, but it is evident that in some patients plasma does have elevated amounts of this antigen present.[38] Experi-

ence will determine its role in diagnosis and management.

STAGING OF PROSTATIC CARCINOMA

The available evidence demonstrates that clinically manifest prostatic carcinoma is uniformly understaged. Since no restrictions are placed upon me with regard to the considerations that relate to staging, the following system includes a consideration of data usually available to the physician when evaluating a patient with prostatic carcinoma. It is obvious that a means of classification is essential and gross differences are easily appreciated. However, the diagnostic armamentarium, while extensive, is scarcely adequate to assign a precise extent of tumor and/or a decision regarding survival for many patients. As will be seen shortly, large areas of gray surround each stage. This imprecision detracts from the value of assigning a stage for a patient but not to the extent that staging becomes a worthless practice. The classification which follows is essentially that of the Veterans Administration Cooperative Urological Research Group, except that letters have supplanted numerals to indicate stage, thus avoiding confusion with expressions of grade. I have also added a substage with the intent of improving the precision of the staging system.

Stage A

These patients have no clinical manifestations of prostatic carcinoma. It is found in patients at autopsy in ever-increasing numbers as age increases. Similarly it is found in patients with benign prostatic hyperplasia who undergo prostatectomy because of obstructive symptoms and, as mentioned previously, it is estimated that about 10% of all such surgical specimens will have histologic evidence of carcinoma present.[15,39] When the age of the population is advanced, the incidence of the disease will rise rapidly. An increase in yield will also be realized if more sections are obtained.[14]

There is a question about the management of patients with this stage of disease since it is viewed by many as an unimportant entity.[40-42] By others it represents a threat to the patient and treatment, accordingly, is necessary.[43] A search of the literature to obtain information on these matters is not very revealing. Aside from age and the existence of other disease, one can find two denominators upon which to base the separation of groups with innocuous tumor and those with lethal tumors. These are the degree of differentiation of the cells and their histologic pattern, and the frequency with which fields of tumor are encountered. Greene and Simon[41] reported on 83 patients with Stage A carcinoma whose survival was nearly that of the male population at large. Nearly all of these patients had well-differentiated carcinoma. Byar et al.[42] reported on 148 patients with (Stage A) carcinoma who had been followed for an average of about five years. Seventy-two patients died, but none from prostatic cancer, thus attesting to the poor outlook this selected population had. However, 10 patients showed progression of disease in the form of either elevated serum acid phosphatase and/or the development of bony metastases. Unlike the vast majority of patients in this series, six of the 10 had undifferentiated carcinoma.

Bauer et al.[40] have addressed themselves to both issues and found a striking correlation between differentiation, size of lesions, and whether the tumor was at the margin of the tissue removed (Table 10–2). Those patients with poorly differentiated cancer and those with large tumors had unsatisfactory outcomes, while patients with small, differentiated tumors suffered very rarely from their neoplasm.

From this brief overview it is clear that further data are necessary to establish an hypothesis that involves the proposition that undifferentiated carcinomas and large carcinomas compete effectively with other causes of death in these elderly males and, as a corollary, that a selected group of patients with an estimated risk of death from other diseases, might benefit from radical prostatectomy or radiotherapy.

Stage B

Jewett has defined this stage precisely:[44] "A palpably discrete nodule of firm or stony consistency limited to a part of one lateral lobe, averaging 1 cm or a little more in diameter, with compressible prostatic tissue always on two, and sometimes on three, sides." These patients have no clinical, laboratory or radiologic evidence of dissemination or of local extension of their disease. The authors are not so clear about urinary symptoms,

Table 10–2

Relationship of differentiation, microscopic size and anatomical position to outcome for patients with stage B carcinoma[a]

Differentiation	Size	No. Patients	Outcome; % Favorable
Well	S[b]	19	73.7%
Moderate-poor	S[b]	4	0 %
Well	L	9	66.6%
Moderate-poor	L	20	15 %
Tumor at margin		46	39 %
Tumor not at margin		6	83 %

[a]From Bauer, W. C. et al.[40]
[b]S = small, i.e. 3 or ≤ low power microscopic fields.

stipulating that "none of the nodules had caused symptoms." For purposes of this classification, patients with Stage B disease should have no urinary symptoms. If present, these symptoms should be minimal and consistent with the degree of benign enlargement present.

Since the intent of this paper is not to deal with therapeutic efforts nor their outcome, it is appropriate that I should refer to these events only in terms that apply to the biological relevance of such data. The retrospective selection of the cases incorporated by Jewett et al.[44] and Jewett[45] provide for insight into one facet of this disease. He selected 111 patients who met the criteria cited; eight were lost to follow-up, and 17 were proven histologically to have periprostatic and/or seminal vesicle involvement. None of the 17 patients was cured. In an earlier paper,[46] a similar experience involving 39 patients (two lived more than 15 years) was reported. Clearly then, while radical prostatectomy may control the local disease, in these patients with disease outside the prostate, even microscopically, the stage is such that failure to cure seems almost inevitable.

Returning to those 86 patients with carcinoma limited to the prostate, while 28 (52% of the whole group, 27% of the 103 followed or 33% of those *surgically* staged) survived 15 years, another 21 were not cured. The reasons for this failure are not at all clear. Those who failed did so at a fairly steady rate up to their 15th anniversary.[47] Of those who failed, not many had local persistence of cancer, and so metastases from this source could not have occurred often.[45] One is left with a choice between two explanations: either metastases were present before operation or, as a result of operation. Possibly, both are correct. In any event, these metastatic areas produced no difficulty for many years. Thus, if Stage A carcinoma can lead to Stage B carcinoma, then it is likely that many patients had

prostatic carcinoma for 20 or 30 years before death.[48]

Until we discover better means of measuring growth potentials, particularly in the well-organized carcinomas, we will continue to select therapy without the assurance that it will be curative.

Stage C

These patients usually have symptoms of prostatism, i.e., frequency, nocturia, a weak stream, and on rectal examination there is firm induration or stony hardness that involves the seminal vesicles, lateral pelvic walls, and base of the bladder in varying degrees.

Although it was originally held by Whitmore[49] that these patients might have elevated SAP, this system of classification excludes those patients. Further, while there is no clinical evidence of nodal metastases, it is quite certain that at least half of these patients will have metastases to pelvic nodes.[49-52]

Stage C₁

Patients in this stage represent an extension of Stage C. Again, the SAP is normal. Flocks et al.[51] have shown that there is an increase in the incidence of positive nodes as periprostatic involvement increases, and McCullough, Daly, and I[52] found that of 11 patients whose primary tumors were estimated to be in the 60–70 g range, nine had positive pelvic nodes. Further, we found that multiple nodes and bilateral nodes were more likely to be encountered as the primary tumor increased in size. This correlation would seem to be sufficient cause for separation of Stage C, particularly since there is some evidence which suggests there is a temporal relationship between positive nodes and progression of the neoplastic process. Whitmore and MacKenzie[53] reported on the results of cystectomy in 19 patients who had positive nodes. None survived beyond six years. At variance with this, and due possibly to selection, is the Massachusetts General Hospital experience (McCullough and Leadbetter)[54] where cystectomy and/or radical prostatectomy were performed. Five of 18 patients lived more than five years and three of these, all with positive nodes, lived over 10 years after extensive surgery.

Most of the emerging data suggest that involvement of pelvic nodes is a positive predictor for further progression. Flocks[55] has reported the results of prostatoseminal vesiculectomy and pelvic lymphadenectomy. In each circumstance, areas of induration were injected with 100 mCu ^{198}Au. The tumors were graded by Shelley's classification, and none was found to be well differentiated; 10% were classified as undifferentiated, and the remainder were "average." Of 32 patients with positive nodes, 28 survived five years, but only four patients lived 10 to 15 years. On the other hand, 69 patients with no nodal involvement (decision made in some circumstances by palpation), 51 (74%) survived five years, 44 (63.7%) 10 years, and 19 (27.5%) 15 years. This is, of course, a remarkable experience, and one awaits reports of the results of similar techniques from other centers.

Hilaris et al.[56] provide some further insight into the relationship of involved nodes to progressive disease. It seems that their purpose was primarily to report on a technique for the injection of ^{125}I seeds into the prostates of patients with Stage B and C prostatic cancer. They mention that of 31 Stage C patients, 20 (65%) had positive pelvic nodes and in Stage B (not so rigidly defined as the "Stage B" in this manuscript) six of 29 (21%) had positive nodes. While the authors perform several analyses, they do not separate some items of interest. Distant metastases were present in 10 of 25 patients with Stage C or Grade 3 carcinoma. In 10 patients at risk two years with positive nodes, whether in Stage B or C, six experienced progression

of the disease compared with one of eight who had negative nodes.

The Massachusetts General Hospital experience regarding nodal involvement without reference to therapeutic effectiveness has also been reported in part.[52] The data in Tables 10–3 and 4 have been generated since 1969 except where otherwise noted. All 22 patients with positive nodes were judged to be in clinical Stage C or C_1 prior to surgery. Of the 38 patients with negative nodes 6, 5, and 2 in the well-, moderately, and poorly differentiated groups, respectively, were judged to be in Stage B, and none of these exhibited progressive disease. Three patients had radical prostatectomies in 1949 and 1950. These patients had negative nodes, two with a moderately differentiated primary (1 in Stage B, 1 in Stage C), and 1 with a poorly differentiated primary (Stage C). All three patients survived 11–18 years with no evidence of progression before succumbing to other causes. Each surgeon exercised his own option regarding treatment, so that prostatoseminal vesiculectomy, radiotherapy, hormonal therapy, or no further treatment were employed.

All patients had thorough historical and physical evaluation, enzymatic and radiographic studies, including radionuclide scans for the past three years. Salient positive data were recorded. No patients with a positive scan or positive metastatic series were included, although there were patients in whom these studies were judged equivocal, in which case staging was conducted. No consistent relationship has yet been noted between these equivocal findings and the progression of disease, except for one patient who has progressed.

When the operation was done for staging alone, with the intent of employing radiotherapy, a midline incision was used and nodes from the hypogastric, external iliac, and obturator regions were resected. Very few blood vessels of any size require

Table 10–3

Diagnostic pelvic lymphadenectomy in 38 patients in whom no positive nodes were found

No. of Patients	Differentiation	XRT	Radical Prostatectomy	Disease Progression	Survival	Maximum Follow-up (years)	Comments
14	Well	4	9	0	13	3.5	1 died (pulmonary embolus)
13	Moderate	6	7	0	9	12[a]	3 died (noncancer); 1 lost to follow-up
11	Poor	4	5	2	9	18[a]	2 no therapy; 2 died (noncancer)

[a] Average follow-up, 3.5 years.

Table 10–4

Diagnostic pelvic lymphadenectomy in 22 patients in whom positive nodes were found

No. of Patients	Differentiation	XRT	Radical Prostatectomy	Disease Progression[a]	Survival	Maximum Follow-up (years)	Comments
3	Well	0	1	1	3	2.5	2 Patients rec'd DES
8	Moderate	3	4	1	7	4.5	1 died (prostatic cancer)
11	Poor	4	2	8	7	3.5	3 died (prostatic cancer); 1 died (noncancer)

[a] Average period between operation and evidence of progression: 11 months.

ligation during this nontherapeutic dissection, which has been nearly always bilateral in the past. The sites of obvious nodal involvement have been clipped and more recently we have used fragments of split shot to identify the bifurcation of the common iliac arteries and the upper portions of the prostate (Figure 10–4).

Stage D

Usually there is ample evidence of prostatic carcinoma on digital rectal examination but occasionally, only scant induration or a small nodule may be present. Sometimes the prostate feels entirely normal and the character of the metastases has directed attention to this gland. These patients may have soft tissue metastases that are clinically evident, bony metastases, uni- or bilateral hydronephrosis not due to bladder neck obstruction, and/or elevated SAP.

Justification for the inclusion of patients with only elevated SAP is based on

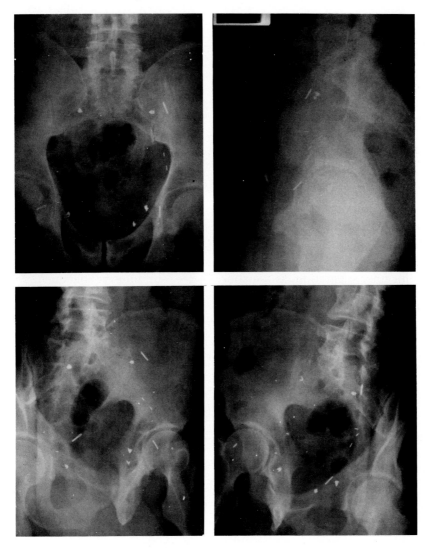

Figure 10–4. Split shot fragments. A, Split shot may be seen at each bifurcation of common iliac artery and two fragments of lead mark anterolateral surface of left side of prostate, and single fragment marks upper lateral extension of gland on the right. B, Oblique projections of same pelvis.

the data of Nesbit and Baum[22] who found that patients with no metastases, but who did have elevated SAP, survived only half as well as those with normal SAP. A similar trend was noted by Ganem,[57] who also showed that hydronephrosis was associated with diminished survival as well. Should a patient have bony metastases, an elevated SAP and hydronephrosis at the time of diagnosis, that patient's outlook for survival approaches zero.[58]

TNM CLASSIFICATION

There has been a concerted, prolonged effort on the part of the International Union Against Cancer and the American Joint Committee on Cancer Staging and End Results to standardize the classification of tumors by site and extent.

A consensus has not been reached regarding such a classification, but its potential advantages are manifest. For instance, in the A,B,C,D staging system, there is no contingency for classifying intraprostatic induration or nodules in excess of 1 cm. Even though the addition of Stage C_1 recognizes the implied difference in extent of disease, the system does not allow for finer separation, as a matter of importance. The descriptive language of the TNM classification requires collection of data and its reproduction in a uniform fashion, thus increasing the precision of communication between centers concerning series of patients. Currently it is virtually impossible to compare series from different institutions where patients are treated by different modalities. Indeed, realistic comparisons can scarcely be made between patients in the same institution.

The following classification outline has been supplied by Dr. F. K. Mostofi of the Armed Forces Institute of Pathology, Washington, D.C.

Rules for Classification

The classification applies only to carcinoma. There must be histologic or cytologic verification of the disease to permit division of cases by histologic type. The following are the minimum requirements for assessment of the T, N and M. categories. If these cannot be met the Symbols TX, NX, or MX will be used:

T Categories: Clinical examination, urography, endoscopy and biopsy (if indicated) prior to definitive treatment.

N Categories: Clinical examination, lymphography and/or urography.

M Categories: Clinical examination, chest x-ray, skeletal studies and determinations of the acid phosphatase level on two or more occasions.

TNM Classification

T, Primary Tumor

The suffix "(m)" may be added to the appropriate T category to indicate multiple tumors, e.g. T2(m).

TX The minimum requirements to assess fully the extent of the primary tumor cannot be met.

T0 No tumor palpable. This category includes those cases of the incidental finding of a carcinoma in an operative or biopsy specimen. Such cases should be assigned an appropriate P, N or M category.

T1 Tumor intracapsular surrounded by palpably normal gland.

T2 Tumor confined to the gland. Smooth nodule deforming contour but lateral sulci and seminal vesicles not involved.

T3 Tumor extending beyond the capsule with or without involvement of the lateral sulci and/or seminal vesicles.

T4 Tumor fixed or invading neighboring structures.

N, Regional and Juxtaregional Lymph Nodes

The regional lymph nodes are the pelvic nodes below the bifurcation of the common iliac arteries. The juxtaregional lymph nodes are the inguinal nodes, the common iliac and para-aortic nodes.

NX The minimum requirements to assess the regional lymph nodes cannot be met.

N0 No evidence of involvement of regional lymph nodes.

N1   Involvement of a single regional lymph node.

N2   Involvement of multiple regional lymph nodes.

N3   There is a fixed mass on the pelvic wall with a free space between this and the tumor.

N4   Involvement of juxtaregional nodes. Subsequent information regarding the histological assessment of the regional lymph nodes may be added to the clinical N category thus: N−(minus) for nodes with no microscopic evidence of metastasis or N+(plus) for nodes with microscopic evidence of metastasis, e.g., N0+, N1−.

M, Distant Metastases

If lymphography indicates extension to the juxtaregional lymph nodes a scalene node biopsy is recommended.

MX   The minimum requirements to assess the presence of distant metastases cannot be met.

M0   No evidence of distant metastases.

M1   Distant metastases present.

M1a   Evidence of occult metastases by biochemical and/or other tests.

M1b   Single metastasis in a single organ site.

M1c   Multiple metastases in a single organ site.

M1d   Metastases in multiple organ sites.

Note: The location of metastases should be specified. The lymph nodes beyond the regional and juxtaregional nodes, and bone, are regarded as single organ sites.

P, Histopathologic Categories

Assessment of the P categories is based on available material whether biopsy, transurethral resection, enucleation or total prostatectomy—the source to be stated.

The suffix "(m)" may be added to the appropriate P category to indicate multiple tumors, e.g. P2(m).

PX   The extent of invasion cannot be assessed.

P0   No tumor found on examination of specimen.

P1   Focal (single or multiple) carcinoma.

P2   Diffuse carcinoma with or without extension to the capsule.

P3   Carcinoma with penetration through the capsule and/or extension to the seminal vesicles.

P4   Extension into adjacent organs.

G, Histopathologic Grading

GX   Grade cannot be assessed.

G0   No evidence of anaplasia.

G1   Low-grade malignancy.

G2   Medium-grade malignancy.

G3   High-grade malignancy.

At present no stage grouping is recommended. Very likely this system will have to be contracted because that which every tumor registry might use should not occupy more than one sheet in any hospital chart.

Whatever the final form, the foregoing system can serve at least as a prototype for a useful and viable system that will allow for uniform classification of both stage and grade in prostatic carcinoma.[59]

References

1. Scott, W. W., and Schirmer, H. K. A.: Carcinoma of the prostate. In Urology. Edited by M. F. Campbell and J. H. Harrison. Philadelphia, W. B. Saunders, 1970, Vol. 2.
2. Marshall, V. F.: Textbook of Urology. 2nd Edition. New York, Hoeber Medical Div., Harper & Row, 1964.
3. Smith, D. R.: General Urology. 7th Edition. Los Altos, Calif., Lange Medical Publishers, 1972.
4. Jewett, H. J.: Significance of the palpable prostatic nodule. J.A.M.A., 160:838, 1956.
5. Biennerhassett, J. B., et al.: Carcinoma of the prostate: Enzyme histochemistry. Cancer, 20:2133, 1967.
6. Kirchheim, D., et al.: Histochemistry of the normal, hyperplastic, and neoplastic human prostate gland. Invest. Urol., 1:403, 1964.
7. Moncure, C. W., et al.: Immunological and histochemical evaluation of marrow aspirates in patients with prostatic carcinoma. J. Urol., 108:609, 1972.
8. Prout, G. R., Jr., and Moncure, C. W.: Prostatic carcinoma. Proc. 6th Nat. Cancer Conf. Philadelphia, J. B. Lippincott Co., 1968.
9. Moncure, C. W., et al.: The immunological detection of prostatic acid phosphatase in dog and man. Fed. Proc., 26:574, 1967.
10. Barnes, R. W.: Survival with conservative therapy. J.A.M.A., 210:331, 1969.
11. Labess, M.: Occult carcinoma in clinically benign hypertrophy of the prostate: A pathological and clinical study. J. Urol., 68:893, 1952.
12. Smith, G. G., and Woodruff, L. W.: The development of cancer of the prostate after subtotal prostatectomy. J. Urol., 63:1077, 1950.
13. Bachman, A. L., and Sproul, E. E.: Correlation of radiographic and autopsy findings in suspected metastases of the spine. Bull. N.Y. Acad. Med., 31:146, 1955.
14. Denton, S. E., et al.: Occult prostatic carcinoma diagnosed by the step-section technique of the surgical specimen. J. Urol., 93:296, 1965.

15. Denton, S. E., et al.: Comparison of the perineal needle biopsy and the transurethral prostatectomy in the diagnosis of prostatic carcinoma: An analysis of 300 cases. J. Urol., *97*:127, 1967.

16. Grabstald, H.: Further experience with transrectal biopsy of the prostate. J. Urol.,, *74*:211, 1955.

17. Veenema, R. J., and Lattimer, J. K.: Early diagnosis of carcinoma of the prostate. Periodic rectal examination is recommended and biopsy of any palpably suspicious area. J.A.M.A., *186*:127, 1963.

18. Kaufman, J. J., et al.: Methods of diagnosis of carcinoma of the prostate: A comparison of clinical impression, prostatic smear, needle biopsy, open perineal biopsy and transurethral biopsy. J. Urol., *72*:450, 1954.

19. Lachman, E.: Osteoporosis: The potentialities and limitations of its roentgenologic diagnosis. Am. J. Roentgenol.,Radium Ther. Nucl. Med., *74*:712, 1955.

20. King, W. R., et al.: Effect of disodium ethane-l-hydroxy-l, l-diphosphonate on bone formation. Clin. Orthop., *78*:251, 1971.

21. Prout, G. R., Jr.: Chemical tests in the diagnosis of prostatic carcinoma. J.A.M.A., *209*:1699, 1969.

22. Nesbit, R. M., and Baum, W. C.: Serum phosphatase determinations in diagnosis of prostatic cancer: A review of 1,150 cases. J.A.M.A., *145*:1321, 1951.

23. Howard, P. J., Jr., and Fraley, E. E.: Elevation of the acid phosphatase in benign prostatic disease. J. Urol., *94*:687, 1965.

24. Woodard, H. Q.: The clinical significance of serum acid phosphatase. Am J. Med., *27*:902, 1959.

25. Schoenfeld, M. R.: High serum acid phosphatase activity in various thromboembolic diseases. Clin. Res., *10*:180, 1962.

26. Oski, F. A., et al.: Use of the plasma acid phosphatase value in the differentiation of thrombocytopenic states. New Engl. J. Med., *268*:1423, 1963.

27. Woodard, H. Q.: Factors leading to elevations in serum acid glycerophosphatase. Cancer, *5*:236, 1952.

28. Fishman, W. H., et al.: Serum "prostatic" acid phosphatase and cancer of the prostate. New Engl. J. Med., *255*:925, 1956.

29. Chua, D. T., et al.: Acid phosphatase levels in bone marrow: Value in detecting early bone metastasis from carcinoma of the prostate. J. Urol., *103*:462, 1970.

30. Bodansky, O.: Serum phosphohexose in cancer. III. As an index to tumor growth in metastatic carcinoma of the prostate. Cancer, *8*:1087, 1955.

31. Baker, R., and Govan, D.: The effect of hormonal therapy of prostatic cancer on serum aldolase. Cancer Res., *13*:141, 1953.

32. West, M., et al.: Serum enzymes in disease. XV. Glycolytic and oxidative enzymes and transaminases in patients with carcinoma of the kidney, prostate and urinary bladder. Cancer, *17*:432, 1964.

33. Prout, G. R., Jr., et al.: Alterations in serum lactate dehydrogenase and its fourth and fifth isozymes in patients with prostatic carcinoma. J. Urol., *94*:451 1965.

34. Shulman, S., et al.: Measurement of prostatic acid phosphatase by gel diffusion methods. J. Reprod. Fertil., *10*:55, 1965.

35. Shulman, S., et al.: Studies on organ specificity. XVI. Urogenital tissues and autoantibodies. Immunology, *10*:99, 1966.

36. Yantorno, C., et al.: Studies on organ specificity. XVIII. Immunologic and biophysical characterization of canine prostatic fluid. J. Immunol., *96*:1035, 1966.

37. Moncure, C. W., and Prout, G. R., Jr.: Antigenicity of human prostatic acid phosphatase. Cancer, *25*:463, 1970.

38. LoGerfo, P., et al.: Demonstration of an antigen common to several varieties of neoplasia. Assay using zirconyl phosphate gel. New Engl. J. Med., *285*:138, 1971.

39. Jordan, W. P., Jr., and Kreager, J. A., Jr.: Incidentally discovered microscopic carcinoma of the prostate. J. Urol., *97*:751, 1967.

40. Bauer, W. C., et al.: Unsuspected carcinoma of the prostate in suprapubic prostatectomy specimens. Cancer, *13*:370, 1960.

41. Greene L. F., and Simon, H. B.: Occult carcinoma of the prostate. Clinical and therapeutic study of eighty-three cases. J.A.M.A., *158*:1494, 1955.

42. Byar, D. P. et al.: Survival of patients with incidentally found microscopic cancer of the prostate. Results of a clinical trial of conservative treatment. J. Urol., *108*:908, 1972.

43. Hudson, P. B., et al.: Prostatic cancer. XI. Early prostatic cancer diagnosed by arbitrary open perineal biopsy among 300 unselected patients. Cancer *7*:690, 1954.

44. Jewett, H. J., et al.: The palpable nodule of prostatic cancer. Results 15 years after radical excision. J.A.M.A., *203*:403, 1968.

45. Jewett, H. J.: The case for radical perineal prostatectomy. J. Urol., *103*:195, 1970.

46. Jewett, H. J.: Treatment of early cancer of the prostate. J.A.M.A., *183*:373, 1963.

47. Jewett, H. J.: Personal communication. April 9, 1970.

48. Hirst, A. E., Jr., and Bergman, R. T.: Carcinoma of the prostate in men eighty or more years old. Cancer, *7*:136, 1954.

49. Whitmore, W. F., Jr.: Hormone therapy in prostatic cancer. Am. J. Med., *21*:697, 1956.

50. Arduino, L. J., and Glucksman, M. A.: Lymph node metastases in early carcinoma of the prostate. J. Urol., *88*:91, 1962.

51. Flocks, R. H., et al.: Lymphatic spread from prostatic cancer. J. Urol., *81*:194, 1959.

52. McCullough, D. L., et al.: Carcinoma of the prostate and lymphatic metastases. J. Urol., *111*:65, 1974.

53. Whitmore, W. F., Jr., and Mackenzie, A. R.: Experiences with various operative procedures for the total excision of prostatic cancer. Cancer,

12:396, 1959.

54. McCullough, D. L., and Leadbetter, W. F.: Radical pelvic surgery for locally extensive carcinoma of the prostate. J. Urol., 108:939, 1972.

55. Flocks, R. H.: The treatment of Stage C prostatic cancer with specific reference to combined surgical and radiation therapy. J. Urol., 109:461, 1973.

56. Hilaris, B. S., et al.: Radiation therapy and pelvic node dissection in the management of cancer of the prostate. Am. J. Roentgenol., Radium Ther. Nucl. Med., 121:832, 1974.

57. Ganem, E. J.: The prognostic significance of an elevated serum acid phosphatase level in advanced prostatic carcinoma. J. Urol., 76:179, 1956.

58. Ganem, E. J.: Carcinoma of the prostate gland. 5-year survival following antiandrogenic treatment. J. Urol., 74:804, 1955.

59. A large portion of this text appeared in Cancer, 32:1096, 1973, under the title, Diagnosis and staging of prostatic carcinoma.

Chapter 11

Growth and Hormonal Response of Prostatic Tumors

ILSE LASNITZKI

Investigations into the effects of hormones on prostatic tumors serve first, to shed light on the role of hormones in the genesis of tumors and second, to evaluate the hormonal response of established tumors and apply the results to their clinical management.

In animal experiments the hormones to be investigated may be partially lost en route to the target organ or reach it in a modified form. Also, the nutritional, immunologic, and hormonal status of the host will alter the basic effects of the hormones and complicate the interpretation of experimental results. These factors are eliminated in an in vitro system, and the direct action of hormones can be studied on the cellular level under well-controlled experimental conditions. The hormone concentration and duration of exposure can be easily manipulated and the reproducibility of the experiments makes it possible to obtain both qualitative and quantitative data. Moreover, in vivo experiments on human prostatic tumors are extremely difficult to quantitate and interpret. They also represent a grave risk to the patient, and for these reasons alone tissue culture systems seem to be the best choice for experimental approach.

Cells or tissues are grown in vitro by various techniques. In earlier experiments, fragments of tissues were cultivated in clots consisting of blood plasma and embryo extract. The explants became surrounded by a halo of cells migrating from the central core of tissue. More recently, the cells were obtained by mechanical or enzymatic dissociation of tissue and grown in monolayer or suspension in semidefined or defined media. In both systems, cellular proliferation serves as the main criterion of effect. Organ culture techniques, on the other hand, aim at preventing the migration of cells from the explants and their replication. To achieve this, organs, or portions of organs, are cultivated on the surface of a plasma or agar clot or on metal rafts while the medium reaches the tissue by passive diffusion. In this way, the differentiated structure of the original tissue and its function are retained in vitro.

STEROID HORMONES AND RAT PROSTATE IN ORGAN CULTURE

Most basic information relating to the effects of androgens and antiandrogens has been obtained using organ cultures of rat prostate glands as experimental models. The organs consist of alveoli lined with secretory columnar epithelium separated by fine strands of fibromuscular stroma. The fine structure of the epithelium is typical of secretory cells and shows channels of rough endoplasmic reticulum, a well-defined Golgi zone and microvilli at the apical surface.[1]

The glands remain androgen-dependent and responsive in vitro. If grown in androgen-free medium, the organs regress in a similar manner as in animals following castration. The alveoli shrink and the epithelium becomes reduced in height, while secretory activity diminishes or is abolished. The rough endoplasmic reticulum collapses, the Golgi apparatus becomes disorganized, and the microvilli disappear. Electron-dense bodies make their appearance. These may be interpreted as autophagic vacuoles involved in the degradation of the degenerate cytoplasmic organelles.[2] Addition of testosterone to the medium prevents the regression and maintains epithelial height, secretory activity, and the fine structure of the cells.

It was discovered that, like the organ in vivo,[3] the isolated gland in culture converts testosterone to various metabolites. The major metabolite was dihydrotestosterone, which is found predominantly in the nuclear fraction. This was, in turn, converted to 3α-androstanediol and 3β-androstanediol. In addition, small amounts of androstenedione, androstanedione, and androsterone were formed.[4,5]

It was not certain whether these metabolites were biologically inactive products or had an activity of their own. Exposure of rat prostate glands in organ culture to the metabolites showed that they all possessed androgenic activity but of varying degree. Dihydrotestosterone was the most active androgen and at doses from 10^{-9} to 10^{-6}M, proved to be 10 times as efficient in preserving the epithelial height and fine structure of the epithelium than testosterone. In addition, the compound promoted the multiplication of the epithelial cells resulting, at higher doses, in epithelial hyperplasia; 3α-androstanediol and androsterone showed similar, though weaker androgenic effects, while 3β-androstanediol maintained cytoplasmic differentiation and stimulated secretory activity but did not promote epithelial cell proliferation even at high doses.[6]

These results suggest that the effect of testosterone is mediated by its metabolites, principally via the formation of dihydrotestosterone which acts at the nuclear level and is involved in both cell differentiation and cell renewal.

The human prostate gland and human prostatic tumors show a similar pattern of testosterone metabolism as the rat prostate.[7] The results obtained in the rat prostate are therefore relevant to the human gland and provide a valuable background and guide for the interpretation of hormonal effects in human prostatic hyperplasia or carcinoma.

BENIGN PROSTATIC HYPERPLASIA AND PROSTATIC CARCINOMA

In an early work, fragments of prostatic adenoma or carcinoma were grown in Carrel flasks on clots of chick plasma and chick embryo extract overlaid with dilute serum. The resulting area of outgrowth was used as a criterion of growth. Allgöwer[8] found that pieces of prostatic adenoma explanted in this way became surrounded by epithelial type cells which liquefied the plasma clot. Such liquefaction is usually associated with very active cellular growth. Röhl[9] studied the effect of androsterone on explants of adenocarcinoma and reported that the hormone promoted growth in some of these. Wojewski and Przeworska-Kaniewicz[10] set up a large number of explants from benign prostatic hyperplasia and adenocarcinoma. Half the number of adenoma explanted, but only 17% of the carcinoma explants showed outgrowth which was mainly fibroblastic. Testosterone (5–25 μg/ml medium) and stilbestrol (20–200 μg/ml medium) inhibited the outgrowth.

Thus, in many explants the tissue remained viable and supported cell migration and division in androgen-free medium. However, it would be difficult to quantify data obtained in this system, and the presence of hormones in the natural medium may complicate the interpretation of results. In cells grown in monolayer, hormonal effects could be more easily quantified and the use of semidefined or defined media would diminish or exclude the interference by other hormones.

Cell Culture

Fraley et al.[11] have established a cell line, MA 160, from a prostatic adenoma. The authors set up a large number of explant cultures which became surrounded by an outgrowth of spindle-shaped and epithelial-like cells. These became confluent and formed a monolayer which could be dissociated and transferred to new culture vessels. The medium used was Eagle's minimal essential medium (MEM),[12] supplemented with glutamic acid and fetal bovine serum. The cells have now been carried through more than 500 passages. They are epithelioid, and their fine structure is characteristic of a secretory cell; the cytoplasm reveals abundant rough endoplasmic recticulum, a well-organized Golgi zone, and microvilli at the cell surface. Examination by the Burstone technique[13] shows that the cells synthesize functional, i.e., tartrate-inhibitable acid phosphatase.[14]

Normally, human adult cells have a finite life span in culture. The long survival of MA 160 in vitro suggests that the cells have undergone spontaneous transformation. This interpretation is supported by the profound change in growth and cytology of the adenoma cells which exhibit all the features characteristic of such transformation: rapid growth, heteroploidy, and most important of all, they form tumors on injection into the cheek pouch of immunosuppressed hamsters.[15] Cells from later passages grew also in nonimmunosuppressed hamsters and induced a high incidence of tumors.[16]

The increased growth potential of MA 160 was associated with a change of testosterone metabolism. Benign prostatic hyperplasia, like the rat prostate, converts testosterone mainly by 5α reduction: the major metabolite is dihydrotestosterone, and only small amounts of androstenedione are formed.[7] Ofner[17] compared the metabolism of testosterone by MA 160 in cells from the 12th and 279th passage. In both, it was reductive, but cells from the later passage formed considerably less dihydrotestosterone than those from the earlier passages. However, in cells from the 400th passage, the metabolism had shifted toward a mainly oxidative pathway, and the major metabolite was androstenedione.[18]

MA 160 grows well in androgen-free medium,[19] but it was thought that steroid hormones might nevertheless influence the growth pattern or cell replication of the cell line. In an attempt to induce structural differentiation, the cells were grown in the presence of testosterone, its 5α metabolites and estradiol-17β, but none of the hormones reversed the anaplastic pattern of growth. On the other hand, cell multiplication was markedly affected by exposure to hormones. The cells were treated with testosterone, dihydrotestosterone, 3β-androstanediol, and estradiol-17β at concentrations ranging from 10^{-9}M to 10^{-5}M and the effect was expressed as increase in cell number over that of the untreated controls after six days' growth.[19]

Physiologic concentrations of testosterone and estradiol alike slightly increased the cell number. Dihydrotestosterone was more active and induced a higher degree of stimulation. In contrast, pharmacologic hormone concentrations severely depressed cell proliferation as their number fell progressively with rising concentrations, and at 10^{-5}M constituted only one-fifth of the control value. Similarly, Ban et al.[14] reported an inhibition of protein and acid phosphatase synthesis in MA 160 by pharmacologic doses of androgens, estrogens, and diethylstilbestrol. Diethylstilbestrol proved to be the most effective inhibitor.

These results clearly indicate that MA 160, although androgen independent, is still hormone sensitive and suggests the presence of androgen and estrogen receptors or their induction by the hormones in the transformed cells.

It has been claimed that MA 160, like other heteroploid cell lines, has been contaminated with HeLa cells.[20,21] The claim is based mainly on the presence of a rapidly moving compound of glucose-6-phosphate and chromosome markers characteristic for HeLa in MA 160 and other cell lines. However, MA 160 shows some features which do not fit HeLa. The cells synthesize functionally tartrate-inhibitable acid phosphatase, and their fine structure is typical of secretory cells. Further, it is not known whether HeLa cells metabolize testosterone, and a comparison of testosterone metabolism of MA 160 and HeLa should provide more decisive evidence for or against the theory of contamination.

Even if contamination with HeLa can be excluded, it is possible that the process of transformation alone may alter the sensitivity of the cells to steroid hormones and short-term cultures may be more suitable to relate hormonal effects in vitro to those of the patient.

Brehmer et al.[22] developed cell cultures from benign prostatic hyperplasia and carcinoma which grew in monolayer in androgen-free medium and remained viable for two to three months. They were established from explant cultures or by trypsinization of the original tumor tissue. The medium used was Eagle's basal medium (BME) with 10% fetal calf serum. The authors expressed cell growth in terms of plating efficiency, i.e., as the percentage of colonies developed from the seeding of single cells.[23] In androgen-free medium, the plating efficiency of cells from the carcinomas was two to four times higher than that of cells from the benign hyperplasia.

Testosterone in low doses increased the plating efficiency of the carcinoma cells; high doses decreased it in cells from the benign hyperplasia but did not affect the growth of the carcinoma cells. Estrone, like testosterone, increased the plating efficiency in both types of cells at low concentrations, while higher doses reduced it. Diethylstilbestrol was more effective than estrone and inhibited the plating efficiency at lower concentrations. With both compounds the inhibition was more pronounced in the carcinoma cells.

Apart from cellular growth the synthesis of functional acid phosphatase is another useful indicator of hormonal effects. Schroeder and Mackensen[24] reported that in cell cultures derived from human prostatic carcinomas, testosterone significantly increased the content of the enzyme in the epithelium.

The cultures consisted of two different cell types: polygonal or rounded cells obviously derived from the prostatic epithelium, and spindle-shaped elements from the fibrous stroma; in cultures derived from an active carcinoma the polygonal type predominated.

The fine structure of carcinoma cells growing in monolayer resembled that of the tumor in vivo.[25] The cytoplasm revealed channels of rough endoplasmic reticulum, free polysomes, and a great number of vacuoles and vesicles. Numerous desmosomes could be observed between adjacent cells as well as intercellular spaces characteristic for prostatic carcinoma cells invading connective tissue.[26]

Since the hormonal response may differ substantially in epithelium and stroma, it would be advantageous to separate the two cell types in culture. Kaighn et al.[27] attempted to produce pure cultures of either epithelium or fibroblasts by cloning cell suspensions of benign prostatic hyperplasia. The clones were grown in F12 K medium with 17% fetal calf serum. Some of them appeared to be epithelial and showed polygonal nonmotile cells with a highly active membrane. If consistently successful, the method would provide a useful model to study the action of hormones and their metabolism on epithelial and stromal tumor elements separately.

Wishnow[28] adapted an SV 40 transformed tumor of the hamster prostate[29] to grow in monolayer and found that the effect of hormones on the tumor cells in vitro was similar to that induced on the tumors in vivo. Pharmacologic concentrations of estradiol-17β and testosterone prolonged the generation time from 20 to 30 hours and decreased intracellular acid phosphatase by 20%. At still higher concentrations, both hormones suppressed cell growth completely and inhibited protein synthesis.

Stonington and Hemmingsen[30] used cells from benign prostatic hyperplasia to produce cytotoxic antibodies. The cells were grown in monolayer and then injected into rabbits, baboons, or human subjects and were associated with human peripheral lymphocytes. If successful, the production of antibodies specific to individual tumors would be an important step toward the control of tumor growth by immunotherapy.

Cells grown in monolayer seem a useful system to evaluate and quantify hormonal effects on cellular growth. But it must be remembered that several weeks elapse between the removal of the tumor from the patient and the establishment of the cells in culture, and during this time a selection of cells best adapted to in vitro conditions takes place. These cells may no longer be representative of the more heterogeneous cell population of the original tumor. Moreover, stromal elements form a substantial part of both the hyperplastic tissue and the carcinomas and the expression of hormonal action may depend on an intact epithelial-stromal relationship.[31]

Organ cultures retain most of the features of the parent tissue and epithelium and stroma, and their anatomic relationship is preserved in vitro. Portions of the hyperplastic tissue or carcinoma can be explanted directly after removal from the patient and the effect of hormones assessed within a few days. The evaluation of hormonal effects in this system is not limited to cellular replication but includes epithelial differentiation and secretory activity as important criteria.

Organ Culture

Schrodt and Foreman were the first to explant prostatic adenomas in organ culture.[32] Fragments of suitable size were grown for up to nine days by a modified Trowell technique[33] on thin slices of agar placed on grids of tantalum mesh. During the first three days, epithelium and stroma were well preserved and most explants showed alveoli lined with columnar secretory cells. The fine structure of the cells resembled that described by Brandes et al. for the fresh tissue.[1] The epithelium showed channels of rough endoplasmic reticulum and was abundant in secretory vacuoles. In the older cultures, the epithelium was often low columnar and occasionally underwent squamous metaplasia. The fine structure of such cells revealed bundles of intracytoplasmic filaments resembling those of tonofibrils in squamous epithelium. Explants treated with testosterone propionate showed large areas of necrosis.

Using a similar technique, McMahon and Thomas[34] examined the effect of testosterone and stilbestrol diphosphate on the growth and maintenance of benign prostatic hyperplasia. The tissue was grown in Eagle's basal medium supplemented with insulin and fetal calf serum. After one week in androgen-free medium, most explants showed well-preserved alveoli embedded in fibromuscular stroma. Some alveoli were lined with columnar, others with cuboidal cells, and in some areas the secretory cells had undergone squamous metaplasia. Addition of testosterone or stilbestrol diphosphate did not alter the morphology of the epithelium or stroma. Harbitz et al.[35] examined the effects of testosterone, dihydrostestosterone, estradiol-17β, progesterone, and cyproterone acetate on human benign prostatic hyperplasia grown in Trowell medium. The epithelium and its enzymes were well maintained in androgen-free medium, and none of the hormones altered epithelial morphology and the normal enzyme pattern or affected DNA synthesis.

McRae et al.[36] studied the effect of testosterone on glucose utilization, and acid phosphatase and DNA synthesis in organ cultures of benign hyperplasia grown in Eagle's basal medium in Leighton tubes. During the first four days, the epithelium was shed into the alveolar lumen and was gradually replaced during the next four days. Glucose utilization was similar in control and testosterone-treated cultures. In contrast, acid phosphatase content was raised in about half the explants, and DNA synthesis was slightly elevated in most explants.

Lasnitzki et al. correlated the effect of testosterone, dihydrotestosterone, 3β-androstanediol, and estradiol-17β on epithelial morphology with that on RNA synthesis.[37] The tissue was grown by a modified Trowell technique in Parker's medium 199[38] supplemented with 10% fetal calf serum. In explants grown in control medium, the epithelium showed evidence of squamous transformation. Testosterone and dihydrotestosterone prevented the squamous changes and preserved the secretory character of the cells; in addition, dihydrotestosterone increased epithelial proliferation beyond that seen in control and the other hormone treated explants. In contrast to the androgens, estradiol-17β caused cellular breakdown including the loss and shedding of the secretory epithelium.

The changes in cytology were reflected in variations of RNA synthesis studied by autoradiographic techniques. Testosterone and dihydrotestosterone raised the incorporation of (^{3}H)-uridine into RNA in both the prostatic epithelium and the cells of the smooth muscle while estradiol reduced it. This effect was more pronounced in the epithelium.

McMahon et al.[39] grew prostatic carcinomas in organ culture for periods from four days to one week. Two of them were poorly to moderately differentiated and showed acinar formation; the third tumor was anaplastic and showed islands of clear cells embedded in the stroma. All three tumors were very well preserved after four days' growth in non-supplemented control medium, and their histologic structure closely resembled that of the tissue of origin. Treatment with testosterone for the same period stimulated the differentiation of the prostatic epithelium. This effect was clearly related to the degree of differentiation of the original tissues. In the moderately differentiated tumors, alveolar formation was promoted and cell height increased due to a hypertrophy of the supranuclear area. In the anaplastic tumor, attempts at alveolar formation were observed, but were in this case accompanied by increased mitotic activity of the epithelium. Exposure to stilbestrol diphosphate did not affect the tissue adversely, and both growth and preservation of the histologic structure were similar to those in explants kept in control medium.

SUMMARY AND CONCLUSIONS

In conclusion, this review shows that under suitable conditions, benign prostatic hyperplasia and carcinoma can be maintained in cell or organ culture.

In contrast to the rodent prostate, which remains androgen-dependent in vitro, cells or tissue from the hyperplastic tissue or from carcinomas grow in medium without added androgens. This growth pattern is not due to the traces of androgens present in the sera used for cultivation.[24] Androgen-independent growth occurs in the transformed cell line MA 160, in short-term cultures from both benign prostatic hyperplasia and carcinomas, and in organ cultures explanted shortly after removal from the patient. Therefore, it is unlikely that this property has been acquired during cell transformation or cell selection or is due to a loss of hormonal receptor sites.

The retention of hormonal receptors is also indicated by the fact that growth can still be affected by treatment with steroid hormones. At pharmacologic concentrations, testosterone inhibits growth in MA 160 and in short-term cell cultures; at physiologic or near physiologic concentrations, the hormone promotes cell replication in the cell line and raises acid phosphatase synthesis in cell cultures derived from carcinomas. Interestingly, estrogens and testosterone produce similar effects: estrone, estradiol, and stilbestrol at pharmacologic concentrations suppress cell growth; estrone and estradiol promote it at physiologic doses.

In organ culture, the effects of hormones are not confined to growth but include maintenance of structural differentiation, of epithelial height and secretory activity as important criteria. Surprisingly, testosterone stimulated differentiation in carcinomas in organ cul-ture and enhanced alveolar formation and epithelial height. In this context it is interesting that Prout and Brewer[40] found that some patients with prostatic carcinoma improved after treatment with testosterone propionate.

In benign prostatic hyperplasia in organ culture, the results relating to androgen independence of growth and maintenance are in close agreement, but those concerned with hormonal response are still controversial. McMahon and Thomas,[34] and Harbitz et al.[35] reported a failure of steroid hormones to modify the growth and morphology of the epithelium and its enzymes. In contrast, preservation of secretory function accompanied by a corresponding increase in RNA synthesis by androgens was demonstrated by Lasnitzki et al.[37] The change in RNA synthesis applied to the epithelium as well as to the cells of the smooth muscle and suggest that the latter is also hormone sensitive.

It is not certain whether the behavior of tumors in vitro reflects that of the tissue in vivo, and many more observations are needed to relate hormonal response in culture to that of individual patients. To simulate the more complex conditions in vivo, it would be important to study the effects of a wide range of hormone concentrations, examine the interaction of androgens with other hormones or factors involved in prostatic growth, and correlate the results with a study of receptors and testosterone metabolism.

References

1. Brandes, D., et al.: Ultrastructure of the human prostate: Normal and neoplastic. Lab. Invest., 13:1541, 1964.
2. Gittinger, J. W., and Lasnitzki, I.: The effect of testosterone and testosterone metabolites on the fine structure of the rat prostate gland in organ culture. J. Endocr., 52:459, 1972.
3. Bruchovsky, N., and Wilson, J. D.: The conversion of testosterone to 5α-androstan-17β-ol-3-one by rat prostate in vivo and in vitro. J. Biol. Chem., 243:2012, 1968.
4. Baulieu, E. E., et al.: Metabolism of testosterone and action of metabolites on prostate glands grown in organ culture. Nature, 219:1155, 1968.

5. Robel, P., et al.: Hormone metabolism and action; Testosterone and metabolites in prostate organ culture. Biochemie, 53:81, 1971.

6. Lasnitzki, I.: The rat prostate gland in organ culture. Some Aspects of the Aetiology and Biochemistry of Prostatic Cancer. In Third Tenovus Workshop. Edited by K. Griffiths and C. G. Pierrepoint. Cardiff, Tenovus Workshop Publication, 1970.

7. Siiteri, P. K., and Wilson, J. D.: Dihydrotestosterone in prostatic hypertrophy. 1. The formation and content of dihydrotestosterone in the hypertrophic prostate of man. J. Clin. Invest., 49:1737, 1970.

8. Allgöwer, M.: The cultivation of human prostate adenomata in vitro. Exp. Cell Res. Suppl. 1:456, 1949.

9. Röhl, L.: Prostatic hyperplasia and carcinoma studied with tissue culture technique. Acta Chir. Scand. [Suppl.] 240:1, 1959.

10. Wojewski, A., and Przeworska-Kaniewicz, D.: The influence of stilbestrol and testosterone on the growth of prostatic adenoma and carcinoma in tissue culture. J. Urol., 93:721, 1965.

11. Fraley, E. E., et al.: Spontaneous in vitro neoplastic transformation of adult human prostatic epithelium. Science, 170:540, 1970.

12. Eagle, H.: Nutrition needs of mammalian cells in tissue culture. Science, 122:501, 1955.

13. Burstone, M. S.: Histochemical comparison of naphthol AS-phosphates for the demonstration of phosphatases, J. Natl. Cancer Inst., 20:601, 1958.

14. Ban, R. W., et al.: Hormonal effects on prostatic acid phosphatase synthesis in tissue culture. Invest. Urol., 11:308, 1974.

15. Fraley, E. E., and Ecker, S.: Tumor production in immune-suppressed hamsters by spontaneously transformed human prostatic epithelium. J. Urol., 106:95, 1971.

16. Richman, A. V., et al.: Heterotransplantation of human prostatic adenoma cells, MA 150, into nonimmunosuppressed hamsters. Cancer Res., 32:2186, 1972.

17. Ofner, P.: Recent developments in the study of hormone effects and metabolism in prostatic tissue. Deutsche Ges. Endokrinol. Sympos., 17:147, 1971.

18. Lasnitzki, I.: Testosterone metabolism in human prostatic tumours. Cancer Res. Camp. Report. In press, 1974.

19. Lasnitzki, I.: The effect of testosterone, testosterone metabolites and oestradiol on the growth of MA 160 (in preparation).

20. Gartler, S. M.: Apparent HeLa cell contamination of human heteroploid cell lines. Nature, 217:750, 1968.

21. Nelson-Rees, W. A., et al.: Banded marker chromosomes as indicators of intraspecies cellular contamination. Science, 184:1093, 1974.

22. Brehmer, B., et al.: Growth and hormonal response of cells derived from carcinoma and hyperplasia of the prostate in monolayer cell culture. A possible in vitro model for clinical chemotherapy. J. Urol., 108:890, 1972.

23. Puck, T. T., et al.: Clonal growth of mammalian cells in vitro. Growth characteristics of colonies from single HeLa cells with and without a "feeder" layer. J. Exp. Med., 103:273, 1956.

24. Schroeder, F. H., and Mackensen, S. J.: Human prostatic adenoma and carcinoma in cell culture. The effects of androgen-free culture medium. Invest. Urol., 12:176, 1974.

25. Kirchheim, D., and Bacon, R. L.: Ultrastructural studies of carcinoma of the human prostate gland. Invest. Urol., 6:611, 1969.

26. Brehmer, B., et al.: Electron microscopic appearance of cells from carcinoma of the prostate in monolayer tissue culture. Urol. Res., 1:27, 1973.

27. Kaighn, M. E., et al.: Clonal Isolation and Characterisation of human prostatic adenoma cells. Abstract, Proceed. Am. Society for Cell Biol, 1974.

28. Wishnow, R. M.: The effect of sex hormones on the growth of SV 40 transformed hamster prostate cells. In Vitro, 6:385, 1971.

29. Fraley, E. E., and Paulson, D. F.: Morphological and biochemical studies on virus (SV 40) transformed prostatic tissue. J. Urol., 101:735, 1969.

30. Stonington, O. G., and Hemmingsen, H.: Culture of cells as a monolayer derived from the epithelium of the human prostate: A new cell growth technique. J. Urol., 106:393, 1971.

31. Franks, L. M., et al.: A comparative study of the ultrastructure and lack of growth capacity of adult human prostate epithelium mechanically separated from its stroma. J. Path., 100:113, 1970.

32. Schrodt, G. R., and Foreman, C. D.: In vitro maintenance of human hyperplastic prostate tissue. Invest. Urol., 9:85, 1971.

33. Trowell, O. A.: The culture of mature organs in a synthetic medium. Exp. Cell. Res., 16:118, 1959.

34. McMahon, M. J., and Thomas, G. H.: Morphological changes of benign prostatic hyperplasia in culture. Br. J. Cancer, 27:323, 1973.

35. Harbitz, T. B., et al.: Benign hyperplasia of the human prostate exposed to steroid hormones in organ culture. Acta Path. Microbiol. Scand. Sect. A. Suppl., 248:89, 1974.

36. McRae, C. U., et al.: The effect of testosterone on the human prostate in organ culture. Br. J. Urol., 45:156, 1973.

37. Lasnitzki, I., et al.: The effect of steroid hormones on the growth pattern and RNA synthesis in human benign prostatic hyperplasia in organ culture. Br. J. Cancer. In press, 1975.

38. Morgan, J. F., et al.: Nutrition of animal cells in tissue culture. I. Initial studies on a synthetic medium. Proc. Soc. Exp. Biol. Med., 73:1, 1950.

39. McMahon, M. J., et al.: Morphological responses of prostatic carcinoma to testosterone in organ culture. Br. J. Cancer, 26:388, 1974.

40. Prout, G. R. Jr., and Brewer, W. R.: Response of men with advanced prostatic carcinoma to exogenous administration of testosterone. Cancer, 20:1871, 1967.

Part III

Management of Prostatic Disease

Chapter 12

Current Status of Therapy in Prostatic Cancer

GERALD P. MURPHY

In the consideration of the treatment of prostatic cancer, both in focal or disseminated conditions, any clinician may be influenced by the limited amount of information available to him. This presentation will primarily address itself to the current evaluation in early 1974 of prostatic cancer as we know it. Before outlining briefly our concepts of this complex problem, most believe it is of some value to consider the basis upon which we currently propose and carry out our clinical endeavors.

PATHOGENESIS AND EPIDEMIOLOGY

Knowledge of the distribution of prostatic cancer based on autopsy results can afford valuable information. Yet in consideration of the data banks or tumor registry information available throughout the United States and elsewhere, it is remarkable that so little has been done in this regard. Examination of the various sites of metastases and coordination of clinical results with the course of the disease can evolve hypotheses which are testable. These hypotheses afford us some knowledge of the routes of dissemination

of cancer. They have been beneficial in studying certain other solid tumor states such as breast cancer.[1] In such an evaluation, one considers the possibility whether the primary tumor metastasizes directly to a metastatic site or indirectly through another intermediate foci such as lymph node or bone. Present studies are now attempting to solve this problem.

There is some indication that prostatic cancer may well directly metastasize in some instances (and these may be a majority) to the bone and from the bone to other secondary organs. Such a hypothesis is based upon a venous route of dissemination. This in no way diminishes concern for the possibility of other pathways such as the lymphatic route. Although recent studies have been attempted in this regard,[2] a comprehensive assessment has not been completed to date. It goes without saying that in the main, prostatic cancer is frequently discovered as an advanced disseminated disease.[3]

Population studies for the identification of high-risk groups have concentrated mostly upon reported changing incidences among blacks, particularly those in the United States, as contrasted to an African population.[4] At the present time, one is unable to utilize this information in individual clinical judgements. However, it should obviously influence, to some degree, our vigilance in detection and surveillance in certain of our patients. It is apparently known by some, and accepted as gospel by others, that certain population groups have a low incidence of prostatic cancer.[5] What is interesting, however, is that the study of such population groups reveals some possible associated changes in incidence with their Americanization or with population moves. Other external factors, such as radiation, are suggestively also responsible for the appearance or detection of certain forms of prostatic cancer.

Whether one is concerned primarily with the biologic potential or latent activity is another matter.[6] On the basis of present established clinical information, many do not think it possible for us to take a position as regards treatment concerning latent prostatic cancer. This is a matter for individual judgement. The reported various detection rates ranging from 2 to 27%[6] will not, at present, entirely resolve the problem. For that matter, such a statement that more study must be done, provides no help to those clinicians faced with this dilemma. Thus, although prostatic cancer is largely a disease of westernized countries, it can be found in the developing world, but the information at present, to our limited understanding, will not affect our treatment considerations. The studies under way sponsored by various cooperative groups including the National Prostatic Cancer Project of the National Cancer Institute will, in the future, lend some further information on this topic in terms of incidence and prevalence rates and perhaps the significance of latent and biologically active prostatic cancer.

Hormonal influences are possibly operative in adult aging males and bear some relationship to prostatic cancer as well as benign hypertrophy. It is known, for example, on the basis of selected and limited studies, that pituitary adenomas occur more frequently in relation to prostatic carcinoma than to other histologic groups.[7] Such autopsy information suggests a hormonal factor that has perhaps not been heretofore considered. These studies can bring to light additional information about prostatic cancer and its hormone-related state and probably provide further insight into benign hyperplastic conditions.[8] Other studies have suggested a relationship with the declining numbers of Sertoli cells in the testes associated with the age of male patients. Unfortunately, however, such studies usually demonstrate some association with benign prostatic hypertrophy alone or with prostatic cancer.[9]

The significant relationship with hyperplasia remains and to my knowledge at this time no definitive studies have evolved a direct association with prostatic cancer. The view that Sertoli cells produce steroid hormones is, of course, well founded but it is not clear at the present time whether these cells in man produce androgens, estrogens, or both, and how these relationships change over time. Other previous studies[7–9] suggest an interaction which could be further explored with benefit in man and undoubtedly contribute to the possible clinical therapy of prostatic cancer, even perhaps to its prevention.

THE ENDOCRINE BASIS FOR TREATMENT

An era of radioimmunoassay and tissue culture studies have afforded us a possibility to study prostatic cancer, perhaps even the isolated prostatic cell. We are, however, unable to make definitive statements at the present time concerning how these factors will influence our clinical decisions. There are additional important effects of hypophysectomy and adrenalectomy that have already been utilized in the clinical state. Because of these and other recent information, it is important that such considerations be reviewed prior to the clinical recommendations for therapy. It is accepted by most that within the various experimental species there are differences, for example, in rat and baboon. However despite this, there is sufficient evidence concerning the peripheral control of hormonal metabolism. Several of the enzymes involved, such as 5-alpha reductase system, may play a regulatory role in the control of important cellular feedback mechanisms.[10] The interruption of such mechanisms by hypophysectomy or perhaps on an androgen influenced state by castration[11] may have heretofore unsuspected and unmeasurable effects that influence the population of prostatic cancer cells in patients that receive objective benefit from such hormonal manipulation.

We are all well acquainted with the importance of the patient's prior cardiovascular status as well as the fluid and electrolyte considerations during certain forms of endocrine treatment such as estrogen administration.[12] At the present time, it is the obvious viewpoint that studies of zinc-binding proteins and the like are suitable subjects for research projects involving benign prostatic hyperplasia but these have not yet progressed sufficiently to merit clinical consideration in prostatic cancer states.[13] Such a situation, of course, could undoubtedly rapidly change with improvement of currently available techniques as well as the availability to study isolated prostatic cells.

Within the past two years, however, considerable information, chiefly from the rat ventral prostate model, has suggested that there are some species related prostatic specific androgen-receptor sites. What is surprising is that these sites can now be identified in the nuclei of prostatic cancer cells as well as in the cytoplasm.[14] Further attempts at isolation of such receptor sites are currently undergoing advanced and sophisticated biochemical characterization.[14] It is, however, not experimentally possible to precisely demonstrate the interaction of steroids in regard to their uptake by individual prostatic cells. Such experimental systems at the present have been confined mostly to the normal or hyperplastic tissues in the dog and the intact rat.[15]

These studies revealed important differences in hormonal sensitivity of normal prostate cells which may possibly be extrapolated to the clinical cancer state. For example, the uptake of progesterone by prostate has not been shown to significantly reduce in vitro ^3H hormonal uptake, e.g., of estrogens.[16] Such endeavors have a most important basis for further clinical therapeutic considerations. Interference with the 5-alpha reductase system[17] appears to be a promising area for categorizing agents, whether they be hormonal or not, in terms of their possible ability to affect abnormal prostatic growth. In this instance, we are concerned with prostatic growth as studied in animal models.

Already, however, correlations are possible between such animal systems and the current therapeutic trials under way by the National Prostatic Cancer Program of the National Cancer Institute involving clinical trials of 5-Fluorouracil (5-FU) and Cytoxan in advanced cases. Such type of chemotherapy screening was initially completed in our own laboratories with the help of many people.[18] This will have to serve as a temporary technique or method of study until further advances are accomplished.

There have been few hormonal studies of the effects of antiandrogens on prostatic cancer states in man.[19] Such studies, of course, have provided some data but do not yet yield sufficient information as to the clinical value of such compounds in the long term state. It would appear at the present time, despite the gaps in research and clinical studies, that a majority of the antiandrogens have some sort of biochemical activity as a common denominator for their biologic effects directly or indirectly on the prostate, and that this is usually involved with inhibition of specific steroid activity in cytosol or the nucleus of the prostatic cell.[20] Immunologic studies of such cellular activities also provide further information concerning specific prostatic antigens which may or may not be androgen dependent.[21] Were such information clinically available today, our recommendations for therapy would be profoundly altered and perhaps, may well be in the future. Newer types of antiandrogens that have been studied by others and also in our own laboratories[22] may well act, not as the molecule is conceptualized in the laboratory or administered to the subject, but as a result of unknown in vivo metabolic alteration and perhaps inactivation.[22]

We have not yet stated that there are other analogs of stilbestrol available for possible utilization.[23] Such analogs under clinical trial may provide further worthwhile information to conduct clinical treatment of both prostatic cancer and hyperplasia. Examples of these are studies that reveal potentially important changes in the tissue receptiveness to estrone, estradiol-17 beta, estriol and the like.[24] For that matter, it is experimentally possible now on a dose-base relationship to show that the simultaneous administration of estradiol and testosterone may have a dose-related effect that has not heretofore been understood.[25] While such studies may provide some insight into the appropriateness of our current forms of clinical therapy, they are not yet improved to the point of making other practical clinical suggestions.

One cannot discuss the current changing facets of the treatment of prostatic cancer without considering these features at some point. Recommendations have been recently made for monitoring plasma testosterone as an accurate monitor of the adequacy of hormonal treatment.[26] While such studies can be done as a result of current improvements in radioimmunoassay and while they may indicate some helpful clinical data, they really do not reflect to an accurate degree the hormonal status of the patient. Studies of hypophysectomized and adrenalectomized patients in our own laboratories reveal that the state of androgenicity of any prostatic cancer patient is more accurately reflected by measurement of 11-deoxy fraction of the 17-ketosteroids in the urine on a 24-hour basis.[27,28] With the availability of gas-liquid chromatography such studies are practical and provide meaningful quantitative data.

The consideration of only the plasma compartment of the available androgen supply in the dynamic state of man does not reflect such turnover rates and may lead to inappropriate conclusions considering the adequacy of perhaps 1 mg of stilbestrol versus a higher dose. One does not think such studies based on plasma hormonal assays, particularly that of testosterone, are therefore totally adequate. They are, however, an improvement over what was available for many. If others had measured the urinary androgens as noted,[27,28] further clinical observations relevant to the state of prostatic cancer therapy and its management could doubtless have been achieved. We have said nothing of the clinical-pharmacologic studies under way which provide important and new observations with reference to the use of hormonal agents as vehicles to achieve intracellular prostatic chemotherapy.

A recent study describing the use of an antiprostatic agent, Estracyt [estradiol-3bis(2-chloroethyl)carbamate-17-dihydrogen phosphate] (A. B. Leo Company, Hälsovägen, Sweden) has been published.[29] This also reflects a whole new area of therapy which is only now under way and perhaps by the time of the publication of this book may be further evolved. Review of present animal models[30,31] does suggest that both individual chemotherapy and additional combinations can be screened through such systems. These screening procedures have been of proven benefit in some forms of leukemia and solid tumors. We do not, however, at the present time have an animal tumor model that is immediately relevant to the clinical state of prostatic cancer.

Diagnostic Considerations

The therapy we undertake for prostatic cancer patients today has been profoundly influenced by certain advances in clinical diagnostic techniques. One cannot discuss the treatment of prostatic cancer without some reference to the improvement in screening patients for occult bony metastases.[32] Such studies in addition to those concerned with measurement of acid and alkaline phosphatases are of considerable benefit. We have not fully developed assay methods that utilize biochemical techniques concerned with isozyme measurement of acid phosphatases.[33] Such information is available and may well provide another technique for purification and characterization of prostate specific acid phos-

phatase enzymes. Occult or latent prostatic cancer in the individual patient remains a clinical dilemma. Such problems may be further benefited by mass screening techniques for detection of prostatic cancer based upon such immunoassay availability. These studies have not yet been totally settled in the laboratory nor have the application of such endeavors been fully achieved. It is hoped, however, that this will be the case.

Other limitations concerned with prostatic biopsy, LDH measurements and the like have been recently adequately reviewed.[34] Tumor specific or tumor associated antigens are not totally accepted by all and remain, at present, an area of clinical prostatic cancer investigation. They are, however, being developed and cannot be ignored even at the present time, for with some improvement, they may be available for additional diagnostic considerations.

We thus have a number of biochemical tests for prostatic cancer, some of which are established, others of which are under evaluation (Table 12–1). These may be of help in the patient initially seen with prostatic cancer and evaluating him for his hormonal therapy or for primary operative treatment or for radiation therapy. If one, however, considers the patient who has relapsed from conventional hormonal therapy in a state of advanced disease, the diagnostic correla-

Table 12–1

Biochemical tests for prostatic cancer

1.	Serum acid phosphatase
2.	Bone marrow acid phosphatase
3.	Alkaline phosphatase
4.	Alkaline phosphatase isoenzyme
5.	Lactate dehydrogenase
6.	Lactate dehydrogenase isoenzyme
7.	Plasma carcinoembryonic antigen
8.	Urinary androgen fractionation
9.	Urinary androgen ratio of deoxy and oxy 17-ketosteroids
10.	Total urinary cholesterol

tions with other parameters in the progression of the disease are not always consistent.

As shown in Table 12–2, acid phosphatase, the 11-deoxy-oxy urinary androgen ratio as well as urinary cholesterol seems to achieve some limited consistency which is, however, not uniform. The same is true for patients in correlating these various parameters with the regression of their disease after relapse and after conventional therapy (Table 12–3). Since

Table 12–2

Correlation of certain biochemical factors and progression of disease in prostatic cancer patients who have had prior endocrine therapy

Group	Change in Parameter			
	Acid Phosphatase	Androgen Ratio[a]	Urinary Cholesterol	No. of Patients
1	↑ [b]	↑	↑	1
2	↑	—	↑	5
3	↑	↓	↑	4
4	↑	↑	—	1
5	↑	—	↑	3
6	↑	—	↓	1
7	—	—	↑	1
8	↓	—	↓	1
			Total	17

[a]Ratio of deoxy to oxy urinary 17-ketosteroids
[b] ↑ : Increase, ↓ : Decrease, —: Stable in normal range

Table 12–3

Correlation of biochemical tests with regulation of disease in patients with advanced prostatic cancer who have received new investigational drugs

Group	Change in Parameter			
	Acid Phosphatase	Androgen Ratio[a]	Urinary Cholesterol	No. of Patients
1	↓ [b]	↓	↓	4
2	↓	↓	↑	2
3	↓	↓	—	1
4	↑	↓	↓	4
5	—	↓	↓	3
6	↓	↑	↓	3
7	↓	—	↓	1
8	—	—	↓	1
9	↑	↓	↑	1
10	—	↓	—	1
11	↑	↓	—	1
12	—	—	—	2
13	—	—	—	1
			Total	25

[a]Ratio of deoxy to oxy urinary 17-ketosteroids
[b] ↑ : Increase, ↓ : Decrease, —: Stable in normal range

most of these patients are in a state of disseminated disease which is obviously clinically widespread to some degree and who have received prior endocrine therapy, these new parameters are of help in evaluating such new agents as Estracyt or, for that matter, other forms of chemotherapy currently under clinical trials by the National Prostatic Cancer Project of the National Cancer Institute.

Current Status of Clinical Therapy of Prostatic Cancer

We have previously alluded to a lack of data base concerning the treatment of prostatic cancer in our own geographic regions as well as perhaps some limitations on a national American scope. One is frequently asked "Where are all the prostatic nodules?" In addition, the statement that most patients present with advanced prostatic cancer, has been reasonably questioned by some. The age relationship between diagnosis and first detection of the disease has remained a matter of controversy in the literature and despite this, is still a matter that will influence our therapies whether they be radical surgery, radiation treatment, or chemotherapy.

For the past few years in Western New York, Roswell Park Memorial Institute has assisted in developing a regional tumor registry with a capacity of 42 hospitals. We thus have, at the present time, complete figures for 1972 which give one some idea, for our region, of what prostatic cancer is, not only in terms of what is seen or referred to a categorical center such as Roswell Park, but more importantly, an impression in terms of the many practicing clinicians, surgeons, and urologists throughout the area who are faced with this current dilemma.[35]

Insight into this matter provides an appropriate basis for recommendations for treatment with which we have some experience at our center. If such information were available elsewhere in the

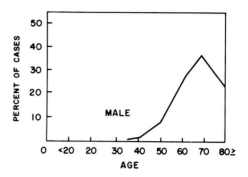

Figure 12–1. Age distribution for males when first diagnosed as having prostatic cancer in Western New York.

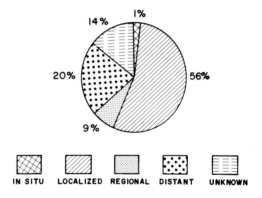

Figure 12–2. Distribution of 1972 prostatic cancer in Western New York.

United States, undoubtedly it would contribute to further resolution of the problem and perhaps less geographic bias. However, since this information, at present, is the only one of its kind, it is appropriate to include it in a discussion about the treatment of prostatic cancer. As shown in Figure 12–1, the majority of patients seen in Western New York, when first diagnosed with prostatic cancer, are above 60 years of age. This suggests some limitations concerning the suitability of patients available for the radical operation. Equally important, however, is the distribution of the stage of prostatic cancer when first diagnosed in our area (Figure 12–2). Less than 1% reflect the so-called nodular localized disease—a small number in view of the many other patients who have regional, distant, or perhaps unknown prostatic cancer states.

On follow-up, we have found most of the "unknowns" were those with diffuse metastases. Thus, as one sees, although there are patients available for the radical operation who have a small Stage B or perhaps even a more multifocal Stage B, there are not a large number of patients presenting who are suitable candidates for one of the modalities of therapy. Faced with this perplexing problem, it is no surprise that, as shown in Table 12–4, when such patients are first seen, they receive a myriad of treatments usually for the relief of symptoms of prostatic obstruction with some variation in hormonal therapy, or radiation treatment, or possibly clinical chemotherapy. Table 12–4 reflects adequately, in our opinion, some of the limitations that we are all experiencing concerning the resolution of the problems that have been reviewed to a limited degree in this chapter.

Despite these limitations, one must make recommendations and certainly those that are suitable for the management of patients. As Jewett[36] has pointed out, the radical perineal operation does not allow for node dissection, but suprapubic lymphadenectomy for involved nodes at the time of his original discourse had never been shown to increase the 15 year survival rate. It has been suggested that lymph node dissection may appropriately follow the perineal operation in suitable cases.[36] Jewett feels that nodes are involved in no more than 7% of the cases in the limited nodule stage. In his opinion, it seems likely that when pelvic retroperitoneal and hypogastric nodes have been involved, more distant spread already existed.[36] On the basis of an evolving study not yet completed at Roswell Park Memorial Institute, we would concur with this viewpoint. Generally, most agree with Jewett's viewpoint and limit the operation to those patients having a good prospect for cure as has been outlined. Lattimer has recently stated that he does not do pelvic lymph node dissections except for diagnostic purposes and to possibly mark palpable nodes for future radiotherapy.[37]

Table 12–4

An example of the variety of treatments given in 1972 to western New York cancer patients[a]

Treatment	Local[b]	Regional	Distant	Unknown	Total
Surgery	80	2	10	12	104
Radiation	—	1	1	—	2
Surgery, radiation	2	—	—	—	2
Surgery, chemotherapy	1	—	—	—	1
Radiation, chemotherapy	1	—	—	—	1
Hormone	13	6	24	11	54
Surgery, hormone	59	10	13	14	96
Radiation, hormone	—	1	2	1	4
Surgery, radiation, hormone	—	—	2	—	2
Chemotherapy, hormone	—	—	1	—	1
Surgery, chemotherapy, hormone	—	1	2	—	3
None	29	8	12	8	57
Total	185	29	67	46	327

[a]327 cases; 5.5% of cases in Lakes Area Regional Tumor Service Registry.
[b]Includes in situ.

On the other hand, Flocks has shown in a series of 91 patients who had extraprostatic extension but did not have any evidence of metastases, that a combination of total prostatectomy plus interstitial radiation gave an incidence of four patients with local recurrence in a period of over 10 years.[38] In contrast, where simply microscopic extraprostatic extension was present, the incidence of local recurrence was 25% in three series followed five years or more. In Flocks' opinion, therefore, interstitial radiation and possibly also external radiation may be utilized satisfactorily in combination with local removal of the entire prostate.[38] Interstitial radiation can be utilized to treat recurrences after 6000 to 7000 rads of external radiation by placing radioactive seeds or the liquid colloidal solution of radioactive gold into the area where the recurrence is taking place.[38] Adenocarcinoma of the prostate can also present as rectal tumors with intestinal obstruction. It is well appreciated that radiation in these situations can afford suitable palliation and local tumor destruction.[39]

Thus, a combination of surgery and node dissection following radiation of the prostate has been prescribed by some. Review of current urologic practice in most major comprehensive centers does not, however, suggest that this program is under intensive pursuit.[40] The knowledge of it, of course, and of its benefit, must not go unrecognized. On the other hand, we are all aware of the complications of such radiation therapy with or without surgery, as has been recently reported.[41] External radiation, in addition to relieving a rectal obstruction, may provide benefit to patients in an objective fashion in terms of relieving ureteral obstruction.[42] In our present review, we are thus discussing all the various forms of adenocarcinoma of the prostate.

The limited information concerning sarcomas[43] or other such variants of prostatic cancer[44] are so rare that one does not feel that commentary concerning their role in the treatment of prostate cancer is appropriate. Undoubtedly, as is relevant, they will be covered in other chapters in this presentation. Equally true are the rare and unusual presenting metastases in prostatic cancer.[45,46] While these may afford important clinical information, they do not provide suitable generalizations for clinical management of local disease.

Thus far in the clinical management of the primary tumor of what would be equivalent to Stage B or, in the opinion of some, Stage C, we have reviewed the current status of radiation therapy to some degree in combination with a radical operation as well as other forms of treatment. Additional reviews provide follow-up information for the management of both primary and metastatic carcinoma of the prostate from the viewpoint of the radiotherapist.[47] A limited number of patients are available for treatment with excision of localized nodules or some form of radical surgery. The role of radiation therapy has been discussed and controversy concerning its complications and the histologic persistence of tumor as evidenced by biopsy in subsequent years, still rages.

Rather than be concerned with radiation therapy as the sole modality, it is more appropriate, in the opinion of some, to consider the types of radiation therapy that have been described as being beneficial, whether they be external radiation therapy, interstitial implant, or equally importantly, other types of linear acceleration therapy that have shown some clinical response. The majority of studies have suggested that radiation therapy at a high dose to the pelvis may provide some benefit. There is disagreement as to how long this benefit lasts or in what stage it can be provided. A comprehensive program has been instituted by Bagshaw and associates and sponsored by the National Prostatic Cancer Project. This program is concerned with alternating radiation therapy to the axial skeleton with pelvic lymph node biopsy in order to suitably stage and histologically grade both the primary tumor and its possible dissemination. Radiation of the pathways for metastases, whether they be bony or lymphatic, has not yet been subjected to controlled clinical trials.

Despite disagreement, the present clinical results would suggest that such trials may provide more information about the role and rate as well as the topographic areas of radiotherapy of prostatic cancer that can be of help in the management of the early form of the disease and possibly contribute to increased survival. The national statistics pertaining to prostatic cancer do not reveal any change in mortality for over 30 years. We must therefore await such additional studies with interest and an open mind. The ongoing experience of Bagshaw and associates will be of some help.[48] Other approaches utilizing newer forms of interstitial therapy for the prostate are currently under way and must also be kept in mind for their possible employment in the early stage of the disease.[49]

TREATMENT AND PALLIATION OF ADVANCED PROSTATIC CANCER

Contrary to other studies, our results for palliative therapy of patients with advanced prostatic carcinoma, regardless of the estrogen dosage or the presence or absence of orchiectomy, have not revealed a large number of cardiovascular deaths (Table 12–5).[35] In our own study, these patients were all followed until death or for a minimum period of about 14 years. There were few dropouts or crossovers and the patients were without a significant degree of prior liver disease. However, as shown in Table 12–5, death from causes related to prostatic carcinoma remains an important factor and on occasion can pose a significantly greater threat to patients with localized disease than to those patients with advanced prostatic carcinoma.[35]

Our own general guidelines for conventional hormonal therapy in patients with advanced untreated prostatic carcinoma are: (1) Withhold the therapy until the patient's symptoms or general condition warrants treatment. (2) Generally use castration alone although some physicians utilize stilbestrol either with or without castration. (3) When stilbestrol is administered following symptomatic or clinical relapse after castration, limit the dose to 1 mg daily. As mentioned previously, there is some suggestion based on plasma testosterone studies that 3 mg a day may provide better androgen suppression of certain patients. This has not been our experience. (4) High dose estro-

Table 12–5

Cause of death by primary treatment[a]

Cause of Death	Orchiectomy Alone (69 patients)	Estrogen plus Orchiectomy (256 patients)
Prostatic carcinoma	47.4	64.7
Other neoplasms	32.8	6.0
Cardiovascular diseases	13.2	22.9[b]
Other, mainly respiratory diseases	6.6	6.4

[a]Excluding patients who are alive or have died from unknown causes.[48]
[b]Not statistically significant.

gen therapy (natural or synthetic source) is not recommended except for selected use in short term, acute situations, for example, involving concern for spinal cord compression and possible conversion of an inoperable state to that of operability.

Hypophysectomy is of significant palliative benefit in patients with relapsed advanced prostatic carcinoma previously treated by conventional methods.[50] Studies by Scott have shown that hypophysectomy has additional effectiveness in terms of ratio of response, relief of pain, and survival of the patient. Open hypophysectomy, admittedly, is a hazardous procedure and can be associated with morbidity rates and operative loss up to 20%.[28] The recently advocated transsphenoidal cryosurgical hypophysectomy has proven more satisfactory in our hands and less hazardous.[28] In fact, this particular approach has demonstrated that it is unnecessary to achieve complete and total ablation of the pituitary.[28]

The results of adrenalectomy for prostatic carcinoma have been reviewed most recently.[27] Based on these and other ongoing studies, we have found that patients who have relapsed after some form of palliation for advanced prostatic carcinoma will generally exhibit a good response if the adrenalectomy is performed within six months of the event of clinical relapse. This is associated with measurable decrease in the 11-deoxy androgen metabolites in the urine. Such decreases correlate well with the clinical course of the patient. As with hypophysectomy patients or, for that matter, patients responding to other forms of hormonal therapy, decreases in acid phosphatase and prolonged decreases in alkaline phosphatase provide objective clinical correlation which is predictable and suitable. One cannot, at the present time, predict which patients will do best with adrenalectomy or hypophysectomy, although there are some suggestions that the quality of survival as measured by an objective score is relatively equal in both forms of surgery as well as that of oral chemotherapy. These will provide equal quality of survival in limited series which may permit some relative comparison in the near future between adrenalectomy and hypophysectomy, but such information at the present time on a national basis is not available.

It has been a clinical maxim that younger patients generally do better than older patients. There are differences of opinion on this matter. Generally our own patients are older (Figure 12–1). Although this may be true in terms of the initial diagnosis of the disease, the information is not available at the present time to state whether that remains true throughout the clinical course of the disease, especially in the disseminated states, that is, those beyond C involving D_1 or D_2 according to the classification of Whitmore.[51] Additionally, there is insufficient information available to enable us to come to conclusions about tumor differentiation in response to endocrine therapy as regards metastatic lesions. However, some peripheral sites of metastases do not consistently correlate with the clinical course of the patient's disease.[52] For example, lung metastases, when things are going well, may provide positive clinical information. However, when there are other sites of advanced progressive disease with lung metastases, this does not correlate with the response to endocrine therapy.

For some unknown reason, however, lung lesions generally show response that is associated with surprising improvement of the patient following adrenalectomy or successful hypophysectomy. Short term palliation in patients with widespread bony metastases has also been achieved by the injection of radiolabeled phosphorus, but there are several limitations to this form of treatment. Initial priming with successive doses of testosterone can, on occasion, contribute to severe morbidity, exacerbation of the patient's pain, and produce unsatisfactory results.

Other studies utilizing parathyroid hormone have exhibited less patient morbidity. However, both forms of therapy usually do not bring about long-term palliation. Another limiting feature of the use of radiolabeled phosphorus is its tendency to produce an associated anemia. In most patients with disseminated prostatic cancer, such anemia may well already be present and limit the use of this therapeutic modality. The drug L-Dopa has been found, in the hands of some, to be of possible benefit for the relief of bone pain in patients with relapsing breast cancer. It has been used in patients with carcinoma of the prostate and the results are not yet reported or evaluated. If such results show some promise, they might well identify those patients that would be best benefited by hypophysectomy. The place of palliative cryosurgery for patients with prostatic cancer must be further evaluated.

Repeat cryosurgery may have a possible influence on the presence of distant metastases. Some patients have undergone measured remission but widespread documentation and other immunologic testing of this is not available in the literature. Studies of cryosurgery that deal with antibody response of man and animals to a variety of tissue preparations will not resolve this problem. Concurrently, in such limited anecdotal reports, little or no attention has been paid to cellular immune responses. In vitro and in vivo investigations of clinical materials must be designed in order to quantitate possible humoral responses associated with these beneficial results. In all of our palliative therapy at the present time, it must be reemphasized that such palliative therapy does not ultimately prolong life. Our main concern for evidence of benefit

is the relief of pain. This is true particularly when patients have advanced disease and are treated with estrogen and castration and are compared with those treated at an institution where this therapy is not available. Such results can only be regarded as palliation.

Complex clinical cooperative trials dealing essentially with hormonal therapy must keep this important fact in mind. Such hormone control of prostatic cancer is only *palliative* in nature. Apparent discrepancies between the effect of estrogen or castration on the palliation of patients with prostatic cancer will likely be further resolved with further knowledge of the prostatic cancer cell, its hormonal receptor sites, and/or peripheral conversion of hormones. These factors are known to exist normally in man and indeed may be altered in the advanced prostatic cancer state. As mentioned previously, a suitable animal model is lacking. The National Prostatic Cancer Project and other cooperative groups are conducting controlled trials (phase I and II) to determine if available antiandrogens may be an alternate form of hormonal therapy. There is some suggestion that these forms may be of benefit but limited clinical information is available. At present, BCG therapy is also limited to clinical trials.[53] Such trials are suitable and appropriate in terms of evaluating the immunologic status of the patient; however, they are not the sort of thing one recommends for widespread general clinical utilization.

As mentioned, estradiol mustard (Estracyt) will likely be used for future chemotherapy of prostatic cancer. Phase I and phase II studies with the oral preparation are presently limited in this country. However, in Europe, chiefly under the leadership of Jönsson and Högberg, intravascular parenterally administered Estracyt has produced a reasonable number of apparent clinical responses in patients with advanced prostatic disease following other forms of conventional palliation.[54]

Further results of chemotherapy in patients with prostatic carcinoma are still awaited. Flocks and associates have described the largest number of patients receiving either 5-FU or Cytoxan with some apparently good results.[55] A survey from the National Cancer Institute on a limited number of prostatic cancer patients that have received a diverse number of agents suggests benefit with a number of possibilities including 5-FU and Cytoxan. For this reason, and because of other animal and in vitro experimental models, a current therapy program is under way throughout the United States as an extramural organ task force on prostatic cancer. This is sponsored by the National Cancer Institute and involves treatment centers in Seattle, Washington; Houston, Texas; Iowa City, Iowa; Baltimore, Maryland; and Boston, Massachusetts. The early results of this endeavor are most encouraging but cannot be published in a definitive form at this time. Such studies suggest that single agent chemotherapy may have some activity against prostatic carcinoma.

In other tumors, drugs in combination have also been shown to be effective, and some attempt is now under way to apply this experience to prostatic cancer. Combinations of Cytoxan and Adriamycin have been applied, but again the results are far too early to discuss either routes of administration or specific responses,[56] as also recently summarized in Memorial Hospital drug trials in which some activity against prostatic cancer was observed. Objective responses in such patients were observed with nitrogen mustard, cyclophosphamide, and 5-FU, and analine mustard was also found to be of such benefit. These endeavors confirm the suitability and appropriateness at the present time for further assessment of chemotherapy in advanced prostatic cancer states.[56]

Throughout this discussion, we have not mentioned the relationship between prognosis for the patient and the grade of the primary tumor. Some comments have been provided about clinical stage which by inference suggest that limited stages are associated with longer survival. Such material has been published and will not be reiterated at this time.[35] These studies have affirmed that patients die of prostatic cancer with increasing frequency as the clinical stage of the disease progresses. They also affirm that the initial grade of the tumor has some influence on the course of the disease. This is a limited amount of information and the clinical observations obtained at the present time should not be prejudiced by this approach. On the other hand, further information must be sought in the future and will undoubtedly contribute towards advancements in the management of clinical therapy of prostate cancer.

One does not think a summary or a conclusion of this present situational analysis of prostatic cancer therapy is warranted. We are in a static state of progression which is showing signs of improvement. The morbidity rates of prostatic cancer have been relatively unchanged to date. Newer investigations and their progress lend one hope for improvement in the near future. Diverse modalities have been employed in the past. The present approach seems to be designed towards consideration of the biologic potential of prostatic cancer and correlating this with the clinical stage of the disease and tumor grade. Factors involving androgenic and immunologic responsiveness will in the future doubtless be manipulated in accordance with the status of the patient. One is convinced that other forms of radiation therapy, single agent and combined chemotherapy, will also have their appropriate place in addition to other hormone concerns.

References

1. Viadana, E., et al.: An autopsy study of some routes of dissemination of cancer of the breast. Br. J. Cancer, 27:336, 1973.

2. McCullough, D. L., et al.: Carcinoma of the prostate and lymphatic metastases. J. Urol., 111:65, 1974.

3. Nussbaum, M.: Carcinoma of prostatic origin. Metastatic to cervical lymph nodes. N.Y. State J. Med., 73:2050, 1973.

4. Dodge, O. G., et al.: Tumours of the male genitalia. Recent Results Cancer Res., 41:132, 1973.

5. King, H., and Haenszel, W.: Cancer mortality among foreign- and native-born Chinese in the United States. J. Chronic Dis., 26:623, 1973.

6. Bean, M. A., et al.: Prostatic carcinoma at autopsy in Hiroshima and Nagasaki Japanese. Cancer, 32:498, 1973.

7. Haugen, O. A.: Pituitary adenomas and the histology of the prostate in elderly men. An analysis in an autopsy series. Acta Pathol. Microbiol. Scand., 81:425, 1973.

8. Haugen, O. A.: Distribution of pituitary cell types in relation to the histology of the prostate in elderly men. An analysis in an autopsy series. Acta Pathol. Microbiol. Scand., 81:411, 1973.

9. Harbitz, T. B.: Morphometric studies of the Sertoli cells in elderly men with special reference to the histology of the prostate. An analysis in an autopsy series. Acta Pathol. Microbiol. Scand., 81:703, 1973.

10. Herrmann, W. L., et al.: Peripheral control of hormone metabolism. Am. J. Obstet. Gynecol., 117:679, 1973.

11. Turgeon, J. L., and Barraclough, C. A.: Pulsatile plasma LH rhythms in normal and androgen-sterilized ovariectomized rats: Effects of estrogen treatment (37902). Proc. Soc. Exp. Biol. Med., 145:821, 1974.

12. Kontturi, M. J., et al.: Body fluid and electrolyte balance during estrogen therapy of prostatic cancer. J. Urol., 111:652, 1974.

13. Heathcote, J. G., and Washington, R. J.: Analysis of the zinc-binding protein derived from the human benign hypertrophic prostate. J. Endocrinol., 58:421, 1973.

14. Nozu, K., and Tamaoki, B.: Incorporation of ^{131}I-labeled androgen-receptor into nuclei of rat prostates. Biochem. Biophys. Res. Commun., 58:145, 1974.

15. Chance, H., et al.: Isolation of a rat ventral prostate chromatin fraction exhibiting a singular melting profile. Biochem. Biophys. Res. Commun., 58:66, 1974.

16. Ghanadian, R., and Fotherby, K.: Interaction between steroids in regard to their uptake by rat prostate. Steroids Lipids Res., 3:363, 1972.

17. Massa, R. and Martini, L.: Interference with the 5 α-reductase system. A new approach for developing antiandrogens. Gynecol. Invest., 2:253, 1971/1972.

18. Saroff, J., et al.: Effects of chemotherapy on the ventral prostate of the rat. Presented at the San Antonio Meeting on "Normal and Abnormal Growth of the Prostate," Southwestern Foundation for Research and Education, San Antonio, Texas, Feb. 28–March 3, 1973.

19. Schoonees, R., et al.: The hormonal effects of anti androgen (SH–714) treatment in man. Invest. Urol., 8:635, 1971.

20. Geller, J., and McCoy, K.: Biologic and biochemical effects of anti-androgens on rat ventral prostate. Acta Endocrinol., 75:385, 1974.

21. Rao, S. S., et al.: Immunological studies with rat prostate: Antigenic localization and effect of hormones. Biol. Reprod., 8:29, 1973.

22. Liao, S., et al.: Action of a nonsteroidal antiandrogen, Flutamide, on the receptor binding and nuclear retention of 5α-dihydrotestosterone in rat ventral prostate. Endocrinology, 94:1205, 1974.

23. Danutra, V., et al.: Studies with stilboestrol analogues in relation to prostatic function. J. Endocrinol., 58:xxviii, 1973.

24. Shimazaki, J., et al.: Testosterone metabolism in prostate; formation of Androstan-17β-OL-3-one and Androst-4-ENE-3, 17-dione, and inhibitory effect of natural and synthetic estrogens. Gunma. J. Med. Sci., 14:313, 1965.

25. Karr, J. P., et al.: Effects of testosterone and estradiol on ventral prostate and body weights of castrated rats. Life Sci., 15(3):501, 1974.

26. Shearer, R. J., et al.: Plasma testosterone: An accurate monitor of hormone treatment in prostatic cancer. Br. J. Urol., 45:668, 1973.

27. Schoonees, R., et al.: Bilateral adrenalectomy for advanced prostatic carcinoma. J. Urol., 108:123, 1972.

28. Murphy, G. P., et al.: Hypophysectomy and adrenalectomy for disseminated prostatic carcinoma. J. Urol., 105:817, 1971.

29. Kirdani, R. Y., et al.: Studies on the antiprostatic action of Estracyt, a nitrogen mustard of estradiol. Cancer Res., 34:1031, 1974.

30. Kline, I.: Potentially useful combinations of chemotherapy detected in mouse tumor systems. Cancer Chemother. Rep., 4:33, 1974.

31. Griswold, D. P., et al.: Approaches to combination chemotherapy in rat, mouse, and hamster tumors. Cancer Chemother. Rep., 4:99, 1974.

32. Bisson, J., et al.: Bone scan: In clinical perspective. J. Urol., 111:665, 1974.

33. Li, C. Y., et al.: Acid phosphatases in human plasma. J. Lab. Clin. Med., 82:446, 1973.

34. Murphy, G. P.: Prostatic malignancy. Current Diagnosis, 4:815, 1974. Edited by H. F. Conn and R. B. Conn, Jr. Philadelphia, W. B. Saunders.

35. Schoonees, R., et al.: Prostatic carcinoma treated at categorical center. Clinical and pathologic observations. N.Y. State J. Med., 72:1021, 1972.

36. Jewett, H. J.: Radical perineal prostatectomy in the treatment of carcinoma of the prostate. In Current Controversies in Urologic Management, Volume 1. Edited by R. Scott. Philadelphia, W. B. Saunders, 1972.

37. Lattimer, J. K.: Radical retropubic prostatectomy in the treatment of carcinoma of the prostate. In Current Controversies in Urologic Management, Volume 1. Edited by R. Scott. Philadelphia, W. B. Saunders, 1972.

38. Flocks, R. H.: Curative radiotherapy for car-

cinoma of the prostate. In Current Controversies in Urologic Management, Vol. 1. Edited by R. Scott, Philadelphia, W. B. Saunders, 1972.

39. Mir, M., et al.: Carcinoma of the prostate presenting as obstructive carcinoma of the rectum. Am. Surg., 39:582, 1973.

40. Gill, W. B., et al.: Radical retropubic prostatectomy and retroperitoneal lymphadenectomy following radiotherapy conversion of stage C to stage B carcinoma of the prostate. J. Urol., 111:656, 1974.

41. Green, N., et al.: Radiation therapy of inoperable localized prostatic carcinoma: An assessment of tumor response and complications. J. Urol., 111:662, 1974.

42. Megalli, M. R., et al.: External radiotherapy in ureteral obstruction secondary to locally invasive prostatic cancer. Urology, 3:562, 1974.

43. Melicow, M. M., et al.: Sarcoma of the prostate gland: Review of literature; table of classification; report of four cases. J. Urol., 49:675, 1943.

44. Michaels, M. M., et al.: Leiomyoma of prostate. Urology, 3:617, 1974.

45. Drake, W. M., Jr., and Burrows, S.: Papillary carcinoma of prostatic ducts. Urology, 3:621, 1974.

46. Kovi, J., et al.: Solitary epididymal metastasis from carcinoma of prostate. Urology, 3:644, 1974.

47. Rodriguez-Antunez, A., et al.: Management of primary and metastatic carcinoma of the prostate by the radiotherapist. Am. J. Roentgenol. Radium Ther. Nucl. Med., 118:876, 1973.

48. Bagshaw, M. A., et al.: Linear accelerator supervoltage radiotherapy, VII. Carcinoma of the prostate. Radiology, 85:121, 1965.

49. Hilaris, B. S., et al.: Radical radiation therapy of cancer of the prostate: A new approach using interstitial and external sources. Clin. Bull., 2:94, 1972.

50. Scott, W. W.: Endocrine management of disseminated prostatic cancer, including bilateral adrenalectomy and hypophysectomy. Trans. Am. Assoc. Genitourin. Surg., 44:101, 1945.

51. Whitmore, W. F., Jr.: The natural history of prostatic cancer. Cancer, 32:1104, 1973.

52. Varkarakis, M. J., et al.: Lung metastases in prostatic carcinoma. Clinical significance. Urology, 3:447, 1974.

53. Merrin, C., et al.: Immunotherapy of prostatic cancer with Bacillus Calmette-Guérin and purified protein derivative. Preliminary results. Urology, 2:651, 1973.

54. Jönsson, G., and Högberg, B.: Treatment of advanced prostatic carcinoma with estracyt (R). Scand. J. Urol. Nephrol., 5:103, 1971.

55. Flocks, R. H., and Cheng, S.-F.: Combination therapy for prostatic carcinoma with special emphasis on the role of chemotherapy. J. Iowa Med. Soc., 58:125, 1968.

56. Yagoda, A.: Non-hormonal cytotoxic agents in the treatment of prostatic adenocarcinoma. Cancer, 32:1131, 1973.

Chapter 13

VACURG* Studies on Prostatic Cancer and Its Treatment

DAVID P. BYAR

The reports by Huggins and Hodges in 1941[1-3] that prostatic cancer was responsive to estrogen therapy or to orchiectomy ushered in a new era in the treatment of this disease. These authors showed that there was often a prompt relief of pain following estrogen therapy or orchiectomy in patients with advanced prostatic cancer. They did not, however, demonstrate that survival of patients with prostatic cancer was increased by either of these treatments. Nevertheless, it became common practice in the decades following their discovery for urologists to treat patients with estrogens, or orchiectomy, or both, as soon as prostatic cancer was discovered in the hope that these treatments would slow down the progression of the disease and perhaps lead to longer survival. The assumption that survival must be prolonged as a consequence of treatment which was so effective in alleviating symptoms of disease was not seriously questioned for some time. However, there was interest in knowing whether it was necessary or beneficial to

*The Veterans Administration Cooperative Urological Research Group.

perform an orchiectomy in addition to giving estrogen.

In 1950, Nesbit and Baum published data on 1818 patients in an attempt to answer this question.[4] Their study showed that the combination of orchiectomy and estrogen was superior to either alone. Although it might at first seem that such a large study must be very authoritative, many urologists failed to recognize that this was a retrospective study of hospital records and thus subject to all the biases inherent in interpreting data retrospectively as opposed to the advantages of a randomized prospective clinical trial. In addition, Nesbit and Baum directed their attention mainly to deaths due to cancer of the prostate, paying less attention to deaths due to other causes. The nonhormonal controls consisted of a group of 795 patients diagnosed between 1925 and 1940 before the beginning of the endocrine era[5] and thus may have differed from the patients treated with estrogen, orchiectomy, or their combination in important respects other than the absence of hormone manipulation from their therapy. If there are biases present in

Table 13–1

Membership in the Veterans Administration Cooperative Urological Research Group

Hospital	Investigator	I	II	III	Focal
Atlanta	*Dr. Earl Haltiwanger	139	49	63	3
Bronx	Dr. Paul Gonick (retired)	—	23	—	—
	Dr. Vincent A. Ciavarra				
Buffalo	Dr. Maurice Gonder	—	—	19	—
Cincinnati	*Dr. George T. Mellinger	112	—	—	4
	Dr. Michael Glucksman				
	Dr. Asher O. Hoodin				
	Dr. Venancio Quiambao				
Des Moines	*Dr. Lino J. Arduino (retired)	237	56	119	11
	Dr. K. H. Moon				
	Dr. Robert E. H. Puntenney				
East Orange	*Dr. Maxwell Malament (deceased)	135	47	69	13
	Dr. Andrew Sporer				
Fort Howard (Loch Raven)	Dr. Howard C. Kramer	116	21	75	3
Houston	Dr. Prince Beach	—	—	58	—
Kansas City	Dr. Winston K. Mebust	—	—	58	—
Lake City	Dr. W. Pope Jordan, Jr.	—	19	—	6
Long Beach	*Dr. Arthur J. Bischoff (retired)	219	37	156	31
	Dr. John Ravera				
Louisville	Dr. Henry I. Berman (retired)	161	33	—	5
	Dr. Mohammad Amin				
Madison	Dr. Paul O. Madsen	—	29	80	5
Manhattan	*Dr. A. Hardy Ulm (deceased)	157	—	—	5
Memphis	Dr. W. Pope Jordan, Jr.	—	9	96	—
Minneapolis	*Dr. Roger Haglund	417	130	269	24
	Dr. George T. Mellinger				
	Dr. Clyde E. Blackard				
Oakland (Martinez, Palo Alto)	Dr. James S. Elliot	127	32	43	3
Oklahoma City	*Dr. William L. Parry	112	33	—	—
Omaha	Dr. Francis F. Bartone	—	7	87	—
Portland	Dr. Robert S. Higgins	182	—	—	—
Syracuse	*Dr. William L. Parry	50	—	—	—
	Dr. Otto M. Lilien				
	Dr. Lloyd S. Rogers				
Tucson	Dr. David A. Parker	—	—	17	—
Wadsworth (Leavenworth)	Dr. Leslie E. Becker	149	36	45	35
Total		2313	561	1254	148

CONSULTANTS: *Dr. Lyndon E. Lee, VA Central Office Liaison Officer

Referee Biochemists:
  *Dr. Richard P. Doe, Minneapolis VAH
    (currently working at U. of Minn. Hosp.)
  Dr. Ulie Seal, Minneapolis VAH
  Dr. John R. Kent, Long Beach VAH
  Dr. James Smith, VAH, Wash., D.C.

Referee Biostatisticians:
  *Dr. Edmund A. Gehan, NIH
    (currently working at U. of Texas)
  Dr. Alan J. Gross, NIH
  Dr. John C. Bailar, III, NIH
  Dr. David P. Byar, NIH

Referee Pathologists:
  *Dr. F. K. Mostofi, AFIP, Wash., D.C.
  Dr. Donald Gleason, Minneapolis, VAH
  Dr. Raymond Yesner, West Haven, VAH

Statistical Assistants:
  Mrs. Marjorie M. Greenberg, NIH
  Mrs. Eileen P. Kessler, NIH
  Mrs. Anna J. Watkins, NIH

Referee Radiologists:
  *Dr. Erich Spiro, Cincinnati VAH
  Dr. Joseph Jorgens, Minneapolis VAH
    (currently working at Los Angeles VAH)
  Dr. Jeannette Hovsepian, Palo Alto VAH

*Original Members
All affiliations refer to period when involved in VACURG studies.

retrospective studies, a large sample size is no protection against them.

Because of dissatisfaction with these results and because of the great importance of the questions involved, the Veterans Administration Cooperative Urological Research Group was formed in 1959 with the expressed purpose of studying the treatment of urologic cancers in the setting of large randomized prospective clinical trials. It was hoped that formal study designs could facilitate assembling a large set of data not subject to the biases and other sources of error inherent in retrospective studies and that these data might be useful in answering questions about the treatment of prostatic cancer. Although the main studies of this group have been concerned with prostatic cancer, there have been two smaller studies of treatment of bladder cancer as well.

In this chapter I wish to place major emphasis on what has been learned about prostatic cancer rather than present detailed data on treatment comparisons. The principal results of treatment comparisons are summarized.

DESIGN OF THE STUDIES

The original group designated as the Veterans Administration Cooperative Urological Research Group (VACURG) consisted of full-time urologists at 14 Veterans Administration Hospitals in various parts of the country.[6] Over the past 14 years additional hospitals have been added and some hospitals have not been included in all of the studies. There have been three main prostate studies designated as I, II and III and, in addition, a smaller study referred to as the Focal Carcinoma Study. The hospitals, principal investigators, consultants, and numbers of patients involved in these studies are shown in Table 13–1 where asterisks indicate the original members; Dr. George T. Mellinger has been the group chairman since the beginning. In all these studies only newly diagnosed, previously untreated patients with a positive histologic diagnosis of prostatic carcinoma were admitted. In all studies patients are followed for fifteen years or until death. In some instances the principal investigators have died or have moved to other hospitals, but provisions have been made to continue following patients in these hospitals. The staging system used in these studies is indicated in Table 13–2. The stage composition of the three main prostate studies (the Focal Carcinoma Study included only patients in stage I) is shown in Table 13–3; note that the stage composition has been remarkably constant for the past 14 years—about 5% each in stages I and II, 50% in stage III and 40% in stage IV. Since the three main studies

Table 13–2

Veterans Administration Cooperative Urological Research Group staging system

STAGE	RECTAL EXAMINATION	PROSTATIC ACID PHOSPHATASE	EVIDENCE OF METASTASES X-RAY OR BIOPSY
I	NO INDURATION	$\leqslant$ 1.0 K.A.U.	0
II	LOCALIZED NODULE	$\leqslant$ 1.0 K.A.U.	0
III	EXTRA-PROSTATIC EXTENSION	$\leqslant$ 1.0 K.A.U	0
IV	ANY FINDINGS	> 1.0 K.A.U. OR	+

Table 13–3

Patients admitted by stage

Stage	Study I		Study II		Study III	
	Number	% of total	Number	% of total	Number	% of total
I	120	5.2	32	5.7	41	4.1
II	179	7.7	21	3.7	45	4.6
III	1104	47.7	294	52.4	479	48.5
IV	910	39.3	214	38.1	423	42.8
All Stages	2313	100.0	561	100.0	988	100.0

are consecutive in time and the patients are drawn from cohorts representing veterans from the major armed conflicts, we find that the age distributions shift toward older ages as we progress from Study I to Study III (Figure 13–1). In addition we can see that the majority of the patients correspond to young personnel in World War I, but that local modes in the younger age group probably correspond to veterans of World War II and the Korean conflict. The average age of stage III and IV patients is roughly 70.

Veterans Administration Hospitals provide an ideal setting for clinical trials of this disease because there is a large patient population at risk for prostatic cancer, treatment in the various hospitals is reasonably similar, and follow-up of patients is facilitated by the availability of free medical care and the possibility of tracing patients through their VA claim numbers.

It has been suggested that the VA population is not representative of the general population of patients with prostatic cancer, but rather represents a "distressed" population, presumably suggesting that the excess of cardiovascular deaths observed on estrogen treatment would not have been found in the general population. Recent evidence suggests that, if anything, a lower overall death rate from cardiovascular (as well as other) causes would be observed in veterans

AGE DISTRIBUTIONS, STAGES III & IV

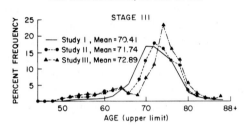

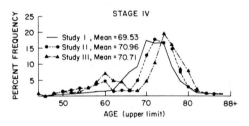

Figure 13–1. Frequency distributions for age at the time of diagnosis for the three main VA clinical trials for patients in stages III and IV.

because the medical examination on entry to the Armed Forces serves to select healthier individuals. An analysis of the subsequent mortality experience of 85,491 veterans of the second World War showed marked deficits in the numbers of deaths due to vascular lesions, arteriosclerotic heart disease, and other cardiovascular disease compared to the US death rates for white males in the same calendar years.[7] Although these deficits were more marked in the years soon after the war (1947–51), the effects of favorable selection were still evident over 20 years later in the data for 1967–69.

Table 13-4

Number of patients and treatments assigned by stage of disease in the VACURG clinical trials

Stage	Study I[a] (1960–67) N[e]	Treatments[f]	Study II[b] (1967–69) N	Treatments	Study III[c] (1969–74) N	Treatments	Focal[d] (1962–67) N	Treatments
I	60 60	Px+Pcb Px+DES (5.0)	18 14	Pcb Px+Pcb	18 23	Pcb Px+Pcb	39 36 38 35	Pcb DES (5.0) Orch+Pcb Orch+DES (5.0)
II	85 94	Px+Pcb Px+DES (5.0)	10 11	Pcb DES	20 25	Pcb Px+Pcb		
III	261 264 55 266 258	Pcb DES (5.0) Orch Orch+Pcb Orch+DES (5.0)	75 73 73 73	Pcb DES (0.2) DES (1.0) DES (5.0)	125 119 114 121	Prem (2.5) Prov (30) Prov+DES (1.0) DES (1.0)		
IV	223 211 57 203 216	Pcb DES (5.0) Orch Orch+Pcb Orch+DES (5.0)	53 52 55 54	Pcb DES (0.2) DES (1.0) DES (5.0)	105 104 105 110	Prem (2.5) Prov (30) Prov+DES (1.0) DES (1.0)		
All Stages	2313		561		988		148	

[a] Patients admitted from March 1960 through March 1967.
[b] Patients admitted from April 1967 through May 1969.
[c] Patients admitted from June 1969 through December 1974.
[d] Patients admitted from July 1964 through March 1969.
[e] N = number of patients.
[f] Treatment abbreviations: Pcb = placebo; Px = radical prostatectomy; DES = diethylstilbestrol; Orch = bilateral orchiectomy; Prem = Premarin; Prov = Provera; daily doses in milligrams are given in parentheses following the treatment abbreviations.

In all VACURG studies the diagnosis has been confirmed by a referee pathologist and all acid phosphatase determinations have been made at a central reference laboratory. The data have been sent to the National Cancer Institute for coding and analysis in the Biometry Branch. Since the beginning, these studies have been a joint venture of the Veterans Administration and the National Cancer Institute.

The treatments studied in the various protocols are summarized in Table 13–4.

NATURAL HISTORY OF PROSTATIC CANCER

Relationship of Metastasis to Acid Phosphatase

The large amount of data collected in the studies under uniform protocols has permitted careful correlation of the relationship between the pretreatment prostatic acid phosphatase levels and the presence of soft part and bony metastasis. Data from all three main studies combined are shown in Table 13–5. It is evident that there is a regular progressive increase in the probability of metastasis as a function of the initial acid phosphatase level. From these data we can determine that despite the high correlation between probability of metastasis and the initial acid phosphatase level, 18% of patients with metastasis at diagnosis had normal acid phosphatase ($\leq$1.0 King Armstrong Units), whereas only about 39% of those with an elevated acid phosphatase had metastasis. Separate analyses have shown that the prognosis for patients with an elevated acid phosphatase without metastasis is better than that for patients with bony metastasis. Survival of patients with bony metastasis but normal acid phosphatase is better than that for patients with both osseous metastasis and elevated acid phosphatase. Additional analysis has shown that for estrogen-treated patients, an increase of over 50% in the acid phosphatase in the first six months is associated with a worse prognosis compared to that of patients whose acid phosphatase remains within 50% of its original value. It was also noted that patients whose acid phosphatase decreased by at least 50% have better

Table 13–5

Relationship of pretreatment prostatic acid phosphatase to presence of detectable metastases, Studies I, II and III combined

Level of pretreatment acid phosphatase[a]	Total patients	Bone metastases	Soft part metastases	Both bone and soft metastases	All metastases
0.0– 0.5	1539	43 (2.8)[b]	16 (1.0)	4 (0.3)	63 (4.1)
0.6– 1.0	1131	41 (3.6)	13 (1.1)	10 (0.9)	64 (5.7)
1.1– 2.0	416	56 (13.5)	6 (1.4)	4 (1.0)	66 (15.9)
2.1– 5.0	350	72 (20.6)	17 (4.9)	8 (2.3)	97 (27.7)
5.1– 10.0	189	72 (38.1)	8 (4.2)	6 (3.2)	86 (45.5)
10.1– 20.0	127	57 (44.9)	7 (5.5)	8 (6.3)	72 (56.7)
20.1– 50.0	166	77 (46.4)	12 (7.2)	17 (10.2)	106 (63.9)
50.1–100.0	71	43 (60.6)	1 (1.4)	8 (11.3)	52 (73.2)
100.0+	114	65 (57.0)	4 (3.5)	17 (14.9)	86 (75.4)
Unknown	25	1 (4.0)	0 (0.0)	0 (0.0)	1 (4.0)
All levels	4128	527 (12.8)	84 (2.0)	82 (2.0)	693 (16.8)

[a]King-Armstrong Units (Normal levels $\leq$1.0 KAU)
[b]Number (percentage)

prognosis than those who stayed within 50% of the pretreatment value or increased by more than 50% after treatment.

Pathology

In Study I, all patients in stages I and II were subjected to radical prostatectomy. An analysis of 208 prostate specimens removed at operation and studied by the step-section technique revealed that in 85% of the cases the disease was multifocal.[8] It was almost always found in the periphery of the gland or in the periphery and the central portion; in only one case was it found in the central portion alone. Correlation between the finding on the rectal examination and the pathologic examination was poor except that when the tumor had extended beyond the confines of the prostate, the agreement on the presence of extension was about 75%. Extension beyond the prostate or invasion of the seminal vesicles was the most important prognostic finding because it signified that disease clinically staged as II would be found on later pathologic examination to be stage III.

Dr. Donald Gleason has done extensive work on grading prostatic carcinoma. Recognizing that in many specimens a variety of patterns of growth will be found, he identified a primary and a secondary pattern which he combined with a patient's stage to obtain a final prognostic category.[9-11] In general, he has found a high degree of correlation between the prognostic category and the probability of cancer death. In addition

Table 13–6

Percent of cases with metastases at autopsy by site and histologic pattern of initial biopsy, all stages and treatments combined, studies I, II, and III

Site	Sum of Primary and Secondary Pattern						All Patterns % POS
	2–4 % POS	5 % POS	6 % POS	7 % POS	8 % POS	9–10 % POS	
Bone	8	10	29	45	56	59	35
Lung	4	2	18	27	24	24	17
Lymph nodes	4	7	20	40	44	51	27
Spleen	0	0	0	7	3	0	1
Liver	0	2	12	13	17	22	12
Stomach	0	0	0	0	1	0	0
Pancreas	0	0	2	2	4	5	2
Duodenum	0	0	0	0	0	0	0
Ileum	4	0	0	0	1	2	1
Colon	0	0	0	0	1	2	1
Rectum	0	0	2	2	6	12	4
All G.I.	4	0	4	5	10	22	7
Kidney	0	0	2	2	2	5	2
Bladder	0	3	13	20	28	29	16
Seminal Vesicle	0	1	7	17	15	22	10
Other G.U.	0	1	1	2	4	5	2
All G.U.	0	5	18	38	38	37	23
Adrenals	4	2	8	10	9	24	9
C.N.S.	0	1	4	0	5	10	4
Other	0	1	7	7	12	22	8
Any site	16	20	40	67	76	83	50
Total patients	25	87	245	40	138	41	576

the prognostic category has been useful in comparing treatments. A study of autopsy reports submitted for patients who died in these studies showed a remarkably constant relationship between Gleason's prognostic categories and the probability of metastasis at autopsy in all the major sites (Table 13–6). The concept of the biologic determinism of prostatic cancer appears to be eloquently supported by these data, that is, that tumors have differing degrees of malignancy and that these can be identified to some extent by examining the histologic material obtained at the time of diagnosis. This observation is of great importance in determining individual prognosis and in making valid treatment comparisons, either within or between studies.

Progression of Untreated Cancer

The inclusion of placebo-treated groups in the various protocols allows us to make comparisons between the course and progression of prostatic cancer in untreated and treated patients. In the Focal Carcinoma Study, all patients had stage I carcinoma; however, because they were too old or too ill or refused operation, none of these patients was treated by radical prostatectomy. To date only 14 of the original 148 patients (9.5%) have shown evidence of progression of disease as judged by the appearance of bony metastasis or elevations in the acid phosphatase, and only one patient has died of prostatic cancer. These data may be compared to similar figures for patients in stage I of Study I, where all patients underwent radical prostatectomy.

In this group 13 of 120 patients (10.8%) have shown similar evidence of progression of disease suggesting that occult foci of potentially malignant cells must have been present before the radical prostatectomies were performed. However, the comparison of stage I patients from Study I with Focal Study patients is not a randomized comparison. We can study

the progression of disease in randomized comparisons for patients in Studies II and III, although the period of follow-up is not so long. In combining the data for stage I from Studies II and III, we find that 13.5 percent of the patients treated by radical prostatectomy have evidence of progression versus 19.4 percent in the placebo-treated controls. The figures for stage II for the two studies combined are 30.6% vs 26.7% for prostatectomy and control respectively. In neither stage is the difference statistically significant. These data raise serious questions as to whether or not radical surgery is justified.

The notion used to justify radical prostatectomy that "no harm can come from a cancer if all of it is preserved in a glass jar"[12] appears to be illusory; these data suggest that those cancers which could truly have been removed entirely by operation may well have lain dormant for years anyway, and those which were destined to spread had already done so silently before the operation. Urologists in

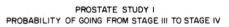

PROSTATE STUDY I
PROBABILITY OF GOING FROM STAGE III TO STAGE IV

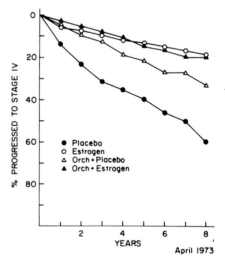

Figure 13–2. Actuarial plots of the probability of progression from stage III to stage IV. The event, progression to stage IV, is defined as the development of bone or soft part metastasis and/or prostatic acid phosphatase greater than 1.0 King Armstrong Unit.

Table 13-7

Relationship between sum of primary and secondary histologic patterns and progression[a] from stage III to stage IV, studies I, II, and III combined[b]

Sum of primary and secondary histologic patterns	2–4	5	6	7	8	9–10	All Patients
Total number of patients	61	284	586	115	166	44	1256
Number who progressed from stage III to stage IV	8	43	101	24	58	17	251
Total months of followup	2506	11995	19872	3328	4908	784	43393
Total months of followup for those who progressed	167	2411	2991	620	1215	272	7676
Probability of progression	0.131	0.151	0.172	0.209	0.349	0.386	0.200
Rate of progression for all patients (progression/1000 patient-months)	3.19	3.59	5.08	7.21	11.82	21.68	5.78
Rate of progression or those who progressed (progressions per 1000 patient-months)	47.90	17.84	33.77	38.71	47.74	62.50	32.70

[a]Progression is defined as the development of bone or soft part metastasis and/or prostatic acid phosphatase greater than 1.0 King-Armstrong unit.
[b]Only about half of the stage III tumors in Study I have been graded.

various parts of the country disagree sharply on the value of radical prostatectomy, particularly with regard to stage I disease.

Data on the progression of stage III disease as judged by the occurrence of elevated acid phosphatase or bony metastasis show that estrogen therapy or orchiectomy is effective in retarding progression of the cancer (Figure 13–2) and give some idea of the rate of progression in untreated patients. In the stage I and II data just presented, there is some suggestion that a higher pathologic grade predisposes to progression of the disease; in stage III the numbers are large enough to permit direct examination of this hypothesis.

Table 13–7 shows the relationship between the sum of the primary and secondary histologic pattern reported according to the method of Dr. Gleason (see Chapter 9) and the progression from stage III to stage IV of the disease. It is apparent from studying this table that the probability of progression is highly dependent upon the histologic appearance of the tumor. Note, for example, that the probability of progression for patients whose tumor biopsy shows a sum between 2 and 4 was only 0.131 compared to 0.386 for those whose tumors were graded 9 and 10, an almost three-fold increase in the probability of progression. The probability of progression is simply the proportion of all patients who were observed to progress, but the statistic fails to take into account the rate at which progression occurred. Also shown in Table 13–7 is an estimate of the rate in terms of number of progressions per 1000 patient-months of observation, and here the results are even more striking; comparing the same two groups we find that the rate of progression, 3.19 versus 21.68, is increased by about 6.8 times. This remarkably clear-cut pattern is even preserved if we confine our examination of the rates of progression to those patients who progressed,

except that the small group of only eight patients who progressed in the 2–4 category gives us an unreliable estimate of the rate of progression; excluding this group there is a regular trend of the increasing rate of progression, the higher the sum of the histologic patterns. These data again emphasize the remarkable degree to which a prognosis in prostatic cancer is dependent upon the individual characteristics of the tumors at the time of diagnosis.

PROGNOSTIC VARIABLES

For Predicting Deaths Due to Prostatic Cancer

I have already indicated that the grade of the primary tumor is a powerful prognostic variable in predicting death due to prostatic cancer. Additional data on this subject will be found in Chapter 9. I have also indicated that the prostatic acid phosphatase is another prognostic variable and that changes in this enzyme in the first six months of treatment with hormones or orchiectomy provide additional prognostic information. Recently we have learned that the pretreatment values of serum 17-hydroxycorticoids provide information about prognosis.[13] The physiologic basis of this finding is not yet understood, but the results of our analysis indicate that in general there is a negative correlation between the level of 17-hydroxycorticoids and the length of survival. Further details are presented in a later section.

Recent work has also shown that the size of the primary lesion, as judged by rectal examination, is important in predicting survival. The primary lesion is drawn on the standard diagram and its surface area estimated in square centimeters. Figure 13–3 shows the relationship between the size of the primary lesion and the probability of death due to prostatic carcinoma.

Another variable which has been

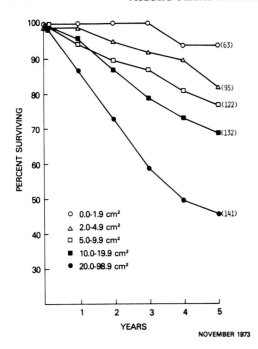

Figure 13–3. Actuarial survival curves based on cancer deaths only by the size of the palpable area of carcinoma. The data are from Study II, all stages and treatments combined.

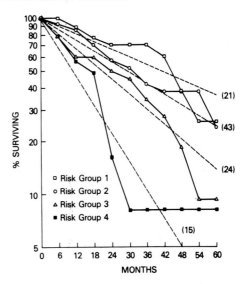

Figure 13–4. Actuarial survival curves (solid lines) and predicted survival (dashed lines) based on the exponential survival model with extent of metastasis in lung, pubis-ischium, and femur as covariates. Curves were constructed for cancer deaths only; deaths from other causes were treated as withdrawals at time of death. Number of patients in each risk group shown in parentheses. Data are taken from Study I for 103 patients who had bone metastasis at time of diagnosis.

shown to affect survival is the extent of metastasis detectable by x-ray examination. The extent of metastasis on a four-point scale was estimated in each of eight major sites. Analysis of data recorded in this way for 103 patients who had metastasis at time of diagnosis showed that these eight sites were involved according to the following percentages: shoulder (upper humerus, clavicle, and scapula), 39%; rib, 53%; lung, 24%; thoracic spine, 60%; lumbosacral spine, 71%; pubis-ischium, 78%; ilium, 83%; and femur, 48%. In addition there was a positive correlation between the height of the acid phosphatase and the number of sites involved. Because of the high degree of correlation between the various sites with respect to presence of metastasis, it was found that prognostic risk groups could be constructed on the basis of extent of involvement in only three sites with little loss of information. Those chosen to give

the best predictions were lung, pubis-ischium, and femur. Risk groups were constructed on the basis of findings in these three sites, and theoretical curves were drawn. These were compared to the observed actuarial curves for these patients (Figure 13–4); the observed curves were in good agreement with the mathematical model for samples of these sizes and showed remarkable differences in the probability of death due to prostatic cancer as a function of the extent of metastatic involvement.

For Predicting Deaths Due to Cardiovascular Causes

The unexpected increase in cardiovascular deaths for patients treated with estrogen in the first VA study has led to a search for variables which might help identify patients at high risk in advance. To date, the most important findings are that a previous history of cardiovascular disease and age greater than 75 are factors which increase the probability of cardiovascular death for patients treated with 5.0 mg of diethylstilbestrol (DES) daily. In addition we have recently noted that the excess cardiovascular mortality in estrogen-treated patients in Study I, stage I, was confined to that group of patients who had two operations within a short period of time. Generally these two operations consisted of transurethral resection followed within a period of two months by radical prostatectomy. This finding is currently undergoing further study; tentatively it seems plausible to hypothesize that major surgical operations alter the coagulation system in some manner so that it is sensitive to estrogen.

Multivariate Risk Factor Models

In addition to studying variables for prognostic importance one at a time, we have constructed multivariate risk factor models based on the exponential survival distribution. These models allow us to introduce many variables simultaneously and increase our ability to make accurate predictions of survival. This approach has been used to analyze the data for patients in stages III and IV of Study I. The relative importance of the various variables can be judged from the magnitude of their regression coefficients in Table 13–8. Combining the information for individual patients, risk groups could be constructed. The actuarial and predicted survival for patients in these risk groups is shown in Figure 13–5. Mathematical details of this approach are shown in references 14–16. These methods allow us to examine the effects of prognostic variables when they act jointly, to predict survival with greater accuracy, and lead to methods of adjustment which allow us to make more reliable treatment comparisons. In addition they illustrate that large differences in survival can be attributed to the pretreatment characteristics of the patient; in fact, these differences are frequently greater than those which can be attributed to the various treatments. Further analysis along these lines, as yet unpublished, permits us to identify subgroups of patients who benefit from various forms of treatment which might be harmful or without effect in other sub-

Table 13–8

Estimates of regression coefficients and their standard deviations, stages III and IV and all treatments combined, study I

No.	Variable	B_j[a] (1)	Std. Dev. (2)	Ratio (1)/(2)
0	Force of mortality	7.88	0.64	12.31
1	Pain due to cancer	−.20	1.75	−0.11
2	Acid p'tase[b] 1.1–2.0	4.15	1.40	2.96
3	Acid p'tase 2.1–5.0	6.94	1.93	3.60
4	Acid p'tase >5.0	11.04	2.09	5.28
5	Ureteral dilatation	4.68	2.31	2.03
6	Metastasis[c]	7.36	1.91	3.85
7	Partially bedridden	11.18	2.39	4.68
8	Totally bedridden	21.55	8.48	2.54
9	Weight <130 pounds	3.50	1.34	2.61
10	Hemoglobin <12 gm %	5.44	1.49	3.65
11	Age ≥ 70 years	3.02	0.85	3.55

[a]Expressed in deaths/1000 patient-months followup.
[b]Acid phosphatase, expressed in King-Armstrong Units.
[c]Osseous or soft part metastasis.

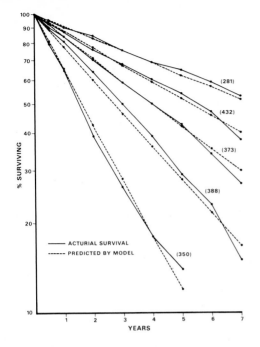

Figure 13–5. Actuarial survival curves (solid lines) and theoretical predicted survival curves (dashed lines) based on mixture of exponential distributions for five risk groups. Data are taken from Study I for patients in stages III and IV, all treatments combined. All causes of death are considered. See reference 14.

groups of patients. This work represents a major step towards the desirable goal of individualizing the patients' therapy, recognizing that patients in a single stage of the disease represent a heterogeneous population with respect to various risk factors.

RESULTS OF TREATMENT COMPARISONS

Radical Prostatectomy

In the first VACURG study, all patients in stages I and II were treated by radical prostatectomy and in addition were randomized for estrogen therapy (5.0 mg DES daily) versus placebo. This study alone allows us no opportunity for judging the efficacy of radical prostatectomy; however, no patients in the Focal Carcinoma Study were treated with radical prostatec-

tomy, either because they were too old or too ill or refused the operation. Some information on the value of radical prostatectomy can be gained by comparing the stage I patients from Study I with the Focal Study patients.[17] Because the patients in the Focal Study were generally older than patients in Study I, the comparison must be made after age-adjustment. When such comparison was made (Figure 13–6) the actuarial curves revealed that five year survival rates for the Focal patients were about 50% compared to 67% for the Study I patients treated by radical prostatectomy; however, the differences were not statistically significant. When we consider that many patients in the Focal Study were sicker than those in Study I, it is probable that the differences would have been even less noteworthy had we been able to adjust for degree of illness in addition to age. Since this comparison is not a randomized one, we can only take the results as suggestive that the role of radical prostatectomy should be reexamined. For this reason, patients in stages I and II of the second and third VA studies were randomized

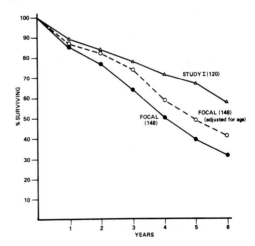

Figure 13–6. Comparison of crude and age-adjusted survival curves for Focal Study and stage I of Study I. (Number of patients in parentheses.) All patients in Study I stage I received radical prostatectomy, whereas no patients in Focal Study received radical prostatectomy. Differences in survival are not significant after age-adjustment.

between radical prostatectomy and placebo. Thus far, no significant difference between those treated with radical prostatectomy versus those treated with placebo has been detected, but the period of followup is short and the number of patients is small. Some comparison of these treatments with respect to progression of disease has already been discussed in the section on the natural history of prostatic cancer.

Orchiectomy

Orchiectomy was studied only in the first VA study; it was compared in a random fashion to placebo, 5.0 mg. DES daily, and orchiectomy plus 5.0 mg DES daily. These treatments were compared in both stage III and stage IV patients. In stage III patients, the only significant differences in survival curves for all causes of death combined indicated that orchiectomy plus estrogen was worse as initial treatment than placebo or orchiectomy plus placebo.[18] There were no significant differences in the survival curves for patients in stage IV; there were, however, significantly more cancer deaths in the two nonestrogen groups in both stages. Otherwise there were no appreciable differences between the three hormonal treatments.[18-20] We concluded from these data that estrogen is more effective than orchiectomy in preventing cancer deaths, and the addition of orchiectomy to estrogen does not offer a clear-cut advantage over either treatment alone; therefore, it appears that if treatment becomes necessary because of development of symptoms from metastatic cancer, initial treatment with estrogen is preferred.[21]

Diethylstilbestrol (DES)

By far the most important contribution of the VA studies to date has been the unequivocable demonstration of the cardiovascular hazards of DES in treating some patients with prostatic cancer when 5.0 mg doses are used daily. This finding

first reported in 1967[18] was as much of a surprise to the investigators in these studies as it was to the urologic and medical world in general. However, the data could not be ignored even though this finding seemed to be inconsistent with medical thinking at that time. Part of the disbelief and controversy that resulted from the report of these findings can be attributed to the then popular belief that, if anything, estrogen should prevent cardiovascular complications in men. Indeed 5.0 mg daily of Premarin (conjugated estrogen) was under study in the Coronary Drug Project as treatment for men who had already suffered one myocardial infarction in the hope that it would be shown to prevent further attacks. Later this treatment had to be discontinued in that project because of excess cardiovascular toxicity,[22] confirming and strengthening the conclusions reached in the VA study. Some hint of the VA results might have been obtained from the paper by Nesbit and Baum[4]; although not referred to in the text of their paper, the data in their Tables 1 and 2 show an increased percentage of deaths not due to carcinoma among patients treated with DES.

Since the results of the first VA study were not anticipated, little information was collected on the patients' pretreatment cardiovascular status. The absence of these data was particularly referred to in the controversy that followed publication. However, a retrospective analysis of the pretreatment cardiovascular status— including such conditions as obesity, diabetes, hypertension, and abnormal electrocardiograms—was carried out in the hospital which had contributed the most patients. This study revealed findings similar to those reported for the whole study, but failed to find any bias indicating worse pretreatment characteristics in the estrogen-treated group.[23]

Additional criticisms were that the dose of DES used was too high and that a natural estrogen such as Premarin should have been used rather than the synthetic estrogen, diethylstilbestrol. It was also suggested that the VA population represented "a distressed patient group," which would be likely to have a high incidence of cardiovascular death. Finally, suspicion was aroused that urologists participating in this study were not well suited to managing cardiovascular complications and that this may have contributed to the results. However, the results of the Coronary Drug Project would suggest that this criticism is probably without firm basis. In any event, the second VA study was designed, partially in response to these criticisms and suggestions, to explore further the relationship between estrogen treatment for prostatic cancer and cardiovascular complications. For this reason, two lower doses of estrogen (1.0 and 0.2 mg daily DES) were compared to the 5.0 mg dose and placebo in stages III and IV. The results of this study[19,20,24] indicated that the 1.0 mg dose of DES was as effective as the 5.0 mg dose in controlling cancer in either stage III or IV, but, in stage III, there were substantially fewer cardiovascular deaths on the 1.0 mg dose compared to the 5.0 mg dose. In both stages the two higher doses were superior to the 0.2 mg dose or placebo in controlling the cancer. It thus appears that there is a dose-dependent dissociation between the toxic effects of DES on the cardiovascular system and its therapeutic effects.

Other Hormones

In the third VA study, the 1.0 mg dose of DES is being compared to Premarin (conjugated equine estrogens, Ayerst) at 2.5 mg daily; Provera (medroxyprogesterone acetate, Upjohn) 30 mg daily; and the combination of Provera 30 mg daily and 1.0 mg DES daily. To date no significant differences in survival in either stage III or stage IV have been detected, but these patients will continue to be fol-

lowed. At present it may be said that none of the treatments studied provides any advantage over 1.0 mg DES alone.

EFFECT OF TREATMENT ON BIOCHEMICAL AND PHYSIOLOGIC PARAMETERS

Biochemical Parameters

In the first VA study, the only biochemical parameters on which data were collected were hemoglobin and acid phosphatase. Treatment with 5.0 mg daily of DES resulted in a significant but minor drop in the hemoglobin at 6 months averaging about 1.0 gram percent in stage III. Orchiectomy had no effect on the hemoglobin. The effect of these treatments on the acid phosphatase agreed with many previously published reports; both orchiectomy and estrogen treatment produced a prompt drop in the acid phosphatase levels for patients whose values were elevated at the time of diagnosis. A drop of at least 50% of the initial values was observed at 6 months in over 85% of the patients treated by orchiectomy, estrogen, or the combination of the two. In the placebo group only 21% showed a decrease of at least 50% by 6 months. In contrast, 40% of the placebo patients showed an elevation of at least 50% above their initial value compared to 4%, 3% and 1% respectively for DES, orchiectomy plus placebo, and orchiectomy plus DES.

In the second and third VA studies a number of additional laboratory measurements were included in an attempt to find out if some of these measurements could help us in selecting patients who might be unusually prone to cardiovascular death if treated with estrogens. These additional assays included alkaline phosphatase, cholesterol, triglycerides, 17-hydroxycorticoids, haptoglobin, plasminogen, fibrinogen, ceruloplasmin, testosterone and corticosteroid-binding globulin. It is beyond the scope of this

Table 13-9

Summary of 3-month changes in laboratory values by treatment, Study II

	Stage III				Stage IV			
	Placebo	DES .2 mg	DES 1 mg	DES 5 mg	Placebo	DES .2 mg	DES 1 mg	DES 5 mg
Acid p'tase[b]		(2)[a] →	(3) →	(3) →			(3) →	(3) →
CBG		(3) ←	(3) ←	(3) ←		(3) ←	(3) ←	(3) ←
Plasminogen		(3) ←	(3) ←	(3) ←			(3) ←	(3) ←
Fibrinogen	(2) →	(2) →	(3) →	(3) →		(1) →	(3) →	(1) →
17-OH		(2) ←	(3) ←	(3) ←			(3) ←	(3) ←
Alk p'tase[b]		(2) ←	(3) →		(2) ←		(1) →	
Cholesterol[b]		(2) ←	(3) ←				(1) ←	
H.S. Alk p'tase[c]								
Ceruloplasmin		(3) ←	(3) ←	(3) ←		(2) ←	(2) ←	(2) →
Haptoglobin		(3) →	(3) →	(3) →		(2) →	(3) →	(2) →
Testosterone			(2) →	(2) →				

[a]Significance code for two-tailed t-test of paired differences; 1 = p<.02; 2 = p<.01; 3 = p<.001.
[b]Significance test done after logarithmic transformation to correct for skewed distribution.
[c]Heat stabile alkaline phosphatase (presumed to arise mainly from bone as opposed to liver).

Table 13-10

Summary of 3-month changes in laboratory values by treatment, Study III

	Stage III				Stage IV			
	Premarin	Provera	Prov + DES	DES 1 mg	Premarin	Provera	Prov + DES	DES 1 mg
Acid p'tase[b]	(3)[a] →	(3) →	(3) →	(3) →	(3) →	(2) →	(3) →	(3) →
CBG	(3) ←		(3) ←	(3) ←	(3) ←		(3) ←	(3) ←
Plasminogen	(3) ←		(3) ←	(3) ←	(3) ←		(3) ←	(3) ←
Fibrinogen	(3) →	(3) →	(3) →	(3) →	(3) →	(1) →	(3) →	(3) →
Triglycerides			(3) ←	(3) ←	(3) →		(3) ←	(3) ←
17-OH	(1) ←		(3) ←	(3) ←	(2) ←		(3) ←	(3) ←
Alk p'tase[b]			(3) →	(3) →			(3) →	
Cholesterol[b]	(2) ←							(3) ←
H.S. Alk p'tase[c]				(1) →				
Ceruloplasmin		(3) →	(3) →					
Haptoglobin	(3) →		(3) →	(3) →	(3) →		(3) →	(3) →

[a]Significance code for two-tailed t-test of paired differences; 1 = $p < .02$; 2 = $p < .01$; 3 = $p < .001$.
[b]Significance test done after logarithmic transformation to correct for skewed distribution.
[c]Heat stabile alkaline phosphatase (presumed to arise mainly from bone as opposed to liver).

chapter to describe the response of each of these serum measurements to the treatments in Studies II and III in detail; however, Tables 13–9 and 10 show in summary form the response of these measurements after three months of treatment based on paired analysis. The arrows in the table indicate whether the values rose or fell compared to pretreatment levels and the significance codes indicate the levels of certainty about these changes. The analysis was performed on three month values because this period of time is sufficient for changes to occur in all these parameters and the comparisons are not confused by the progression of the disease itself. I will now present some highlights of the analyses of the individual assays.

Prostatic Acid Phosphatase

I have already indicated the effects of orchiectomy and the 5.0 mg dose of DES on the acid phosphatase. In order to study mean changes in acid phosphatase as related to dose of estrogen it is necessary to perform a double logarithmic transformation of the acid phosphatase levels because this distribution is so extremely skewed to the right. After such a transformation, however, one can see a clear-cut pattern consisting of an almost linear dose-response curve for the three doses of DES studied. This means that while all three doses of DES affect the prostatic acid phosphatase, the 5.0 mg dose has a greater effect than the 1.0 mg dose which, in turn, has a greater effect than the 0.2 mg dose. This analysis is currently being prepared for publication. The data from Study III indicate that while Premarin and Provera in the doses studied lead to significant falls in the acid phosphatase, they are not as effective as 1.0 mg DES in this regard. It is also noteworthy that Premarin is more effective than Provera in lowering the prostatic acid phosphatase.

Alkaline Phosphatase

Unlike acid phosphatase, alkaline phosphatase is not pathognomonic of metastasis due to prostatic carcinoma. However, it is useful in some instances as a measure of the extent of bony metastasis. In some recent analysis we have found pretreatment level to be a valuable prognostic variable. The response of the alkaline phosphatase to treatment is more difficult to understand. It has generally been said that estrogen treatment usually produces an increase in the alkaline phosphatases, possibly followed by a later decrease. This behavior may be reflected in our data at three months where we see an inconsistency between the 1.0 and 5.0 mg doses with respect to this variable. With the exception of the placebo-treated group, when we have observed significant changes in the hormonal treatment, they have always been decreased compared to the pretreatment values. In addition to measuring the total serum alkaline phosphatase we have also measured a heat stable portion defined as that portion of the activity which remains after heating the serum to 52° C. It is thought that this measure will be useful in distinguishing between bone involvement and hepatic involvement. Detailed analysis of these data correlated with autopsy findings is planned.

Corticosteroid-Binding Globulin

This variable shows a rather precise dose-related response to estrogen and has therefore been useful in monitoring adherence to the study protocol. When the value falls below that appropriate for the specified dose of estrogen, then we know the patient has stopped taking his medication; conversely, if the value rises inappropriately, we suspect an intake of estrogen not assigned on the protocol. This has permitted us to encourage more careful adherence to the study design. Readers interested in more detail about this serum protein can consult references 25–28.

Plasminogen and Fibrinogen

These variables were included in the hope that they might shed some light on the clotting mechanism as related to cardiovascular deaths on estrogen treatment. In addition it was known that fibrinogen was an acute phase reactant which would be expected to increase in any condition characterized by general stress, such as acute illness or a major operative procedure. This perhaps explains why a significant fall in fibrinogen has been noted in placebo-treated patients. Apparently some acute process, not necessarily the carcinoma of the prostate, brought the patient to the hospital. We have also noted that pretreatment values are generally higher in stage IV patients compared to stage III patients in both Studies II and III; these differences disappear if we omit from the analysis those patients known to be suffering from intercurrent illnesses. In general, fibrinogen has been observed to fall on hormone treatment although the pattern is not entirely clear-cut. Plasminogen, on the other hand, shows a dose-related increase except that the 1.0 mg dose shows as great an increase as the 5.0 mg dose, indicating a plateau in the dose-response curve. Premarin at the 2.5 mg daily dose shows less increase than 1.0 mg DES, and Provera does not apparently affect the serum plasminogen.

An analysis of the relationship between pretreatment values of plasminogen and fibrinogen and death rates has shown that both measurements provide useful prognostic information. Specifically, high initial fibrinogen values were associated with higher death rates for all causes and for prostatic cancer, but not for cardiovascular disease. For plasminogen, low initial values were associated with higher death rates for all causes and for cardiovascular causes, but not for prostatic cancer.

Cholesterol and Triglycerides

These lipids were studied because of the considerable literature suggesting that they are risk factors for cardiovascular death. The mean pretreatment cholesterol levels for these patients were 196 ± 1.3 mg per 100 ml (mean $\pm$ S.E.). This value is significantly lower than that reported for non-cancer controls of similar age. Significant increases in serum cholesterol occurred in some of the estrogen treatments, but the pattern was not entirely consistent; there were no significant declines in cholesterol for any other treatments studied. Pretreatment triglyceride levels were similar to those reported for non-cancer controls of a similar age. One milligram of DES produced a significant increase at three months in both stages III and IV. A smaller increase was noted for Premarin, but this was only present in stage III; Provera at the dose used had no effect on the serum triglycerides. Analyses performed to date have not revealed cholesterol values as being useful in prognosis; however, serum triglycerides have shown the paradoxical result that prognosis is worse if they are in the normal range than if they are either above it or below it! This peculiar finding is being studied in more detail.

Ceruloplasmin and Haptoglobin

These two serum proteins were studied because it was hoped that they might provide some information about severity of disease. Both are known to be acute phase reactants which, in addition, are hormone-responsive. Ceruloplasmin shows a dose-related response to estrogens similar to that for plasminogen, that is, the increase seen with the 1.0 and 5.0 mg doses of DES are equivalent. This variable was not measured in Study III. Haptoglobin, on the other hand, shows a dose-related fall on estrogen therapy. Provera evidently has no effect on haptoglobin; the response to 2.5 mg daily of Premarin is similar to that for 1.0 mg DES.

17-Hydroxycorticoids

The 17-hydroxycorticoids, like the corticosteroid-binding globulin, show a dose-related response to DES. A significant increase was also seen with Premarin, but to a lesser extent than that seen with 1.0 mg DES. Provera appears to be without effect. A detailed analysis[13] has shown that the initial value of the 17-hydroxycorticoids provides useful information about prognosis: in general, the higher the initial value, the worse the prognosis. The 17-hydroxycorticoids did not predict the cause of death but rather were only useful in predicting death from all causes combined. For this and other reasons, it appears that the serum level of the 17-hydroxycorticoids represents a generalized measure of stress. In order to study the relation of this variable to other variables known to be important in the prediction of death such as age, treatment and stage of disease, a logistic regression analysis was performed. Analysis for Study II revealed that all variables except the pretreatment 17-hydroxycorticoids could be eliminated without seriously affecting our ability to predict death at one year. In Study III, however, treatment could be eliminated but stage and age were necessary in addition to 17-hydroxycorticoids to avoid a significant loss of predictive ability for death in the first year.

Testosterone

Testosterone was not measured routinely in either Study II or III, although assays were performed on a limited number of patients. Analysis of these data[29] shows that neither placebo nor 0.2 mg of DES daily caused significant decreases in the serum testosterone levels at three or six months. The 1.0 mg dose of DES did cause a significant decrease in serum testosterone by three months. However, this effect was only observed in stage III. The 5.0 mg dose of DES caused a significant fall by three months in both stages III and IV and the magnitude of this fall was somewhat greater than that for the 1.0 mg dose in stage III. The failure of 1.0 mg of DES to uniformly suppress the serum testosterone may be explained in two ways: (1) the dose is not sufficient to suppress the testosterone in all patients; or (2) not all patients on the 1.0 mg dose were adhering to the assigned treatment at the time the measurements were made. In a recent article, Shearer et al. have suggested that 1.0 mg of DES is not sufficient to suppress the serum testosterone in all patients; however, they found that the 3.0 mg dose was adequate.[30] In the two new VA protocols it is anticipated that testosterone measurements will be performed at all follow-up visits for all patients. These data should be useful in helping to provide a more definitive answer concerning the adequacy of the 1.0 mg dose of DES in suppressing testosterone. In selecting treatment it is important to remember that we are not treating the serum testosterone—we are treating the patient's cancer. It may be that less than maximal suppression of serum testosterone is sufficient.

Zinc

There has been increasing interest in the role of zinc in the prostate, since it is known that the zinc concentration of the prostate is higher than that of any other organ in man. Most of the zinc is concentrated in the epithelium, but its function is unknown. However, several reports have indicated that there is less zinc in prostatic carcinoma than in normal epithelium and, in addition, it is known that the zinc concentration of the prostate is under hormonal control.[31] Because of this interest, the VACURG has been conducting some studies of zinc in plasma, hair, and needle biopsy specimens from the prostate in conjunction with their clinical trials. The data on plasma and hair have not yet been analyzed in detail, but the study of needle biopsy specimens has confirmed that the concentration of zinc in cancer epithelium is much lower than that in normal or hyperplastic epithelium by a factor of about 17-fold.

Physiologic Parameters

Pain and Clinical Status

On the basis of various kinds of evidence we have recommended withholding estrogen therapy until it is required for relief of the patient's symptoms. However, we have frequently been asked if the clinical status of the patient initially treated with placebo and later changed to estrogen was as good as that of the patient who was given estrogen at the time of diagnosis. This is a difficult question to

study since assessment of pain and clinical status is more difficult than recording survival experience. However, since the beginning of our studies we have recorded information on pain and clinical status. Initially, and at each follow-up visit, pain was classified into one of the following categories: no pain, mild pain, moderate pain, or severe pain. By mild pain, we mean the patient complains, but no narcotics or nerve destructive procedures are required. By moderate pain, we mean that the pain is easily controlled with narcotics or surgical procedures. Severe pain is that which is difficult to control even with narcotics and surgical procedures.

In addition the patients' clinical status was rated on a four-point scale as follows: normal activity; some symptoms but patient needs to be in bed less than 50% of the daytime; patient must stay in bed more than 50% of the daytime; patient is

Table 13–11

Average percent of time in pain by stage and treatment, Studies I and II

Stage	Treatment[a]	Number of patients	Average % time in pain
	A. Study I		
	Placebo	262	6.2
III	DES[b]	265	3.7
	Orch+Pcb	266	4.2
	Orch+DES	257	3.5
	Placebo	223	27.0
IV	DES	211	22.5
	Orch+Pcb	203	23.7
	Orch+DES	216	20.2
	B. Study II		
	Placebo	75	3.2
III	0.2 mg DES	73	4.0
	1.0 mg DES	73	0.2
	5.0 mg DES	73	1.3
	Placebo	53	16.7
IV	0.2 mg DES	52	29.1
	1.0 mg DES	55	14.8
	5.0 mg DES	54	14.1

[a]Treatment abbreviations: DES = diethylstilbestrol; Orch = bilateral orchiectomy; and Pcb = placebo.
[b]The dose of DES in Study I was 5.0 mg.

unable to get out of bed. Detailed analysis of these variables indicated that in neither Study I nor Study II were patients initially assigned to placebo more likely to suffer pain or impaired performance, provided their treatment could later be changed when required because of symptoms. In addition we have found that the four treatments in each of the two studies differed more with respect to pain than with respect to performance. However, these two variables are highly correlated.

In Table 13–11(A) the four treatments in stage III and IV patients in the first study are compared with respect to the average percentage of time spent in pain. We note that in stage III the average percentage of time spent in pain is quite low, roughly 5% or less. It is true that the percentage of time for placebo is greater than that for the other three treatments, but the differences are not great. In stage IV, patients were in pain roughly 20 to 27% of the time and again placebo appears to be only slightly inferior to the other treatments.

Similar data for Study II are presented in Table 13–11(B). Note that in both stages III and IV, patients were in pain less than in the first study. We have no ready explanation for this apparent difference, but it may be related to more careful management of patients. In this study, in both stages III and IV, the 0.2 mg of DES was associated with slightly more pain than the other three treatments. Possibly, this may be explained by the clinician's reluctance to change a patient's treatment if he was receiving 0.2 mg of DES; this dose is sufficient to cause breast changes in about one third of the patients, but it is not sufficient to control prostatic cancer. Since this was a double-blind study, the clinicians may have mistakenly assumed that the patient was receiving one of the higher doses of DES; this error would not have occurred with placebo since breast changes would seldom have been noted. The equivalence of the 1.0 and 5.0 mg doses of DES in controlling pain is

apparent, but neither was much better than placebo. We concluded that these results, with respect to pain and performance status, are in good agreement with those based on survival, i.e. (1) the patient's welfare is not jeopardized by initial therapy with placebo and (2) the 1.0 and 5.0 mg doses of DES appear to be equivalent in their ability to relieve the symptoms of prostatic cancer.

Our data also suggest that patients may show a better response when treatment is delayed until it is required.[32] It is true that patients whose initial treatment is placebo require a change of treatment more often than patients who are started with estrogen or orchiectomy. However, if we compare the time placebo patients spent in pain after their treatment had been changed with that of patients started on more active therapy, we find that placebo patients generally did better. Unfortunately our data are insufficient to establish this point with certainty, but the concept that the response may be improved by delaying therapy should be taken into account when trying to decide whether to treat patients at the time of diagnosis or to delay treatment until it is required for the relief of symptoms. In any event, the results of Study I and II for stage III patients indicate that initial treatment with placebo, that is, delaying estrogen treatment until and if it is needed to control symptoms, did not adversely affect the overall survival compared to initial treatment with estrogen.

Blood Pressure

Analysis of data from Study II has revealed that there is a small but significant dose-related change in pulse pressure due to estrogen treatment. The possible relationship of this finding to the excess cardiovascular deaths on estrogen treatment is being explored and will be the subject of a future publication. It is not likely, however, that much of the excess cardiovascular hazards can be explained in this way because the cardiovascular deaths have resulted from a variety of causes including myocardial infarction, pulmonary emboli, cerebrovascular accidents, and congestive heart failure. Estrogen treatment of women treated with contraceptive pills has also been implicated in causing an increase in blood pressure.[33]

Breasts

It is well known that breast changes characterized by subareolar thickening and sometimes accompanied by pigment change and tenderness occur in males treated with estrogens. The degree of response is variable, but the condition often progresses to full-scale gynecomastia. The data in Studies II and III permit us to examine the effects of different doses of estrogen on these changes. It may be that minimal changes are difficult to detect because we have had breast changes reported after six months of placebo therapy in 10 of 93 patients in stages III and IV of Study II. This was of course a double-blind study, so the investigators were not aware of the drug being received by the patient. In tabulating these figures we removed patients who were known not to be adhering to the assigned study treatment, but it is possible that some of these ten patients may have received exogenous estrogens from some source unknown to us. The 0.2 mg dose of DES produced breast changes at six months in about a third of the patients while the 1.0 and 5.0 mg doses produced breast changes in roughly two-thirds of the patients.

After six months of treatment there is no difference in the probability of breast changes between the 1.0 and 5.0 mg doses. In the third VA study, breast changes were noted by six months in about two-thirds of the patients treated with 2.5 mg of Premarin daily, but in only about 10% of the patients treated with Provera, 30 mg daily. In this study only a

little more than 75% of the patients on 1.0 mg daily DES showed breast changes at six months. A slightly greater percent was observed for patients receiving both 1.0 mg DES and Provera.

It is known that breast changes can be avoided in patients treated with estrogen by prior irradiation of the breasts. This procedure might well be worth consideration in future studies, particularly if it is desirable to avoid bias in changing patients' therapy in a double-blinded study. For example, the breast changes in Study II in effect allowed the investigators to identify the treatment the patients were receiving in a large number of instances at least so far as distinguishing between placebo and estrogen therapy. Of course another advantage of prior irradiation might be sparing the patient the tenderness and possible embarrassment consequent to gynecomastia.

Edema

Pedal edema has not been a major problem in these studies. In Study II, pedal edema was observed more frequently in stage IV than in stage III when evaluated after six months of therapy. In stage III, the percentages of patients showing edema at six months were 8.3 for placebo and 3.7, 10.9, and 11.8 for 0.2, 1.0, and 5.0 mg DES, respectively; in stage IV, the corresponding figures were 12.1, 14.7, 12.8 and 34.3. These data suggest that the 5.0 mg dose of estrogen causes fluid retention in some stage IV patients. In stage III, the three doses of DES do not differ significantly from placebo with respect to this side effect, and in stage IV, the 0.2 and 1.0 mg doses caused fluid retention no more often than placebo. In the third VA study, pedal edema was found at 6 months in about the same proportion of patients for 2.5 mg of Premarin and 1.0 mg of DES. Pedal edema was no more common in those patients treated with Provera plus 1.0 mg DES than those treated with 1.0 mg DES alone.

Provera alone was associated with pedal edema at six months in less than 4% of the patients, lower than the rate for placebo in Study II. Since pedal edema would be expected in some portion of the patients in this age group even without any drug therapy, it is difficult to relate hormone therapy to development of pedal edema, except perhaps in stage IV patients treated with 5.0 mg DES.

Size of the Primary Lesion

I have already noted, in the discussion on prognostic variables, the importance of the primary lesion size. In addition, when the primary tumor is rectally palpable, it provides a good opportunity for measuring the effectiveness of hormonal therapy. It has of course been known since 1941 that estrogens cause the primary tumor to regress.[1-3] Our studies provide additional information of a somewhat more quantitative nature on the effects noted with differing doses of DES and with Premarin and Provera. In both studies, the primary tumors averaged about 10–12 sq. cm. in stage III and about 16–20 sq. cm. in stage IV. In Study II no significant change was noted at six months in the placebo-treated groups. The 0.2 mg dose of the DES showed insignificant or minimal changes; however, the 1.0 and 5.0 mg doses were comparable in the changes effected in the size of the primary lesion. The reduction at six months in stage III was about 6–7 sq. cm. compared to about 9 sq. cm. in stage IV. In Study III, Provera showed little effect on the size of the primary lesion; the effect of Premarin was equivalent to that of 1.0 mg DES. The combination of Provera and 1.0 mg DES was no more effective than 1.0 mg DES alone in reducing the size of the primary tumor.

FUTURE PLANS

At the time of this writing (December 1974) two new protocols are almost completed and it is anticipated that the entry of patients into the third VA study will terminate early in 1975 when the new protocols are activated. The first of these two protocols, designated as Study IV, is planned as a natural sequel to the preceding three main studies described in this chapter. In all these studies the staging system shown in Table 13–2 has been used. In Study IV the first major innovation will be to assign treatment on the basis of the combined stage-grade category rather than according to the more or less classic staging system shown in Table 13–2. Details of the stage-grade category can be found in Chapter 9. Patients in category 3–8 will be randomly assigned to one of the following three treatments: (1) no treatment, (2) DES, 1.0 mg daily, or (3) DES, 3.0 mg daily, plus aspirin, 300 mg twice a day. It is hoped that aspirin may possibly further reduce the cardiovascular complication in patients with carcinoma of the prostate, since it is known that aspirin can reduce platelet aggregation and may thus be of value for preventing arterial thrombosis. In addition, aspirin has been shown to prevent venous thrombosis in postoperative patients. Patients who fall into categories 9–15 will be randomly assigned to one of the following three treatments: (1) DES, 1.0 mg daily; (2) Flutamide, 250 mg three times a day; or (3) a combination of DES and Flutamide. Flutamide (Schering 13521) is a new antiandrogen which probably exerts its effect on prostatic cancer by a mechanism different from that of estrogens.

It is thought that the antiandrogen blocks the growth effects of testosterone and other androgens on prostatic epithelial cells, possibly by inhibiting the formation of an essential dihydrotestosterone-protein-chromatin complex in the prostatic cell nucleus. Flutamide is a nonsteroidal drug which is apparently devoid of estrogenic, progestational, androgenic or adrenal cortical activity. In addition antiandrogens are not known to affect the cardiovascular system adversely; therefore, these agents are potentially ideal for the treatment of prostatic carcinoma. This drug has not yet been tested in a large-scale clinical trial.

In addition to changes in the design of the protocol, in Study IV more hormonal assays will be performed routinely. It is anticipated that prolactin, FSH, and LH will be measured along with testosterone, estrogens, and a number of the more interesting assays described for Studies II and III.

The second new protocol, to be designated as the Chemotherapy Study, is designed to admit patients who are in relapse from previous hormone therapy or orchiectomy. Patients from all previous studies will be eligible for this study when they relapse in addition to the patients who have never been in the previous studies. Also it is anticipated that patients will be admitted from 12 additional VA hospitals connected with the newly organized Cooperative Urological Radiotherapy Research Group. Here patients will be randomized to one of the following three treatments: (1) intravenous diethylstilbestrol diphosphate (Stilphosterol) followed by oral Stilphosterol, (2) oral Estracyt, and (3) L-phenylalanine mustard (L-PAM). Stilphosterol is widely used in the treatment of late-stage prostatic cancer patients in relapse, and will therefore serve as the reference group. Estracyt is a new urethane-type nitrogen mustard, a derivative of estradiol which has been used with some success both in Sweden and to a lesser extent in this country.

It is known that the drug has very low toxicity for a nitrogen mustard-type compound, and it is assumed that the drug is transported to its target site in an inactive form, being guided, as it were, by the estrogen moiety. Following hydrolysis into its two separate components at the target site, both the estrogen and the alkylating portion are free to act on the cancer cells. The third drug, L-PAM, is a nonestrogen and a noncell-cycle–specific alkylating agent. Its structure is that of a cytoxic group attached to a carrier molecule of phenylalanine. This drug may be administered orally. Unlike most nitrogen mustards, it is characterized by minimal toxicity confined for the most part to myelosuppression which is usually dose-related. Occasional transient nausea and vomiting controllable with antiemetics has been encountered, but skin rashes and alopecia are rare and hepatic and renal toxicity have not been reported. This drug has recently been used with success as adjuvant therapy in treating post-mastectomy breast cancer patients who have positive lymph nodes and are therefore at increased risk of early recurrence. The logic of the chemotherapy protocol is to compare a pure estrogen (Stilphosterol), an estrogen bound to a nitrogen mustard (Estracyt), and a pure (nonestrogenic) nitrogen mustard derivative (L-PAM).

CLINICAL TRIALS IN PROPER PERSPECTIVE

In this chapter I have tried to illustrate the benefits to be obtained from large randomized prospective clinical trials. It should be apparent that a wide variety of questions have been answered, including many which were not anticipated when the studies were originally designed. Of course the main goal in any clinical trial is to compare treatments in as unbiased a fashion as possible, but in addition, large amounts of data are collected in a uniform way at regular intervals; here these data have been found useful in answering a variety of questions about the nature of prostatic cancer and the effects of treatment on its course. Nevertheless, it is important to remember that even these large studies can only provide answers to a limited number of questions, since only a limited number of specific treatments were studied and the patient population under study is not necessarily representative of all patients with prostatic cancer.

With this caveat in mind, one is still free to speculate about general truths regarding this disease.

The work described in this chapter represents the dedicated contributions of a great number of people over a long period of time. This work will continue and should provide the medical world with valuable information to supplement the knowledge gained in other research settings. Clinical trials are only one of the many ways of obtaining scientific information about the nature of a disease and its treatment. Their interpretation is likely to be more fruitful when combined with careful clinical observations, with detailed laboratory investigations in small series, and the accumulated experience of critical and observant clinicians.

References

1. Huggins, C, and Hodges, C. V.: Studies on prostatic cancer. I. The effect of castration, of estrogen and of androgen injection on serum phosphatases in metastatic carcinoma of the prostate. Cancer Res.,1:293, 1941.
2. Huggins, C., et al.: Studies on prostatic cancer. II. The effects of castration on advanced carcinoma of the prostate gland. Arch. Surg., 43:209, 1941.
3. Huggins, C., et al.: Studies on prostatic cancer. III. The effects of fever, of desoxycorticosterone and of estrogen on clinical patients with metastatic carcinoma of the prostate. J. Urol., 46:997, 1941.
4. Nesbit, R. M., and Baum, W. C.: Endocrine control of prostatic carcinoma. J.A.M.A., 143:1317, 1950.
5. Nesbit, R. M., and Plumb, R. T.: Prostatic carcinoma—a follow-up on 795 patients treated prior to the endocrine era and a comparison of survival rates between these and patients treated by endocrine therapy. Surgery, 20:263, 1946.
6. The Veterans Administration Co-operative Urological Research Group: Carcinoma of the prostate: A continuing co-operative study. J. Urol., 91:590, 1964.
7. Seltzer, C. C., and Jablon, S.: Effects of selection on mortality. Am. J. Epidemiol., 100:367, 1974.
8. Byar, D. P., et al.: Carcinoma of the prostate: Prognostic evaluation of certain pathologic features in 208 radical prostatectomies—examined by the step-section technique. Cancer, 30:5, 1972.
9. Gleason, D. F.: Classification of prostatic carcinoma. Cancer Chemother. Rep., 50:125, 1966.
10. Mellinger, G. T., et al.: The histology and prognosis of prostatic cancer. J. Urol., 97:331, 1967.
11. Gleason, D. F., et al.: Prediction of prognosis for prostatic adenocarcinoma by combined histological grading and clinical staging. J. Urol., 111:58, 1974.
12. Huggins, C.: The treatment of cancer of the prostate. Can. Med. Assoc. J., 50:301, 1944.
13. Blackard, C. E., et al.: Correlation of pretreatment serum nonprotein-bound cortisol and total 17-hydroxycorticosteroid values with survival in patients with prostatic cancer. N. Engl. J. Med., 291:751, 1974.
14. Byar, D. P., et al.: An exponential model relating censored survival data and concomitant information for prostatic cancer patients. J. Natl. Cancer Inst., 52:321, 1974.
15. Bayard, S., et al.: An analysis of treatment data from patients with prostatic cancer using an exponential model relating survival to concomitant variables. Cancer Chemother. Rep., 58:845, November/December 1974.
16. Greenberg, R. A., et al.: Selecting concomitant variables using a likelihood ratio step-down procedure and a method of testing goodness of fit in an exponential survival model. Biometrics, 30:601, 1974.
17. Byar, D. P., et al.: Survival of patients with incidentally found microscopic cancer of the prostate: Results of a clinical trial of conservative treatment. J. Urol., 108:908, 1972.
18. The Veterans Administration Co-operative Urological Research Group: Treatment and survival of patients with cancer of the prostate. Surg., Gynec. & Obstet., 124:1011, 1967.
19. Byar, D. P.: Treatment of prostatic cancer: Studies by the Veterans Administration Cooperative Urological Research Group. Bull. N.Y. Acad. Med., 48:751, 1972.
20. Byar, D. P.: The Veterans Administration Co-operative Urological Research Group's studies of cancer of the prostate. Cancer, 32:1126, 1973.
21. Blackard, C. E., et al.: Orchiectomy for advanced prostatic carcinoma: A reevaluation. Urology, 1:553, 1973.
22. The Coronary Drug Project Research Group: The Coronary Drug Project—Initial findings leading to modifications of its research protocol. J.A.M.A., 214:1303, 1970.
23. Blackard, C. E., et al.: Incidence of cardiovascular disease and death in patients receiving diethylstilbestrol for carcinoma of the prostate. Cancer, 26:249, 1970.
24. Bailar, J. C., III, et al.: Estrogen treatment for cancer of the prostate: Early results with 3 doses of diethylstilbestrol and placebo. Cancer, 26:257, 1970.
25. Seal, U. S., and Doe, R. P.: Purification and properties of transcortin, the cortisol-binding globulin from patients with cancer of the prostate. Cancer Chemother. Rep., 16:329, 1962.
26. Seal, U. S., and Doe, R. P.: Corticosteroid-binding globulin. I. Isolation from plasma of diethylstilbestrol-treated men. J. Biol. Chem., 237:3136, 1962.

27. Seal, U. S., and Doe, R. P.: Corticosteroid-binding globulin: Species distribution and small-scale purification. Endocrinology, *73*:371, 1963.

28. Doe, R. P., et al.: Estrogen dosage effects on serum proteins: A longitudinal study. J. Clin. Endocrinol. Metab., *27*:1081, 1967.

29. Kent, J. R., et al.: Estrogen dosage and suppression of testosterone levels in patients with prostatic carcinoma. J. Urol., *109*:858, 1973.

30. Shearer, R. J., et al.: Plasma testosterone: An accurate monitor of hormone treatment in prostatic cancer. Br. J. Urol., *45*:668, 1973.

31. Byar, D. P.: Zinc in male sex accessory organs: Distribution and hormonal response. *In* Structure and Function of the Male Sex Accessory Organs. Edited by D. Brandes. New York, Academic Press, 1973.

32. Hurst, K. S., et al.: An analysis of the effects of changes from the assigned treatment in a clinical trial of treatment for prostatic cancer. J. Chron. Dis., *26*:311, 1973.

33. Weir, R. J., et al.: Blood pressure in women taking oral contraceptives. Br. Med. J., *1*:533, 1974.

Chapter 14

Radiation Management of Cancer of the Prostate

W. D. RIDER

After more than half a century of being in the wilderness, radiotherapy is now coming to the fore as a potent weapon in the management of prostatic cancer.

It is perhaps germane to examine, at least from an historical point of view, why and how this change has occurred. In the early days of radiotherapy, the equipment available was generally of very low voltage by today's standards, the physics of radiation was primitive, and radiobiology was in its infancy. These three factors combined to create an impression that cancer of the prostate was an "inherently" radioresistant cancer. Unfortunately, before this misconception could be corrected, the era of hormone management came on the scene and dominated thinking for a quarter of a century.

Interest in the radiation management of prostatic cancer was reawakened by Flocks in 1952,[1] when he reported on the use of radioactive colloidal gold injections. In 1962 Bagshaw reported, at the International Congress of Radiology in Montreal, the experience of the Stanford group using their new linear accelerator.[2] Both reports were encouraging and stimulated great interest. Many reports since have confirmed that the classic prostatic cancer is indeed a radioresponsive tumor, but that regression rates are quite variable. Thus, some tumors will have vanished before the completion of a course of irradiation, but the majority require months and even years before the gland has either reverted to normal, or disappeared altogether.

It has been pointed out that regression rates, or disappearance rates after irradiation, have almost nothing to do with the eventual "radiocontrol."[3] This is a very important concept, since in the past, the assessment of radiation has, to a large degree, been based on early impressions of the disappearance of the tumor. Likewise, assessment of radiation effect has relied on histopathologic interpretation of biopsies taken some time after the event. On morphologic grounds alone, opinions have been expressed as to the viability of the tumor. As has been shown by modern radiobiology, there are no reliable morphologic criteria on which to base such an opinion. At present, only time will tell if a cancer is radiocontrolled

—by its biologic behavior and not by its appearance under a conventional microscope.

The management of prostatic cancer should be a multidisciplinary approach. The indiscriminate use of estrogens by urologists is to be condemned as much as the treatment of all prostatic cancers by the radiation oncologist. For instance, the treatment of a 50-year-old virile buck should not necessarily be the same as that for a 90-year-old priest. While prostatic cancer occurs commonly, it is often not the cause of the patient's death. Nature often intervenes, and occasionally she is helped by the female hormone, or misdirected irradiation.

SELECTION OF THE PATIENT FOR IRRADIATION

Any method of therapy is bound to have bias, based on the author's personal experience.

The question of potency looms large in the minds of many these days, and for the younger individual is very important, but for the older patient it may be of no consequence. Some assessment of the biologic virulence of the disease is essential, and this can only be appreciated by serial clinical observations. Thus an enlarged hard gland found on routine examination and shown to be malignant should not necessarily be treated. Cancer, particularly prostatic cancer, is often a chronic disease and should be handled along lines similar to the treatment of other chronic diseases. Far too many patients have been crucified on the cross of "cure."

Perhaps the most important decision to be made is to treat or not to treat. Obviously, the younger the patient the more likely is active treatment going to be advised. A period of observation is usually not out of place, since growth of the gland and the state of symptoms can only be assessed by several observations.

Once a decision has been made to treat, the next step is how, and here, valued judgement is required. First of all a critical assessment of the extent of the disease must be made.

PRINCESS MARGARET HOSPITAL— PRETREATMENT ASSESSMENT

1. History, physical examination with particular attention to facts which may lead to an assessment of growth rate of the tumor.
2. Biochemical evaluation—particularly acid and alkaline phosphatase measurements of serum.
3. Hematologic evaluation. Hb., WBCs, platelets, and so on.
4. Bone marrow examination where indicated.
5. Search for distant metastases by means of X-ray studies and/or radioisotope investigation.
6. Renal function studies as measured by blood urea and intravenous pyelograms. Ureteral obstruction is no contraindication to irradiation, be it radical or palliative. More than 50% of patients with ureteral obstruction recover function following irradiation.
7. Lymphography can be a useful investigation.
8. Examination under anesthesia and cystoscopy. This is one of the most important assessments of all and must be carried out by the radiation oncologist if he is to be responsible for treatment of the patient. Of course, this does not exclude urologic participation in the examination. Ideally, a collaborative assessment leads to agreement on the size, extent, and fixation of the tumor. The information gleaned from this assessment must then be transferred to suitable radiographs so that the radiation planning will be accurate. It is hoped that some of the newer developments in radiology will help to make this evaluation

more accurate, e.g., computerized tomography.

Once all this information has been collected the most important decision of all has to be made: to treat or not to treat, and if to treat, how.

Some hints regarding the philosophy of treatment have been given and will not be repeated. It is assumed that treatment is indicated. Should this be radical or palliative, but how radical or how palliative?

All irradiation *must* be done with supervoltage equipment.

RADICAL IRRADIATION

Doses, times, and techniques in radical irradiation have, on the whole, been poorly described in the literature. Doses, in particular, have been grossly overestimated on the old assumption that this is a radioresistant cancer. Much iatrogenic damage has been produced, and this has caused discredit of a valuable method of therapy.

The experience of the Princess Margaret Hospital leads to the belief that treatment with doses in excess of 5000 rads in four weeks, by conventional techniques, controls as many patients as does treatment with higher doses, and is associated with very low morbidity and zero mortality. Regression rates may be lower than with the more commonly practiced U.S. dose levels, but this appears to be of no consequence in the long run. In the early P.M.H. experience, radiation was confined to the prostate gland using rotation techniques similar to those described by Bagshaw.[2] However, it was not long before it became clear that we were facing the same problems as had been surmounted many years before in the treatment of bladder cancer; the development of gross metastases in regional lymph nodes. This experience and past philosophy lead to the standard "radical irradiation" program, which consists of a regional lymph nodal irradiation plus what is fashionably called a "boost" in the

prostatic gland itself. The regional irradiation dose is 3500 rads in three weeks and the "boost" 1500 rads in one week. At the moment the need for the prostatic booster dose is not absolutely clear. Some patients in whom it has been omitted have fared as well as those who have had it. Further evaluation is clearly needed.

How regional should the lymph node irradiation be? In the past 15 years the region irradiated for both bladder and prostatic cancer has been getting larger and larger. Initially it was strictly confined to the pelvic lymph nodes, then the lower paraaortics were added, and currently the total regional lymphatic chain to the level of the diaphragm is included in the area treated. Lymphography has demonstrated that far more paraaortic lymph nodes are involved than previously suspected. This increased radiation volume puts an additional strain on the patient in terms of small bowel morbidity, but with the use of X rays generated at 15 to 25 Mev, this morbidity can be greatly reduced, particularly if the overall time for this part of the treatment is extended to four weeks, and the booster dose is increased to 2000 rads in one week. With this program, the prostate receives 5500 rads in a period of five weeks. It is important not to exceed these dose levels. The details of the techniques are illustrated in diagrammatic form (Figure 14–1).

A word of warning—the "rad" may not yet be internationally reliable—local experience and custom must be taken into account in the planning of a treatment program.

The postirradiation followup is of paramount importance. Assessment of the size of the gland has a very high error rate in the conscious patient, but the hope of accurate evaluation by newer radiologic means may well give us better information on the rates of regression after irradiation and thereby produce some useful data with which to plot "dose

Cancer of Prostate—P.M.H. Radical Irradiation

(1) Regional lymph node irradiation
    (a) Irregular A.P. and P.A. fields
    (b) Minimum energy Co[60] ideal 15–25 Mev X-rays
    (c) Dose-midplane 3500 rads in 20 fractions
                                 –26 days
(2) "Boost" dose to prostate
    (a) Technique depends on tumor size
      (i) Small—360-degree rotation
      (ii) Large—opposed fields
    (b) Dose—1500–2000 rads tumor dose

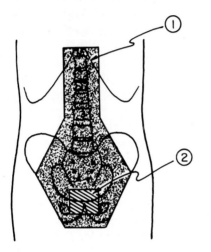

(3) Important anatomic landmarks
    (a) Obturator fossae
    (b) Diaphragmatic level for paraaortic lymph nodes
    (c) Wide enough to include all iliac lymph nodes

Figure 14–1. Cancer of prostate—PMH radical irradiation.

response" curves. One of the clinical pitfalls which has come to light is mistaking the pubic arch for the prostate gland. This pitfall can be avoided if a firm catheter or metal probe is passed into the bladder before the prostate is examined per rectum. All too commonly the issue is confused by different observers, and additional therapy is advised purely on the basis of a single observation with one digit in the rectum! There is only one way to assess radiation failure, and that is to be sure that the gland is growing larger at least six months after irradiation.

The question arises—should patients be treated concurrently with their irradiation by estrogens and/or orchidectomy? Opinions differ on this topic, but Bagshaw's results suggest that the addition of hormone manipulation does not clearly improve the results.[4] It is the Princess Margaret Hospital impression that such manipulation in fact makes the outcome worse. Generally speaking, in the practice of medicine, the use of "blunderbuss" therapy has been condemned, perhaps with the exception of combination cancer chemotherapy, for which there is a reasonably rational basis.

One of the most important decisions to be made by the urologic fraternity is "What is the best primary treatment for prostatic cancer?" One of these days, we will see a truly multidisciplinary approach—the team being headed by an appropriate oncologist.

PALLIATIVE MANAGEMENT

A great deal of medical practice is, in reality, palliation—diabetes is not cured, heart and lung disease are not cured, rheumatology and psychiatry have their failures, and fractured bones often heal if left to nature!

All too commonly in the past, palliation has been equated with "indifferent therapy," be it surgical or radiotherapeutic. In the radiotherapeutic field, any form of therapy using energies less than Co[60] is to be condemned; in North America there is absolutely no justification for the "occasional radiotherapist" to practice palliative irradiation for prostatic cancer with orthovoltage equipment.

A realistic attitude toward palliation in cancer of the prostate must be taken. What are we trying to palliate and where in the scheme of things does our particular brand of therapy have its place? No one denies the dramatic subjective and objective response to either orchidectomy and/or the administration of estrogens, but it is doubtful that this happens more often than in 30% of patients. Much of the credit attributed to hormone manipulation is only the result of the natural history of the disease.[5] The so-called acceptable side effects have been ignored—the large and miserably painful breasts induced by estrogens, the impotence, and the cardiovascular complications all attest to the lack of appreciation of the true value of palliation. Likewise, the radiation trauma to the rectum, with the production of hemorrhagic proctitis, strictures, and fistulas are no credit to those who practice radiation therapy, while the induction of massive radiation fibrosis in the subcutaneous tissues and radionecrotic fractures of the pelvis, in the name of palliation, can no longer be condoned.

What then is the place of irradiation in the palliation of prostatic cancer? Is it real or is it just another medical myth?

Real palliation can be obtained in many circumstances by well-designed plans of irradiation. Some of these are listed below:

"The Obstructed Bladder Syndrome"

When the bladder neck is constricted by cancer and the patient has difficulty in voiding, the best radiation results are achieved when there has been no previous transurethral resection. This is probably because the transurethral resection destroys the muscle of the bladder neck, whereas radiation does not. Any bladder neck incompetence after irradiation is due to muscle destruction caused by the cancer—man repairs only by fibrous tissue, unlike the worm. It is time to "slay the myth" that irradiation commonly causes bladder neck obstruction by edema and that for these reasons it is better to carve out a channel with the hot, or perhaps more fashionably, the cold loop. It is far better to leave in situ a small indwelling catheter during the course of irradiation than to resect the prostate surgically.

The best radiation techniques are "short and sharp." The following prescriptions are good, with a distinct bias for the last mentioned:

1. Using 20 Mev X-rays—3500 rads in 10 fractions over a period of two weeks, with large parallel opposed fields.
2. Using Co^{60}—2000 rads in one week in five fractions also using large opposed fields.
3. Using any form of supervoltage therapy, be it Co^{60} or higher X-ray energies—three doses of 800 rads to the prostate with parallel opposed fields delivered on days 0–7–21 over a period of three weeks. Some of these patients are clinically free of disease at five and more years.

Bleeding from tumor in the prostatic bed can also be treated along lines similar to the obstructed bladder neck, but a single dose of 500 to 1000 rads often permits more critical evaluation, so that future planned irradiation can be carried out more effectively once the hematuria has ceased.

Distant Metastases

A variety of metastatic syndromes exist and each presents problems in management, demanding considerable understanding of the disease and expertise in radiation therapy if the patient is to obtain maximum benefit.

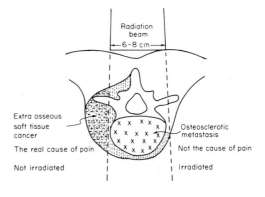

Figure 14–2. The real problem in irradiation of spinal metastases.

It has been said that the predominant metastatic problem is of secondary disease in the pelvis and lumbar spine, due to venous spread via the Batson plexus. This is probably just another "myth," if the problem is viewed from a symptomatic point of view. Most osteosclerotic metastases do not cause pain, but pain may be present with osteosclerotic disease, and the fundamental cause is soft tissue disease, usually in the extradural or paraspinal spaces (Figure 14–2).

Secondary Disease in Bone

The characteristic secondary bone disease in prostatic cancer is osteosclerotic. If osteolytic secondaries are discovered one must consider a "secondary primary." Osteolytic involvement of bone by prostatic cancer does occur, but is almost invariably due to direct extension from

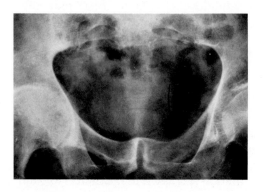

Figure 14–3. Osteolysis from direct invasion of left superior pubic ramus in cancer of prostate.

adjacent soft tissue disease—for example, erosion of the pubic rami directly from the prostate itself or from involved lymph nodes in any site (Figures 14–3 and 14–4). Very occasionally a "free soft tissue metastasis" will erode bone and produce osteolysis. Fortunately, from a therapeutic point of view, these distinctions may not be all that important, but there are occasions when it is vital. Take, for example, the situation of a patient with intractable pain in the lumbar spine. Roentgenograms show osteosclerotic metastases in several vertebrae; irradiation is given, using narrow fields to a relatively high dose, and the pain is not relieved. Ergo, prostatic cancer is radioresistant. A much better explanation for the failure to respond to irradiation is that the paraspinal disease which was really the cause of the pain was not included in the volume treated. Paraspinal secondary disease is probably much more common than is generally realized, and most often missed by "innocent radiotherapy." Thus in the planning of radiotherapy, a cardinal rule is, as always, give a wide margin to cover the inaccuracies inherent on clinical investigation and in the physics of irradiation (Figure 14–1).

Neurologic Problems

There are two clinical situations worthy of comment. The first is spinal cord

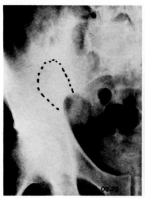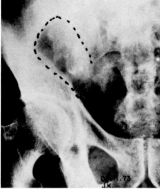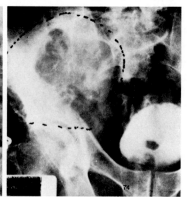

Figure 14—4. Progressive osteolysis from metastatic prostate cancer in internal iliac lymph nodes.

compression with impending paraplegia due to extradural or even intradural secondary cancer. A myelogram can be helpful in locating the anatomic level, but frequently is unnecessary when plain roentgenograms show paraspinal secondary disease. When the level has been localized, irradiation can be used most successfully to relieve the pain and forestall the paraplegia. It is most important, in the radiation plan, that large enough fields are used—rarely anything less than 10 cm wide is sufficient and never less than 15 cm long, however short the lesion may appear radiologically. It is a good working rule of thumb that the largest compatible field should be used. As to dose, any fraction less than 500 rads carries with it a high risk of "radiation edema" which will accentuate the cord compression. A good prescription is 2000 rads tumor dose in 4 fractions or if the patient is mobile 800 rads on days 0–7–21 will permit easy clinical assessment of the neurological status.

For the patient already affected with paraplegia, adequate irradiation can often forestall the need for surgical decompression, provided the neurologic status is monitored carefully. Thus evaluation of the status every 2–4 hours is carried out; if matters get worse, and there is no response either to intravenous mannitol or steroids, then surgical decompression is required.

It has been found that the classic neurosurgical teaching of decompression laminectomy for either paraplegia or complete block on myelography needs revision; it is, in fact, rarely necessary.

Careful followup of patients with prostatic cancer is essential since spinal cord problems can be anticipated and treated most successfully long before the patient becomes a "paraplegic emergency."

The second neurological lesion is intracerebral metastases. Here, the management is along lines similar to spinal cord metastases. Once again neurosurgical decompression is rarely indicated, and

excision of a "solitary metastasis" belongs to anecdotal medicine. The irradiation plan for cerebral metastases must include the whole brain since single metastases are very rare. In a patient with known secondary disease, detailed neurological work-up by arteriography, air studies, and the like are usually unnecessary. A positive brain scan or evidence from computerized tomography, if available, is sufficient indication for irradiation. Radiation techniques are simple—large parallel opposed fields to the whole head to doses identical with those used for spinal cord problems—cover with intravenous mannitol or steroids when necessary.

The results of neurologic irradiation often surprise the most optimistic radiation oncologist and can boggle the neurosurgical mind. The longest remissions, sometimes years, occur usually in patients with the most chronic, low voltage, forms of prostatic cancer—the worst results, symptomatic relief lasting only a few weeks, occur in those unfortunate to have virulent disease.

Hematologic Problems

A major problem of secondary disease in bone, is bone marrow replacement and the attendant anemia. Leukoerythroblastic anemia is a common feature in widespread metastatic prostatic cancer to bone. Its management is one of the most difficult problems faced by oncologists. For the radiation oncologist, who, all too commonly, has to see these patients after all other forms of therapy have been tried, it is indeed a dilemma. On the whole, it is probably best to let the patient die with dignity, but there are occasions when an effort must be made. In recent years a somewhat unconventional and experimental approach has been made in Toronto in the management of advanced metastatic cancer of all kinds. This consists of giving total body irradiation of 800 rads. As is well known, 800 rads in a single whole body dose would be fatal due to ablation of the bone marrow, however, if this dose is given as two half body doses most patients survive, and somewhat paradoxically often get tremendous relief of their symptoms.

Put in very simple terms, the body is divided into two halves at the level of the umbilicus; one half, the most symptomatic half, is irradiated to 800 rads and five to six weeks later the other half is given the same dose. Provided that the bone marrow is not totally destroyed by cancer, the patient will survive, hematologically speaking, because bone marrow stem cells circulate from the unirradiated half to the irradiated half during the period between the doses of irradiation, and at the same time it is believed that the cancer cells, which are more likely to be "fixed," do not.[6] In widespread secondary disease from cancer of the prostate, which is causing great pain and misery, this technique has brought great alleviation in suffering—indeed far greater and with much less morbidity than the use of radiophosphorus. At the present time, it is still in the experimental phase and should not be attempted without the back-up of a complete oncologic institute and for these reasons details of technique will not be given. It may be that the "prophylactic" use of some form of total body irradiation will eventually be incorporated into the plan of management of primary prostatic cancer as has been suggested for cancer of the esophagus.[7]

MISCELLANEOUS DISORDERS

Radiation for Suppression of Estrogen-induced Gynecomastia

Irradiation of the breasts, if given *before* the administration of estrogens, will reduce the probability of this unpleasant complication. Fairly large doses of irradiation are required, for example—1000 rads single dose or its equivalent. Estrogens should not be started earlier than 3–4 weeks after the irradiation to allow time for atrophy of the target cells in the breast.

Benign Prostatic Hypertrophy

Not uncommonly in the radiation management of bladder cancer, the radiation oncologist is faced with the problem of a large benign prostatic hypertrophy causing some degree of obstruction. In the past, because of the risk of edema, it has been the custom to resect the gland transurethrally. Over the years it has proved unnecessary to resect these benign glands surgically because the majority will shrivel under the influence of irradiation. This has led to the use of irradiation as a primary therapeutic modality for the large adenoma of the prostate, with good results. A simple technique of three fractions of 600 rads on days 0–7–21 has produced total ablation of large prostatic adenomas without the necessity of hospitalization.

References

1. Flocks, R. H., et al.: Treatment of carcinoma of the prostate by interstitial radiation with radioactive gold (Au[198]) a preliminary report. J. Urol., 68:510, 1952.
2. Bagshaw, M. A., et al.: Linear accelerator supervoltage radiotherapy. VII Carcinoma of the prostate. Radiology, 85:121, 1965.
3. Rider, W. D.: Radiosensitivity—What Is It? Laryngoscope, LXXXI, 1045, 1971.
4. Ray, G. R., et al.: Definitive radiation therapy of carcinoma of the prostate; a report on 15 years of experience. Radiology, 106:407, 1973.
5. Whitmore, W. F., Jr.: The natural history of prostatic cancer. Cancer, 32:1104, 1973.
6. Fitzpatrick, P. J., and Rider, W. D.: Half-body radiotherapy. Int. J. Radiat. Biol., 1:197, 1976.
7. Rider, W. D.: Innovations in radiation therapy. J.A.M.A., 227:183, 1974.

Chapter 15

Cryosurgery of the Prostate

MYRON S. ROBERTS, EROL O. GURSEL, MAGUID R. MEGALLI, and RALPH J. VEENEMA

Since the advent of cryosurgical equipment first developed by Cooper in 1961,[1] much attention has been centered on the field of cryobiology and the destructive effect of cold on human tissues. In 1964, Gonder et al.[2] first reported on the use of cryoprostatectomy for the clinical management of benign and malignant prostatic diseases. The original purpose of this operation was literally to destroy by freezing, obstructing prostatic tissue, so as to provide for an adequate urinary passageway. However, our experience with this operation since 1964, confirmed by other investigators,[3-8] has led us to the conclusion that the procedure has a very limited application and certainly is not the panacea for prostatectomy that was originally proposed.

As with many clinical experiments and new surgical techniques, the so-called by-products of the technique turn out to be more valuable and of greater clinical importance than the initial procedure itself. This may be the case with cryoprostatectomy, as the immunologic and autoimmune responses that have been observed following destruction of malignant prostatic tissues have opened up an entirely new avenue of cryosurgery research.[9-11]

EQUIPMENT

The cryosurgical equipment consists of a Linde CE-4 cryosurgical unit with a CR 10 prostate cryoprobe (Frigitronics), which is a completely integrated system employing liquid nitrogen as its cooling medium. The unit consists of a vacuum-insulated liquid nitrogen container, feed-line, and probe assembly and is equipped with temperature control devices, including a heater so that at the proper time the probe can be quickly warmed and withdrawn.

The prostate cryoprobe is 8 mm in diameter (No. 24 French) and is shaped very much like a Van Buren urethral sound. Its vacuum insulation allows all but the heat exchange chamber to remain at room temperature. The heat exchange chamber measures 5½ cm in length. A small button is located 1 cm from the exchange chamber, the purpose of which is to allow for easy rectal palpation of the position of the heat exchange chamber at the time of cryoprostatectomy (Figure 15–1A).

277

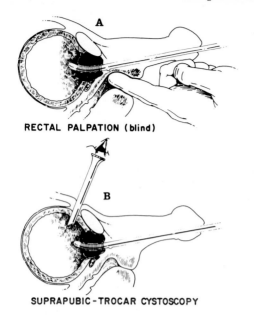

RECTAL PALPATION (blind)

SUPRAPUBIC-TROCAR CYSTOSCOPY

Figure 15–1. Transurethral cryosurgery of prostate.

SURGICAL PROCEDURES

We prepare our patients for cryoprostatectomy as we would for any other type of conventional prostate surgery. The preoperative workup includes an intravenous pyelogram, chest roentgenogram, electrocardiogram, renal function studies, urine culture, serum acid phosphatase, retrograde urethrogram, and cystoscopy. Patients with prostatic carcinoma, in addition to the just-mentioned studies, should also have a bone scan, immunologic profile, and a bone marrow acid phosphatase determination.

Cryosurgery of the prostate can be performed either transurethrally or via the perineal approach.

Transurethral Cryosurgery

The method of treatment is simple and is usually done under a light general or regional anesthesia (Figure 15–1). Cases have been successfully performed without anesthesia as the freezing process itself acts as a local anesthetic. The fact that cryoprostatectomy can be successfully performed without an anesthetic agent must certainly be regarded as one of the great advantages of this procedure. We routinely dilate the urethra with a No. 28 French catheter to facilitate the passage of the cryoprobe. Subsequent to this, either a No. 16 or No. 18 French catheter is passed into the urinary bladder and the bladder is emptied of its content. Then 200 to 400 cc of air is instilled into the urinary bladder, the purpose of which is to hold the bladder wall away from the tip of the cryoprobe. Water cannot be used for this purpose as it too will freeze. The cryoprobe is then inserted transurethrally until the button is palpated rectally at the apex of the prostate. With correct positioning of the cryoprobe, any part of the freezing chamber extending beyond the prostate gland enters the bladder, which is insulated by air.

The process begins by initially freezing the prostate to $-20°$ C. At this temperature the probe is frozen in place. This is a critical temperature as the adjacent tissues, although frozen, are not irreversibly destroyed. It is at this temperature that the position of the cryoprobe is rechecked. If it is not properly placed, the probe can be reheated and repositioned without fear of destroying any important structures, such as the urethra or sphincter. If the probe is properly positioned, the temperature is then lowered to $-180°C$ and the freezing process continued.

During the freezing process, the prostate gland becomes rock hard and swollen and feels very much like a far advanced prostatic neoplasm. The button is engulfed by the swelling of the prostate during the freeze and within a few minutes is no longer palpable.

During the freeze the rectal finger continuously moves the rectal mucosa. If there is any suggestion that the freeze is extending onto the rectal wall, the procedure must be immediately terminated. The proper end point of the freezing process is when all lobes of the prostate are rock hard and a sensation of coolness is transmitted to the rectal finger. Once again, the rectal wall should never be involved in the freezing process. If this happens the chance of producing a rectal fistula is increased.

After freezing, the cryoprobe is heated to 37°C and removed. A No. 22-30 cc three-way Foley catheter is immediately inserted on a stylet into the urinary bladder, and the bladder is irrigated. Variable amounts of hematuria will be noted for the first eight to 12 hours, but this rarely presents a problem.

The postoperative management of the patient is simple. Proper catheter hygiene is essential and the patients are placed on antibiotics. The patients are fully ambulatory by the first postoperative day and pain has not been a major factor.

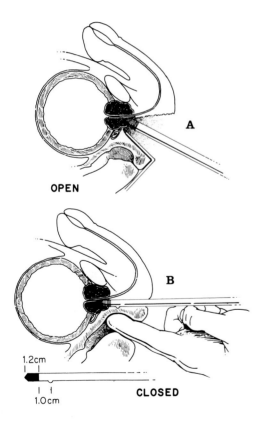

OPEN

1.2cm

1.0cm

CLOSED

Figure 15–2. Transperineal cryosurgery of prostate.

Suprapubic trocar cystoscopy during cryoprostatectomy has been advised by some surgeons as it allows for direct visualization of the freezing procedure and may help prevent accidental freezing of the trigone (Figure 15–1B).[12] We have used this method in 10 patients without complications but have not felt that this is an essential part of the procedure.

Transperineal Cryosurgery

Open Perineal Cryosurgery

This method, first advocated by Flocks et al.,[13] is almost exclusively used in the treatment of prostatic cancer (Figure 15–2A). The prostate gland is exposed via an open perineal procedure and under direct visualization, a pierce point cryoprobe is inserted into the prostate and then frozen. The rectal wall is retracted well away from the field of freezing, allowing for a very thorough freeze of the prostate without fear of producing a rectourethral fistula. We have used this technique successfully in six patients.

Closed Perineal Cryoprostatectomy

This procedure is quite simple and can easily be done under local anesthesia (Figure 15–2B).[14]

Transperineal prostatic cryosurgery is performed by introducing the pierce point cryoprobe through a small stab incision in the perineum. The probe is localized in the prostate by careful rectal palpation. When properly positioned, the prostate gland is then completely frozen, using as the end point of the freeze the same guidelines that are used for transurethral cryoprostatectomy. This technique has been employed in 12 patients with good results. The only complication encountered was a perineal abscess in one patient who responded to conservative management.[15]

It has been advocated by some investigators that cryosurgery in combination with a limited transurethral resection of the prostate gland is advisable.[16] This has been suggested to help reduce the freezing time and to facilitate the functional results of cryoprostatectomy, as it will allow for earlier urethral extubation.

Postoperative Complications

Postoperative complications have been minimal and similar complications have been observed both in patients with benign prostatic hypertrophy and prostatic carcinoma (Table 15–1). The main difficulty encountered with this procedure is the marked adherence of the cryonecrotic prostate tissue in the prostatic urethra. Almost all patients continue to pass pieces of prostatic tissue per urethra for at least three months and sometimes for as long as six months after operation. This explains why many of the patients initially experience difficulties with voiding after the Foley catheter has been removed. As more and more of the prostatic tissue sloughs, the urethral passageway widens. The patients' voiding

habits improve and their residual urine is decreased. Five patients sloughed their entire prostate gland into the bladder, resulting in intermittent urinary retention as a ball-valve type of obstruction. Three of these patients required a suprapubic cystostomy to remove this mass of necrotic debris. In the other patients the tissue was successfully extracted endoscopically.

Bleeding is usually not a problem, although most of our patients have had a mild hematuria for eight to 12 hours after surgery. It is for this reason that cryoprostatectomy is advised for those patients with coagulopathies. Other complications, as listed in Table 15–1, include urinary incontinence, sepsis, transient penile edema, periurethral abscess, urethral perineal fistula, urethral stricture, urethritis, epididymitis, vesicorectal fistula, and vesicoureteral reflux.

Nonurologic complications of cryoprostatectomy are listed in Table 15–2. As noted, cardiopulmonary problems presented the major complications, but it should be remembered that most of the

Table 15–1

Urological complications of (transurethral) cryosurgery

Manifestation	BPH (50 pts.)	Prostatic Cancer (80 pts.)	
Slough retention	4	1	
Required cystostomy	(2)	(1)	
Total urinary incontinence	1	3	
Bilateral hydronephrosis	——	1	
Gram-negative sepsis	4	5	(1 died)
Urinary retention	3	——	
Persistent hematuria	3	1	
Penile edema	3	2	
Periurethral abscess	——	3	
Urethroperineal fistula	——	1	
Urethral stricture	——	2	
Urethritis	2	2	
Epididymitis	1	——	
Vesicorectal fistula	1	1	
Vesicoureteral reflux	1	2	

——, not applicable.

Table 15–2

Nonurological complications of transurethral cryosurgery

Manifestation	BPH (50 pts.)	Prostatic Cancer (80 pts.)
Cardiopulmonary	1	3 (2 died)
Phlebitis	1	——
Intestinal obstruction	1	——
Spontaneous pneumothorax	——	1
Allergic		
Urticaria	4	——
Anaphylactic shock	1	1 (died)

——, not applicable.

patients subjected to cryoprostatectomy were very debilitated and at poor risk.

Four patients developed urticaria during surgery. One was associated with a severe hypotension which responded promptly to steroids and antihistamines. The exact cause of this reaction is not known but it was suspected to be due to a histamine release triggered by the local freezing process. One patient, who had a sequential freeze in the treatment of advanced carcinoma of the prostate, developed anaphylactic shock and expired.

Other nonurologic complications of transurethral cryosurgery include: phlebitis, intestinal obstruction, and spontaneous pneumothorax.

Immunologic Aspects of Cryosurgery

Recently cryosurgery of the prostate has been performed for the management of prostatic cancer, not for the relief of obstructive uropathy, but merely for provoking a possible immunologic response. After observing the production of autoantibodies to rabbit prostatic tissue complex,[17] and noting that repeated freezing of rabbit prostates produced a booster phenomenon,[18] cryosurgery has now been performed in patients with far advanced prostatic carcinoma. The purpose of this technique is to stimulate an isoimmune response. Clinical observations by Soanes et al.[9] suggested that the remission of metastatic lesions in patients with prostatic cancer could be related to the cryosurgery and its induced immunologic response. We have employed this technique in 35 patients with disseminated prostatic cancer, using initially the sequential freezing technique, i.e., freezing the prostate three times, at two-week intervals.

More recently we have used the double-freezing technique at one sitting, freezing for one minute and thawing for 90 seconds, followed immediately by another freeze until the temperature again reaches −160° to −180°C (Figure 15–3). Using this double-freezing technique, we

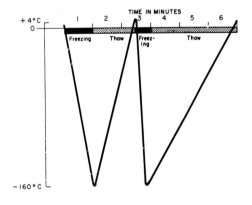

Figure 15–3. Double freeze and thaw cycles during cryotherapy.

have observed palliation of metastatic osseous pain in 20 patients.[10] In one patient regression of osseous metastasis was observed, as evidenced by isotopic bone scanning.[11]

Interestingly, postmortem examinations of three of the eight patients who died more than six months after cryosurgery showed no residual tumor in the prostate.[10] However, no histologic evidence of an immunologically induced response was noted in these autopsied patients.

In conclusion, cryoprostatectomy is a safe maneuver that can be quickly performed with slight blood loss and little postoperative discomfort. This procedure can be performed satisfactorily with minimal or no anesthesia. Postoperative urologic and medical complications have been observed, but for the most part have been minor, even though most of our patients have been very poor surgical risks. It is our opinion that cryoprostatectomy is the procedure of choice for those patients who have a bleeding tendency or in patients who forbid the use of transfusions. The immunologic response induced by a double prostatic freeze and its effect in controlling metastatic bone pain has been commented on.

The main disadvantage of this procedure is the slow postoperative improvement. This is due to the marked adherence of the necrotic prostate tissue and prolonged urethral obstruction.

Cryoprostatectomy, at this time, is not meant to replace any other method of prostatectomy. It is definitely a very useful additional operative technique for the urologists' armamentarium when they treat the very elderly and the poor-risk medical patients, or when they deal with those patients who have far advanced metastatic prostate carcinoma, when all other therapeutic efforts have failed.

References

1. Cooper, I. S., and Lee, A. St. J.: Cryothalamectomy—hypothermic congelation: A technical advance in basal ganglia surgery. Preliminary report. J. Am. Geriatr. Soc., 9:714, 1961.
2. Gonder, M. J., et al.: Experimental prostate cryosurgery. Invest. Urol., 1:610, 1964.
3. Jordan, W., Jr., et al.: Cryosurgery of the prostate: A preliminary report. J. Urol., 98:512, 1967.
4. Ortved, W. E., et al.: Cryosurgical prostatectomy. A report of 100 cases. Br. J. Urol., 39:577, 1967.
5. Roberts, M., et al.: The place of cryoprostatectomy. Trans. Am. Assoc. Genitourin. Surg., 60:58, 1968.
6. Marshall, A.: Cryogenic surgery of the prostate. Proc. R. Soc. Med., 61:1139, 1968.
7. Green, N. A.: Cryosurgery of the prostate gland in the unfit subject. Br. J. Urol., 42:10, 1970.
8. Kishev, S. V., et al.: Late results following cryosurgery of the prostate (A clinical and panendoscopic study of 80 patients). J. Urol., 104:893, 1970.
9. Soanes, W. A., et al.: Remission of metastatic lesions following cryosurgery in prostatic cancer. Immunologic considerations. J. Urol., 104:154, 1970.
10. Gursel, E. O., et al.: Cryosurgery in advanced prostate cancer. Urology, 1:392, 1973.
11. Gursel, E., et al.: Regression of prostatic cancer following sequential cryotherapy of the prostate. J. Urol., 108:928, 1972.
12. Reuter, H. J.: First experience with endoscopic cryosurgery of prostatic adenoma and carcinoma. Int. Urol. Nephrol., 3:31, 1971.
13. Flocks, R. H., et al.: Perineal cryosurgery for prostatic carcinoma. J. Urol., 108:933, 1972.
14. Megalli, M. R., et al.: Closed perineal cryosurgery in prostatic cancer: New probe and technique. Urology, 4:220, 1974.
15. Megalli, M. R., et al.: Closed Transperineal Cryosurgery in Prostatic Cancer. Presented at the 72nd annual meeting of the New York Section of American Urological Association, London, Sept. 19–27, 1974.
16. McDonald, H. P., Jr.: Combined Cryosurgery and Transurethral Resecton for Obstructive Prostate Disease. Presented at International Symposium on Cryosurgery in Urology, Stuttgart, Germany, July, 1973.
17. Shulman, S., et al.: Studies on organ specificity XVI: Urogenital tissues and autoantibodies. Immunology, 10:99, 1966.
18. Riera, C. M., et al.: Studies in cryoimmunology IV: Antibody development in rabbits after isoimmunization followed by freezing. Immunology, 15:779, 1968.

Chapter 16

Surgery of the Prostate Gland

JOHN G. CONNOLLY

The purpose of this chapter is to discuss the role of surgery and to describe the surgical procedures used in the diagnosis and control of prostatic cancer. I have not described the more common urologic procedures such as TUR of the prostate gland or bilateral orchiectomy, as these are discussed in the standard urologic textbooks. In addition, no amount of writing or illustration would facilitate learning the technique of transurethral resection of the prostate gland unless the reader has had adequate training in the basics of the procedure. I have omitted any discussion about the less conventional surgical approaches to the prostate gland such as combined suprapubic and perineal approach. The transsymphyseal approaches have not been discussed. Hypophysectomy and adrenalectomy are infrequently used in prostatic cancer, and the details of these procedures have been omitted.

Prostatic cancer is the leading cause of death in men over 75 years of age, and more men die of this cancer than of any other except bronchogenic and gastrointestinal carcinoma. In 1970, prostatic cancer caused 17,000 deaths in the United States and it was estimated that 35,000 new cases would be recognized in the U.S. in 1972.[1] About 11% of all carcinomas in the male are of prostatic origin and 14 to 40% of men over 50 years of age will have histologic evidence of prostatic cancer at postmortem.[2-4] However, it should be emphasized that many of these tumors are latent, are of no biologic significance, and are recognized as an incidental finding at operation or at postmortem.

While prostatic cancer is rare before the age of 50, its incidence increases rapidly until the age of 80—a phenomenon that may be owing to increased exposure to carcinogens or that may reflect the aging process. The incidence of prostatic cancer shows some remarkable racial and geographic differences: Its frequency in Chinese and Japanese is approximately one-tenth that noted in the Caucasian. It is common in the American Negro and in Alameda County, California. The incidence in the Negro is nearly twice that in Caucasians living in that state.[5]

ANATOMY OF THE PROSTATE

General Relationships

The prostate gland, a firm structure made up of glandular and muscular elements, lies immediately below the bladder neck and surrounds the proximal portion of the urethra. Situated in the pelvis between the symphysis pubis and the rectum, it sits on the deep layer of the urogenital diaphragm. In its nonhypertrophied state in the adult, the gland is about the size of a chestnut and weighs approximately 20 g. It has an anterior, posterior, and two lateral surfaces, as well as an apex and a base. The base, which is directed upward and applied to the neck of the urinary bladder, is pierced by the prostatic urethra, and approximately one-third of the gland lies anterior to this structure. The urethra goes out through the apex of the gland, which is directed downward and lies on the superior fascia of the urogenital diaphragm.

The anterior surface of the prostate lies deep to the symphysis pubis and is attached to it by the puboprostatic ligaments. The broad, flattened, triangular posterior surface, which lies anterior to the rectum, contains a longitudinal midline depression called the median sulcus. The sulcus is more distinct at the base and virtually disappears in the lower portions of the gland. Two ejaculatory ducts enter the prostate gland in a concavity at the junction of the base and the posterior surface. They pass downward and forward through its posterior portion to open at the verumontanum in the apical portion of the prostatic urethra.

The prostate gland is divided into an anterior lobe, a pair of lateral lobes, a median or posterior commissural lobe connecting these two, and a posterior lobe. The last-mentioned structure, which is the most frequent site of prostatic cancer, lies behind the plane of the ejaculatory ducts, whereas the median lobe lies between this structure and the urethra. In man, the individual lobes are not so clearly demarcated as in some other species and, on cross section, it is difficult to distinguish true lobes. However, the anatomist can display two concentric layers of prostatic tissue as Franks origi-

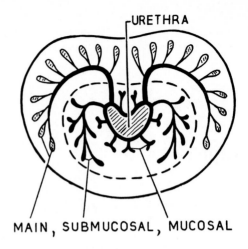

MAIN , SUBMUCOSAL , MUCOSAL

Figure 16–1. Transverse section of prostate. Prostate in transverse section showing three concentric groups of glands. (From Grant's Method of Anatomy, 9th ed., edited by J. V. Basmajian. Baltimore, Williams & Wilkins, 1975.)

nally described them in 1954 (Figure 16–1).[6] The outer concentric layer is thick and composed of long tortuous glands—the prostatic or main glands. Prostatic cancer arises in these structures. The inner glands, which consist of two types—the larger submucosal variety and a small 'mucosal' set immediately underneath the mucosa—are separated from this outer layer by an indefinite capsule. Benign prostatic hypertrophy arises from these inner glands. For the most part, the epithelial cells that make up the prostatic acini are tall, columnar epithelium, and beneath them is a flattened layer of basal cells which is not easy to identify. There is no important histologic difference between the inner and outer groups of glands.

As its outer covering, the prostate possesses a true capsule which consists of a dense, tough, whitish layer. The capsule is composed of both fibrous tissue and smooth muscle fibers that are continuous with the muscular tissue of the bladder and urethra. Because it sends prolongations into the parenchyma, the capsule's attachment to the gland is extremely firm. In addition, outside of the capsule the gland possesses a fascial sheet that is derived from the rectovesical layer of the pelvic fascia. This rectovesical layer passes inward on the superior and lateral surfaces from the side walls of the pelvis. Anteriorly, it sweeps off the gland and is attached to the posterior surface of the symphysis pubis as the puboprostatic ligaments. Beneath and between the puboprostatic ligaments lies the prostatic venous plexus of Santorini. The rectovesical fascia of Denonvilliers', which covers the posterior surface of the prostate gland, is formed by the fusion of the two layers of peritoneum. This fascia covers the seminal vesicles and the ampulla of the vas and fuses with the prostatic capsule at the junction of the ampulla and the ejaculatory ducts.

ARTERIAL SUPPLY

The prostate gland derives its main arterial supply from a branch of the internal iliac artery via the inferior vesical artery. This small artery terminates in two large groups of prostatic vessels—the urethral group and the capsular group. We are indebted to Flocks for much of our knowledge concerning the blood supply of the prostate.[7] The urethral arteries enter the prostate gland at the vesicoprostatic junction to supply the bladder neck and the periurethral portions of the gland (Figure 16–2). The capsular arteries enter the gland laterally and give off four or five branches which supply mainly the periphery of the parenchyma; however, these vessels eventually reach the urethra in the region of the verumontanum.

VENOUS DRAINAGE

The veins draining the prostate communicate with each other, with the deep dorsal vein of the penis, and with other veins to form three venous plexuses. One is located anteriorly and two are lateral to the prostate gland. The venous drainage of the prostate enters the inferior vena cava except for a few posterior tributaries that may enter the portal circulation. The anterior plexus which is important to the surgeon, is in two layers—one superficial and the other deep. The veins in the superficial layer are situated in the fatty tissue of the endopelvic fascia which overlies the prostate and vesical neck. Deep to the superficial veins and within the capsule lies the plexus of Santorini. This plexus receives tributaries from the prostate gland and the bladder and also receives large branches from the deep dorsal vein of the penis.

The deep veins of the anterior plexus constitute venous sinuses which may be perforated during transurethral surgery. The right and left branches of the deep dorsal vein of the penis form the lateral venus plexuses of the prostate (Figure 16–3). These plexuses, which receive tributaries from the prostate gland, take a posterolateral course around the side of the gland and continue on to the bladder base.

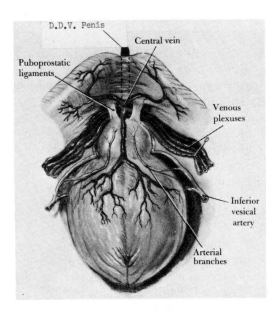

Figure 16–2. Blood supply of prostate gland. (From Weyrauch, H. M.: Surgery of the Prostate. Philadelphia, W. B. Saunders Co., 1959.)

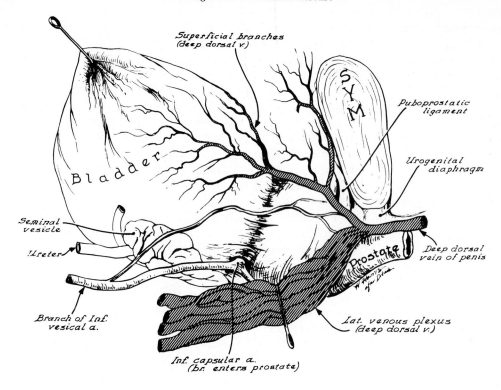

Figure 16–3. Venous plexuses of prostate: lateral view (After Beneventi.) (From Weyrauch, H. M.: Surgery of the Prostate. Philadelphia, W. B. Saunders Co., 1959.)

At the base they receive branches from the seminal vesicles and usually coalesce into one inferior vesical vein which empties into the internal iliac vein. In addition to the anastomosis between the anterior and lateral plexuses, there are many communications with the pubic, pudendal, deep epigastric, and obturator veins and with the hemorrhoidal and vesical plexuses.

LYMPHATICS OF THE PROSTATE GLAND

The many lymph vessels in the prostate gland are arranged as fine capillaries in a network around each glandular acinus. These small capillaries drain into larger vessels which pass toward the periphery of the gland. At the periphery there is a definite periprostatic lymphatic network that eventually forms three or four main

branches lateral to the prostate gland (Figure 16–4). These collecting vessels empty into nodes lying beside the internal and external iliac arteries. In addition to these lymphatic routes, lymph vessels can be found going to nodes in the presacral region, and they make numerous communications with lymphatics of the bladder, seminal vesicle, and rectum.

SURGICAL TREATMENT OF PROSTATIC CANCER

Treatment of this cancer is determined by its stage, by certain biologic properties of the tumor, and by the aggressiveness of the surgeon. Radical surgery can be recommended only for those patients who have a reasonable life expectancy; who have tumor confined to the prostate gland; and who give no radiological or biochemi-

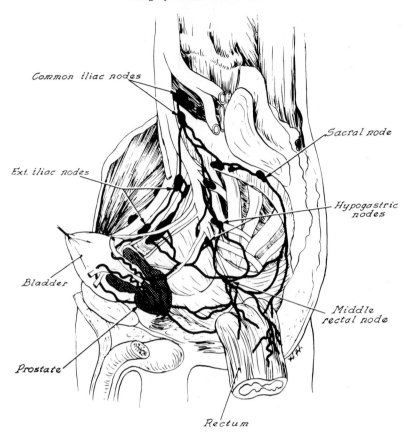

Common iliac nodes

Sacral node

Ext. iliac nodes

Hypogastric nodes

Bladder

Middle rectal node

Prostate

Rectum

Figure 16–4. Lymphatic drainage of prostate. (From Weyrauch, H. M.: Surgery of the Prostate. Philadelphia, W. B. Saunders Co., 1959.)

cal evidence of metastatic disease. The presence of anaplastic tumor should probably be a contraindication to radical surgery. Any discussion of the treatment of prostatic cancer must be based on a method of staging the disease, and the most acceptable method currently is that based on Whitmore's classification.[8]

The principal features of this classification are as follows:

In *Stage A*, there is no clinical evidence of prostatic cancer. The diagnosis is made by the incidental finding of tumor either in a surgical specimen or at autopsy. There is no evidence of local tumor extension beyond the prostate gland and there are no metastases.

In *Stage B*, there is a palpable nodule or an indurated area in the prostate gland. On examination, the tumor is confined to the prostate gland and there is no evidence of metastases.

In *Stage C*, the tumor is easily palpable and there is evidence of extension beyond the prostate gland but no distant metastases. Serum acid phosphatase may or may not be elevated.

In *Stage D*, there is evidence of distant metastatic cancer of the prostate gland.

Early prostatic cancer (stages A and B) can be managed by several methods, including: radical surgery, hormonal therapy, external or interstitial irradiation, or a combination of these approaches. There is much controversy about the best method of treating this stage of the disease.

Patients with well-differentiated stage A cancer of the prostate gland do well regardless of treatment, and the five-year survival approaches normal.[9-11] While it is likely that all clinically active prostatic cancers begin as stage A lesions, not all stage A lesions become clinically manifest. Many are not biologically active. Therefore, if any series advocating the various therapeutic approaches contain a large number of patients with well-differentiated stage A disease, the results will be impressive.

In reviewing the literature on the treatment of early prostatic cancer, the percentage of latent cancers varies from series to series, and it is almost impossible to find truly comparable groups of patients who have undergone different treatments. Hence the difficulty in selecting the optimum treatment. However, while most investigators believe stage A prostatic cancer to be a low-grade disease,[8,12,13] others believe it requires vigorous surgical treatment.[14] There is no question that poorly differentiated stage A lesions—especially if they involve the margins of the tissue removed—have a grave prognosis. Table 16–1 is a summary of the results obtained in treating prostatic cancer by various approaches.

Most series in this table contain patients with stage A cancer. If one examines the 15-year survivals, there appears to be little to choose between the various treatments with the exception of the Mayo series in which 54% survived 15 years (stages B and C). The Mayo series are of some interest in that they laid down rigid criteria for the patients to be included in their prospective study. They represent a highly select group. These results are impressive; however, about 50% of the survivors were on hormonal therapy for metastatic disease.

Those who advocate conservative treatment of early prostatic cancer quote the work of Barnes and Ninan.[15] Thirty-three percent of their patients (many were stage A), treated by hormones and TUR where

indicated, survived for at least 15 years. The proponents of radical surgery refer to the work of Jewett and others.[13,14,16-18] It is of interest to examine the Jewett series in some detail. Of the 86 patients who were shown to have cancer confined to the prostate gland at surgery, 28 were cured but 21 were not cured. It is obvious that either the metastases were present (undetected) before the surgery or they occurred during the surgery. Those patients who failed usually died of metastases. It is quite clear that radical prostatectomy will control local disease; however, our present methods of determining the spread of cancer are crude. We are, therefore, unable to state with certainty that radical surgery will be curative.

DIAGNOSTIC SURGERY—The Prostatic Biopsy

Diagnosis of prostatic cancer is made on the basis of history, general physical examination, and specific examinations of the prostate gland. In most instances, patients with early prostatic cancer have few urologic symptoms, and the only finding is a suspicious area—either a nodule or an indurated area. A discrete nodule, the earliest palpable change, has a 50% chance of being malignant.[19] The obvious reason for performing a prostatic biopsy is to determine whether or not such a nodule is malignant, but a further indication for this procedure may be a patient with an unknown primary who has a metastatic lesion of glandular origin.

The most widely accepted method of obtaining prostatic tissue for histologic diagnosis is by needle biopsy, which may be done by the transperineal or transrectal approach. In early cancers of the prostate gland, transurethral resection (TUR) may be unrewarding because the posterior lobe is relatively inaccessible by this approach. However, if the patient has advanced prostatic cancer and severe urologic symptoms, TUR will establish a diagnosis in more than 90% of patients. In addition,

Table 16–1

Survival rates in prostatic cancer by treatment[a]

Author(s)	Patients	% Survival		Clinical Type of Lesion	Pathologic Staging	Treatment
		10 yr	15 yr			
Emmett et al. (1960)[24]	57	54		Latent	A	TUR only
Barnes and Ninan (1972)[15]	136 108	57	33	Palpably confined and latent	A B	Endocrine ± TUR
Jewett (1970)[17]	103 86	50	35 41	Palpably confined; micro-scopically confined	B C	Surgery ± endocrine
Belt and Schroeder (1972)[16]	464 185	44 55	22 31	All, including latent, microscopically confined	A B	Surgery ± endocrine
Hudson and Howland (1972)[14]	13	62		Microscopically confined including 6 latent	A B	Surgery ± endocrine
Ray et al. (1973)[24]	51 18	41 56		All, including 4 latent palpably confined	A B C / A B	Radiation ± endocrine / Radiation alone
Mayo series (1972)[13]	115 74	72	54	Palpably confined nodules	B C	Surgery ± endocrine

[a]Adapted from Culp, O. S., and Meyer, J. J.[13]

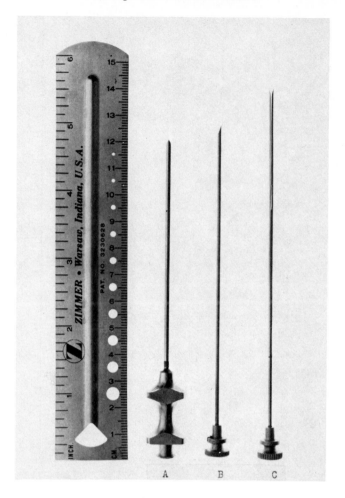

Figure 16–5. Vim-Silverman needle. A, Sheath; B, Obturator; C, Cutting prongs.

10% of patients undergoing prostatectomy for prostatic disease that appears clinically benign will have a malignant focus in the excised tissue, i.e., "latent" prostatic cancer.

In making a percutaneous perineal approach, most surgeons prefer to use the Franklin modification of the Vim-Silverman needle (Figure 16–5). This needle contains a metallic ridge near the tip of the cutting prong to trap a core of tissue. The perineal approach is usually made under general anesthesia; however, some surgeons do it under local anesthesia. With the patient in the lithotomy position,

suitably prepared and draped, the surgeon inserts a well-lubricated finger into the rectum and then introduces the needle into the perineal skin immediately above the anal sphincter. The finger in the rectum guides the needle tip into the suspicious area of the prostate gland. The obturator is then withdrawn, the cutting prongs are inserted, and a long cylinder of tissue is removed. If the suspicious area is less discrete, the surgeon should do multiple biopsies of the suspicious lobe and also take several biopsies from the contralateral lobe.

Complications after perineal biopsy include hemorrhage, occasional febrile episodes, and (rarely) "seeding" of tumor along the needle track. To prevent local sepsis, it is wise to sterilize the patient's urine beforehand and to give antimicrobial prophylaxis after the procedure, e.g., 4 tablets trimethoprim sulfamethoxazole/ day for four days.

Some surgeons use a Veenema cup biopsy through the perineal approach; this is a satisfactory instrument but is not as popular as the Vim-Silverman needle.

Perineal needle biopsy usually provides adequate specimens for diagnosis and has the advantage that the procedure does not disturb the anatomic planes in the event that further surgery is necessary. However, the surgeon faces a problem; if his index of suspicion is high but the tissue obtained is benign he then has the choice of doing an open perineal biopsy or waiting and repeating the procedure in four-to-six weeks. If an adequate specimen was obtained from a highly suspicious nodule and it was benign, the needle biopsy should be repeated in six-to-eight weeks. If the second biopsy is negative and the clinical impression is that the patient has a malignant lesion, the case for an open perineal biopsy should not be undertaken lightly, because it carries a significant risk of impotence, urinary incontinence, and rectal injury.

Transrectal Biopsy with the Franzen Needle

In 1960, Franzen and colleagues described a transrectal aspiration biopsy of the prostate gland using a long, fine needle introduced along a special guide.[20] A ring on the guide fits over the tip of the examining finger which is then placed in the rectum. This arrangement allows the examining finger to palpate the nodule and then pass the needle along the guide and into the nodule for aspiration biopsy. Cytologic examination is done on the aspirate of prostatic material. Such a transrectal aspiration biopsy can be done under general or local anesthesia.

A word should be said about the cytologic studies of fluid obtained by prostatic massage. This is a most unreliable method of obtaining material for diagnostic study, and of course massage of a malignant gland violates certain important surgical principles.

Open Perineal Biopsy

Open perineal biopsy is usually undertaken in suspected early prostatic cancer when one cannot obtain satisfactory biopsy specimens by other means. Open biopsy may be indicated when the index of suspicion is high and when repeated needle biopsies are negative, and when the needle specimens are highly suspicious but not diagnostic. There are several complications associated with open perineal biopsy including impotence, urinary incontinence, and rectal injury. A further difficulty can arise if radical surgery is contemplated and the frozen sections are not diagnostic. The surgeon may be faced with the prospect of closing the incision and waiting for the permanent sections to be read before deciding on further surgery. If the permanent sections reveal that the patient has prostatic cancer and the patient is fit for further surgery, radical prostatectomy by the perineal or retropubic route is technically possible during the first seven days after the diagnostic surgery. If more than this time is allowed to elapse, the intervention should be deferred for at least eight weeks.

Positioning of the patient is very important in perineal prostatic surgery. The perineum must be supported by a perineal elevator (Palmer perineal board, sandbags, or folded towels) and should be elevated so that it is on a plane parallel with the floor. When the proper position is obtained, the perineum projects beyond the end of the operating table.

The operation is begun, after the patient is suitably prepared and draped, by inserting a curved urethral tractor into the bladder and opening the blades. Some

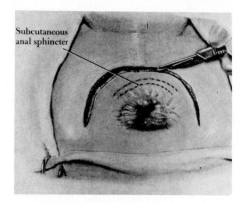

Figure 16–6. Skin incision. (From Hudson, P. B., and Stout, A. P.: An Atlas of Prostatic Surgery. Philadelphia, W. B. Saunders Co., 1962.)

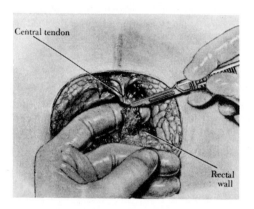

Figure 16–7. Division of central tendon. (From Hudson, P. B., and Stout, A. P.: An Atlas of Prostatic Surgery. Philadelphia, W. B. Saunders Co., 1962.)

surgeons carry out this step later. A curved skin incision is made about 1 inch anterior to the anus and extended between the medial borders of the ischial tuberosities (Figure 16–6). The skin incision is deepened to divide the various layers of fascia in the perineum. Following this the ischiorectal fossa is encountered. By developing this space on either side, it is then possible to elevate the central tendon by inserting the finger under it and to divide it with a scalpel (Figure 16–7). After the central tendon has been severed, the an-

terior rectal wall is protected from injury by a gauze sponge and is depressed with the surgeon's index and middle fingers. This exposes the deep portion of the external anal sphincter which is then separated from the rectum by blunt dissection.

Careful dissection is necessary to elevate the entire external anal sphincter from the rectal wall without injury (Figure 16–8). Sometimes this step is done at an earlier stage in the operation. As the elevation proceeds, the midline separation between the two leaves of the levator ani muscle come into view and by carefully retracting the deep external anal sphincter off the ventral surface of the rectum, the fused leaves of the levator ani are seen. Using blunt dissection, the leaves of the levator ani muscle are elevated and cleared from the rectum. The dissection is begun just above the insertion of the muscle fibers into the anterior rectal wall. It is important at this phase that traction and pressure on the levators be exerted laterally to protect the rectum. Once the levators have been separated, the posterior layer of Denonvilliers' fascia as it covers the prostate gland is seen (Figure 16–9).

During the remainder of the operation, a superior tractor is used to elevate the deep

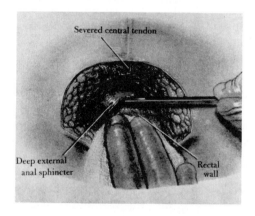

Figure 16–8. Elevation of deep external anal sphincter from rectal wall. (From Hudson, P. B., and Stout, A. P.: An Atlas of Prostatic Surgery. Philadelphia, W. B. Saunders Co., 1962.)

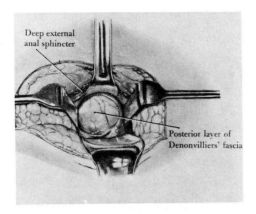

Figure 16–9.   Posterior layer of Denonvilliers' fascia. (From Hudson, P. B., and Stout, A. P.: An Atlas of Prostatic Surgery. Philadelphia, W. B. Saunders Co., 1962.)

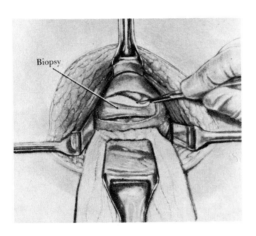

Figure 16–10.   Removal of prostatic biopsy specimen. (From Hudson, P. B., and Stout, A. P.: An Atlas of Prostatic Surgery. Philadelphia, W. B. Saunders Co., 1962.)

external anal sphincter while the rectum covered by heavy gauze is also retracted. The posterior layer of Denonvilliers' fascia is then incised and the potential space between it and the anterior layers is developed by blunt dissection. Having retracted the posterior layer of Denonvilliers' fascia, a prostatic biopsy is carried out over the suspicious area (Figure 16–10).

It is very important that the biopsy specimen contain a full thickness of the posterior portion of the prostate; this means that the depth of the incision should go at least to the level of the periurethral or benignly enlarged portion of the prostate gland. Following the biopsy, interrupted sutures of 00 or 000 chromic are placed through the full thickness of the posterior prostatic capsule. The bleeding edges of the biopsy site should be coagulated and the sutures then tied. Next, 00 interrupted sutures are placed in the levator ani muscles, the operative site is drained, and the skin closed with interrupted sutures.

TOTAL PROSTATOVESICULECTOMY

Before deciding on surgery, the surgeon must be certain that the disease is localized. There should be no evidence of ureteral obstruction on IVP, and examination under anesthesia must confirm that the tumor is confined to the prostate gland. The patient must have a normal serum and bone marrow acid phosphatase level and a normal bone marrow biopsy from the posterior iliac crest. There should be no evidence of metastases on the skeletal survey and technetium bone scan. It is still possible however, by our present methods of assessment, to have disease remain undetected beyond the confines of the prostate gland, especially in anaplastic tumors. Whether or not this picture will be altered with the addition of other investigations, such as carcinoembryonic antigens, remains to be determined. If the tumor in the prostate gland is localized and the patient has a reasonable life expectancy, then the patient should be considered for radical surgery.

Perineal Prostatovesiculectomy

The positioning of the patient and the early operative steps of this procedure were described under open perineal prostatic biopsy.

Once the posterior layer of Denonvilliers' fascia has been incised and reflected from the prostate gland, the fascia and the underlying rectum are then covered with a gauze sponge and retracted. Usually a sponge forceps is used as a retractor to displace the rectum from the operative field. Using blunt dissection, the space between the two layers of Denonvilliers' fascia is developed exposing the dorsum of the seminal vesicles covered by the anterior layer of Denonvilliers' fascia (Figure 16–11).

By elevating the curved urethral tractor and thus the prostate gland, the potential space is opened up, allowing dissection up to the tips of the seminal vesicles. The lateral aspects of the prostate are freed by blunt dissection. By closely following the anatomical capsule of the prostate gland (the anterior layer of Denonvilliers' fascia), the operator avoids the lateral venous plexuses as the dissection proceeds ventrally around the gland. After freeing both lateral aspects of the prostate (and it may

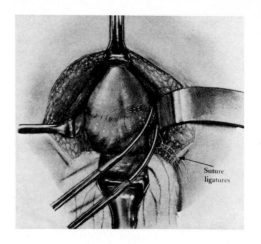

Figure 16–12. Ligation of left vascular pedicle. (From Hudson, P. B., and Stout, A. P.: An Atlas of Prostatic Surgery. Philadelphia, W. B. Saunders Co., 1962.)

be necessary to divide the medial portions of the levator ani to do this), one will encounter resistance posterolaterally owing to the vascular pedicles and their fascial folds as they enter the gland on the lateral aspect to supply the prostate and bladder neck. The arteries are derived from the inferior vesical artery, and the veins belong to the inferior vesical veins. By careful retraction these vascular pedicles are readily outlined, clamped, divided, and ligated (Figure 16–12).

In the next step the apex of the prostate gland and adjacent membranous urethra are cleared. The urethra is then transected as close to the apex of the prostate gland as is possible after removing the curved urethral tractor (Figure 16–13). A Lowsley or Markel straight urethral tractor or Foley catheter is then passed into the bladder and traction is exerted on the prostate gland to expose the puboprostatic ligaments. These ligaments are clamped, divided and ligated to expose the retropubic space and the anterior aspect of the bladder. An incision is then made in the anterior aspect of the bladder neck. Bleeding may be minimized by inserting a

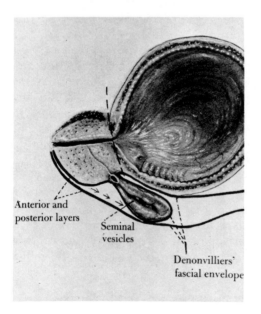

Figure 16–11. Relationship of two layers of Denonvilliers' fascia. (From Hudson, P. B., and Stout, A. P.: An Atlas of Prostatic Surgery. Philadelphia, W. B. Saunders Co., 1962.)

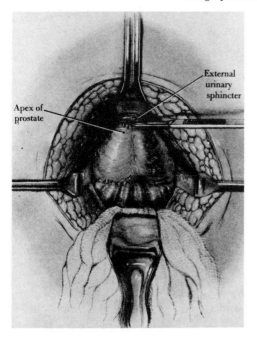

Figure 16–13. Transection of urethra. (From Hudson, P. B., and Stout, A. P.: An Atlas of Prostatic Surgery. Philadelphia, W. B. Saunders Co., 1962.)

series of interrupted 00 chromic atraumatic sutures around the circumference of the bladder in its anterior half before making the incision (Figure 16–14). Division of the anterior bladder wall is begun with a scalpel and is probably more easily continued with scissors.

The entire anterior aspect of the bladder neck is divided from lateral surface to lateral surface, exposing the posterior surface of the bladder neck and the trigone. Using a scalpel, the posterior bladder neck is incised distal to the ureteral orifices, leaving a margin of 1 cm (Figure 16–15). Further traction on the prostate gland is applied, and the posterior bladder neck is lifted with Babcock forceps to expose the subvesical or genital fascia. By blunt dissection in this fascia the vas deferentia are exposed and are clamped, divided, and ligated. By exerting traction on the specimen, and with careful blunt dissection bilaterally, it is

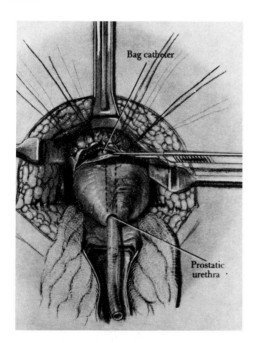

Figure 16–14. Insertion of atraumatic sutures around circumference of bladder to stanch bleeding. (From Hudson, P. B., and Stout, A. P.: An Atlas of Prostatic Surgery. Philadelphia, W. B. Saunders Co., 1962.)

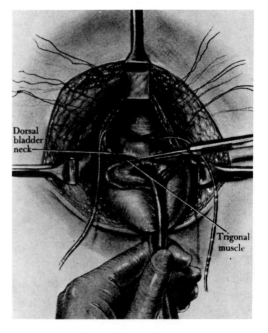

Figure 16–15. Incision of posterior bladder neck distal to ureteral orifices. (From Hudson, P. B., and Stout, A. P.: An Atlas of Prostatic Surgery. Philadelphia, W. B. Saunders Co., 1962.)

possible to remove the few remaining muscle fibers attached to the tips of the seminal vesicles, allowing easy removal of the surgical specimen. A urethral catheter is then inserted through the urethral meatus and brought up to the level of the transected membranous urethra. It is advisable to catheterize both ureteral orifices to determine their patency before proceeding with further surgery.

At this stage, Babcock forceps are applied to the lateral edges of the open bladder and the bladder neck is inspected. It may be necessary to narrow it with interrupted sutures of 000 chromic so that it may be more readily anastomosed to the membranous urethra (Figure 16–16). In order to approximate the membranous urethra to the bladder neck 00 chromic sutures are used and a 20 or 22 Fr Foley catheter is left in place during the procedure and for the postoperative period (Figure 16–17). Some surgeons do not attempt to suture the bladder neck to the membranous urethra but rely on the Vest traction sutures instead. These are in-

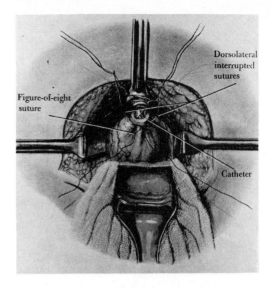

Figure 16–17. Completion of sutures for vesico-urethral anastomosis. (From Hudson, P. B., and Stout, A. P.: An Atlas of Prostatic Surgery. Philadelphia, W. B. Saunders Co., 1962.)

serted as an anterior and a pair of lateral sutures of #1 chromic into the bladder neck. They are then passed beneath the mucosa of the membranous urethra to emerge from the urethra at the bulb.

Traction on these sutures approximates the bladder neck to the membranous urethra. They are then brought out to the skin of the perineum, anterior to the incision, and tied over buttons or gauze swabs. Following the reanastomosis, the remaining pelvic fascia is drawn down and sutured with interrupted sutures of 000 chromic. The operative site is drained and the levator ani are approximated, as is the central tendon of the perineum. The subcutaneous tissues and the skin are closed in the usual fashion.

Retropubic Prostatovesiculectomy

The indications for this operation are similar to those of the radical perineal prostatectomy. An advantage of this approach is that it enables the surgeon to sample some of the lymph nodes draining the prostate gland. If these are shown to

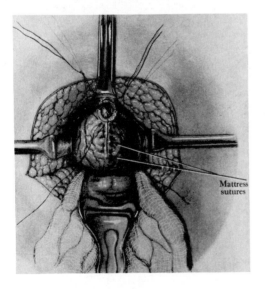

Figure 16–16. Narrowing of bladder neck with interrupted chromic catgut sutures. (From Hudson, P. B., and Stout, A. P.: An Atlas of Prostatic Surgery. Philadelphia, W. B. Saunders Co., 1962.)

contain tumor, most surgeons would consider it unwise to subject the patient to radical surgery. This, of course, is one of the disadvantages of the perineal approach.

The patient is placed on the operating table so that the pelvis is slightly elevated. The table is flexed at the patient's knees to facilitate the steep Trendelenburg position which will be required at a later stage in the operation. It is assumed that the patient has been previously cystoscoped and the bladder clear of any pathology. After preparing the operative field which includes the lower abdomen, the genitalia, perineum, and the medial aspect of the thighs, a Foley catheter is inserted, and the bladder is emptied. The catheter is left in the bladder and protected with a sterile towel. A classic Pfannenstiel incision is made two fingers breadth above the symphisis pubis. Once the retropubic space is exposed, a Millen self-retaining retractor is inserted into the wound. The anterior and lateral surfaces of the prostate are then cleaned by sweeping away the loose areolar tissue from the gland with dental pledgets on long Kelly forceps. In fibrofatty tissue and on the capsule a number of superficial veins will be encountered at this stage, and these are dealt with by electrocoagulation.

Using blunt dissection, the endopelvic fascia on either side of the prostate gland is then incised and these spaces opened up (Figure 16–18). Following this, the puboprostatic ligaments with their accompanying vessels are then divided between clamps and ligated. These structures are intimately related to the dorsal veins and tributaries of the penis and great care must be exercised to prevent serious bleeding (Figure 16–19). Following the division of the puboprostatic ligaments, the urethra is seen and is freed by careful dissection of any fibers of the external sphincter attached to it. Following this, the urethra is transected beyond the apex of the prostate gland and it is

important that no residual prostatic tissue be left attached to the stump.

The apex of the prostate gland is then grasped with Babcock or Allis forceps and drawn upward; or a new Foley catheter is inserted into the bladder and is used for

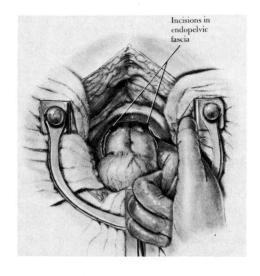

Figure 16–18. Incision of endopelvic fascia on either side of prostate. (From Hudson, P. B., and Stout, A. P.: An Atlas of Prostatic Surgery. Philadelphia, W. B. Saunders Co., 1962.)

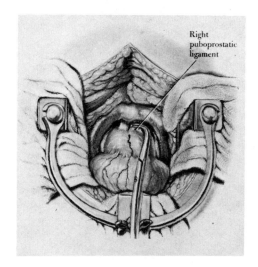

Figure 16–19. Division, clamping, and ligating of puboprostatic ligaments. (From Hudson, P. B., and Stout, A. P.: An Atlas of Prostatic Surgery. Philadelphia, W. B. Saunders Co., 1962.)

the same purpose. A plane of cleavage between the rectum and the apex of the prostate gland is established by dissecting between the two layers of Denonvilliers' fascia. In this plane it is possible to reach the base of the prostate gland without undue bleeding. By retracting the prostate gland cephalad and upward, the seminal vesicles are placed under tension and can be felt extending downward and laterally on either side of the underlying rectum (Figure 16–20).

By maintaining counter traction on the rectum, it is possible to pull the seminal vesicles and the ampulla away from the rectum, the adjacent peritoneum and the lower ends of the ureter. It is usual to start the dissection laterally and free the right seminal vesicle to its upper extremity where it is possible then to divide and ligate the fascial attachments above this point. The next step is to isolate, clamp, divide, and ligate the ampulla of the vas deferens on the same side. A similar

procedure is carried out on the opposite side. The bloc dissection is completed posteriorly by freeing the prostate gland at the vesical prostatic junction.

Next, the bladder is incised anteriorly at the level of the bladder neck and the entire anterior wall of the bladder neck in this area is incised, thus bringing into view the trigone and ureteral orifices. It is wise at this stage to catheterize both ureteral orifices. The posterior bladder neck is incised completely about 1 cm distal to the ureteral orifices. At the conclusion of this incision the bloc removal of the prostate gland, the seminal vesicles, the ampulla of the vas, and the fascial coverings is easily accomplished. The vesical neck is carefully inspected for bleeding, which is controlled by transfixing sutures of fine catgut and by diathermy. A 20 Fr Foley catheter is then inserted through the urethra and into the bladder. The bladder neck may require some tailoring, and this can be done with interrupted 00 chromic sutures—the idea being to make the bladder neck of a satisfactory caliber in order to facilitate the anastomosis between the bladder neck and the urethra.

The vesicourethral anastomosis is carried out using 00 chromic sutures, and these are interrupted sutures between the bladder neck and the urethra (Figure 16–21). Some surgeons do not attempt direct urethrovesical anastomosis but use instead the Vest method of approximating the bladder neck to the urethra.

In this method, three or four mattress sutures of #1 chromic catgut are placed through the vesical neck and are left long. A straight needle is used to carry the suture ends through the genitourinary diaphragm and out into the skin of the perineum posterior to the scrotum. These sutures are brought out into the perineum and are tied over gauze, while the bladder neck is brought into apposition with the genitourinary diaphragm by the operator from above. Rather than direct urethroves-

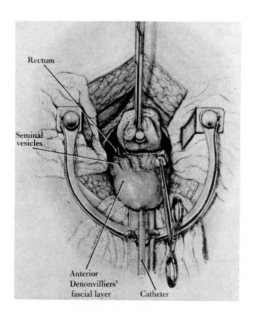

Figure 16–20. Retraction of prostate and downward and lateral extension of seminal vesicles. (From Hudson, P. B., and Stout, A. P.: An Atlas of Prostatic Surgery. Philadelphia, W. B. Saunders Co., 1962.)

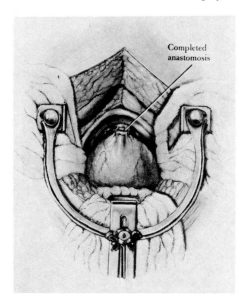

Figure 16–21. Vesicourethral anastomosis. (From Hudson, P. B., and Stout, A. P.: An Atlas of Prostatic Surgery. Philadelphia, W. B. Saunders Co., 1962.)

ical anastomosis, some surgeons suggest holding the bladder neck and urethra in apposition by traction on the inflated Foley balloon catheter. It is probably undesirable to use this method because of the undue traction on the external sphincter. After the urethrovesical anastomosis is completed, a Penrose drain or Hemovac is inserted into the retropubic space and the wound is closed in layers. The Foley catheter is usually attached to closed drainage without continuous bladder irrigation.

Much remains to be done in the management of prostatic cancer. Little progress has been made since the hormonal responsiveness of the tumor was first demonstrated by Huggins et al. in 1941.[21] Current research on an in vitro method of predicting the hormonal responsiveness of prostatic cancer is well advanced.[22] Such a predictive test hopefully will enable one readily to select the nonresponsive tumors and thus stimulate work

therapy, and immunotherapy. Advances are already being made in the field of chemotherapy, and the role of radiotherapy shows considerable promise both in treatment and palliation.[23]

References

1. Silverberg, E., and Holleb, A. I.: Cancer statistics 1972. CA, *22*:2, 1972.
2. Hudson, P. B., et al.: Prostatic cancer. XI. Early prostatic cancer diagnosed by arbitrary open perineal biopsy among 300 unselected patients. Cancer, *7*:619, 1954.
3. McNeal, J. E.: Regional morphology and pathology of the prostate. Am. J. Clin. Pathol., *49*:347, 1968.
4. Moore, R. A.: The morphology of the small prostatic carcinoma. J. Urol., *33*:244, 1935.
5. Franks, L. M.: Etiology, epidemiology and pathology of prostatic cancer. Cancer, *32*:1092, 1973.
6. Franks, L. M.: Benign nodular hyperplasia of the prostate: A review. Ann. R. Coll. Surg. Engl., *14*:92, 1954.
7. Flocks, R. H.: The arterial distribution within the prostate gland: Its role in transurethral prostatic resection. J. Urol., *37*:524, 1937.
8. Whitmore, W. F., Jr.: Hormone therapy in prostatic cancer. Am. J. Med., *21*:697, 1956.
9. Barnes, R. W.: Survival with conservative therapy. J.A.M.A., *210*:331, 1969.
10. Byar, D. P. and the Veterans Administration Coopertive Urological Research Group: Survival of patients with incidentally found microscopic cancer of the prostate: Results of a clinical trial of conservative treatment. J. Urol., *108*:908, 1972.
11. Hanash, K. A., et al.: Carcinoma of the prostate: A 15 year followup. J. Urol., *107*:450, 1972.
12. Bauer, W. C., et al.: Unsuspected carcinoma of the prostate in suprapubic prostatectomy specimens. Cancer, *13*:370, 1960.
13. Culp, O. S., and Meyer, J. J.: Radical prostatectomy in the treatment of prostatic cancer. Cancer, *32*:1113, 1973.
14. Hudson, H. C., and Howland, R. L., Jr.: Radical retropubic prostatectomy for cancer of the prostate. J. Urol., *108*:944, 1972.
15. Barnes, R. W., and Ninan, C. A.: Carcinoma of the prostate: Biopsy and conservative therapy. J. Urol., *108*:897, 1972.
16. Belt, E., and Schroeder F. H.: Total perineal prostatectomy for carcinoma of the prostate. J. Urol., *107*:91, 1972.
17. Jewett, H. J.: The case for radical perineal prostatectomy. J. Urol., *103*:195, 1970.
18. Jewett, H. J., et al.: The palpable nodule of prostatic cancer. Results 15 years after radical excision. J.A.M.A., *203*:403, 1968.
19. Jewett, H. J.: Significance of the palpable prostatic nodule. J.A.M.A., *160*:838, 1956.

20. Franzen, S., et al.: Cytological diagnosis of prostatic tumours by transrectal aspiration biopsy; A preliminary report. Br. J. Urol., 32:193, 1960.

21. Huggins, C., and Hodges, C. V.: Studies on prostatic cancer. I. The effect of castration, of estrogen, and of androgen injection on serum phosphatases in metastatic carcinoma of the prostate. Cancer Res., 1:293, 1941.

22. Mobbs, B. G., et al.: Hormonal responsiveness of prostatic carcinoma. In vitro technique for prediction. Urology, 3:105, 1974.

23. Murphy, G. P.: Cancer of the prostate. Cancer, 32:1089, 1973.

24. Emmett, J. L., et al.: Endocrine therapy in carcinoma of the prostate gland—10-year survival studies. J. Urol., 83:471, 1960.

25. Ray, G. R., et al.: Definitive radiation therapy of carcinoma of the prostate. Radiology, 106:407, 1973.

Part IV

Surgical Pathology of the Prostate

Chapter 17

Histopathology of the Prostate Gland

MYRON TANNENBAUM

This section is devoted to the histopathology of the prostate gland. The format with the pathology text first and then the photomicrographs is intended to guide both the urologist and the beginning surgical pathologist toward the proper diagnostic clinical cache. There are also numerous examples of some of the pitfalls encountered in diagnosing prostate gland pathology. In addition, several important diagnostic problems are often encountered in the routine examination of microscopic slides of urologic surgical specimens. These are (1) artifact or cancer, (2) atypical hyperplasia or cancer, or (3) cancer or seminal vesicle. These topics and various diagnostic criteria for malignancy are considered in this chapter.

UROLOGIC ARTIFACT AND HISTOLOGIC PROCESSING OF TISSUE

There is nothing more disturbing to the surgical pathologist than examining tissue under the microscope and not being able to determine whether histologically it reveals a lesion or is only artifact. This situation presents itself more often with the urology service and its genitourinary specimens, particularly bladder and prostate, than in any of the other surgical specialties.[1]

Clinical Procedures

Tissue artifact occurs because urologists use an electrical cutting current to resect isolated bladder tumor and its associated bases for staging. Microscopically, the same artifact can be seen with a transurethral resection of prostatic urethra or bladder neck. Often when resection procedures are performed by urology residents, and sometimes, even by the more experienced urologists, tissue submitted to the laboratory for histologic evaluation appears cooked or cauterized. Therefore, it is important that the pathologist notify the resectionist of the possibility of artifact in tissue and that greater care be taken when removing tissue. With cooperation between these services, excellent histologic preservation of tissue is possible. Thus, the pathologist should be alerted by the urologist that it may be necessary to use a blended cutting and coagulating current through the loop in order to control bleeding during resection.

At the same time, the urologist should

be aware of structural changes that the pathologist sees when tissue is presented for microscopic evaluation. For staging of bladder tumor this is important so that appropriate therapy can be instituted. Many times in critical cases of bladder tumor, a cold biopsy specimen is taken in order to insure accurate staging without electrical artifact. Of equal importance are the pieces of prostatic tissue which are removed during a transurethral resection. We will address ourselves in this section to this latter situation.

Tissue Processing

All of the transurethral tissue or chips should be submitted for pathologic evaluation in order to diagnose unsuspected carcinoma of the prostate. In cases of suprapubic or retropubic prostatectomy specimens, the prostate gland should be oriented as to what parts of the specimen are close to the posterior prostatic lobe. The weight of the specimen will determine how many sections should be taken from that surface of the prostate specimen closest to the enucleation line or posterior lobe of the prostate. One section should be taken for every 5 g of weight. If sections are taken in this systematic fashion, there will be greater recognition of prostatic carcinomas that have extended from the posterior lobe into the surgical specimens.

If a diagnosis of prostate cancer is made, procedures can then be initiated by the urologist to either control or eradicate the lesion. Therefore, it is essential whenever possible that tissue be free of cautery artifact, so that many of these unsuspected and well-differentiated carcinomas of the prostate can be diagnosed accurately and as quickly as possible. If more sections of the cauterized prostatic tissue, free of artifact, are needed to observe a more characteristic malignant pattern, time delay is evident.

When a transurethral resection is performed, we are in essence removing the core of the apple, and as we approach the skin of the apple or the prostatic capsule, we are more likely to encounter tumor. For this reason, it is crucial that the urologist explain to the surgical pathologist that all of the prostatic chips be placed in as many cassettes as necessary for proper histologic sectioning and detection. It is with this approach that the edge of a carcinoma from the various lobes can be pathologically discerned. In addition, it is important for the urologist to understand the plight of many of the surgical pathologists throughout the country when they examine these sections. If these chips are mutilated by cauterization it does not allow for proper pathologic evaluation. This can best be illustrated by the following examples.

Histology

The first example is taken from a case in which the initial histologic picture was that seen in Figure 17–59. With this picture we cannot be sure whether inflammatory cell infiltrate or prostatic tumor is surrounding the nerve. Further sectioning of this tissue block, which caused a three-day delay in diagnosis, revealed the histologic pattern seen in Figure 17–82. Here there is no cauterization of cells surrounding the nerve. There are numerous carcinomatous glands and few lymphocytes that are not mutilated.

In the second case, illustrated in Figure 17–80, the prostatic tissue revealed numerous distorted and cauterized glands that were suggestive for carcinoma of the prostate, but there was no cellular detail diagnostic for carcinoma. Further tissue levels revealed the picture seen in Figure 17–81. The photomicrograph reveals numerous distorted glands with no cellular detail in the upper half of the picture. However, in the lower portion of picture there are several glands that are intact and indicate cellular detail diagnostic for prostatic cancer. Here the glands are back-to-back, lined by a single row of cells that have nuclei with very prominent nucleoli.

ATYPICAL EPITHELIAL HYPERPLASIA VS PROSTATIC CARCINOMA

Light microscopic scrutiny of prostatic chips obtained from a transurethral resection, or prostatic tissue procured from a supra- or retropubic surgical specimen, will manifest itself as atypical epithelial hyperplasia in approximately 20% of the noncancerous prostates examined. This is frequently seen in cases of prostatic epithelial melanosis, and on many occasions, we have specifically detected an association of atypical epithelial hyperplasia with carcinoma of the prostate.[2] Atypical epithelial hyperplasia can demonstrate numerous histologic glandular formations that are the imagery of the more carcinomatous patterns. These configurations can be of even greater clinical import than of academic interest, for they can possibly represent a biologic state in which the prostatic cell is irrevocably embarked on a journey toward the "cancerous state."

There are numerous examples in uropathologic literature in which a statistical correlation demonstrates that prostatic carcinoma prevails more frequently in prostates associated with nodular epithelial hyperplasia than prostates without hyperplasia.[3] These studies did not, however, connote an etiologic relationship between the two pathologic paradigms. Per contra, there have been myriad studies which have also attested to the frequency of benign epithelial hyperplasia as being similar in the carcinomatous states as in the noncarcinomatous prostates.[4] When the materials and methods of some of these urologic reports were carefully analyzed, one outstanding and glaring deficiency was observed, namely, that many of the surgical specimens were not critically examined from a histopathologic point of view. Only a few sections of tissue were taken and the glands were not geographically blocked out when selective sections were taken on an anatomic and weight basis.

Evaluation of autopsied prostate is likewise fraught with diagnostic difficulty because of the vast time delay in obtaining the prostate gland for formalin fixation. Considerable distortion of the epithelial glands and loss of subtle cellular histologic detail are often seen. There is usually no preservation of nuclear chromatin detail, and there is a concomitant loss of nucleoli. The latter is an important feature in diagnosing prostatic cancer. Moreover, prominent desquamation of cells into the lumen of epithelial glands causes considerable diagnostic difficulty, especially when the pathologic diagnosis of benignity is also contingent on the preservation of a double layer of cells.

In surgically removed material, however, the uropathologist is not always between Scylla and Charybdis, because the prostatic tissue is usually well fixed. Unless there is cautery artifact, the pathologic group of patterns can be easily discerned. Until recently, very little or no attempt had been made to alert the urologic audience to the presence and possible significance of the atypical epithelial hyperplasia.[5]

Pathology

Atypical and normal epithelial hyperplasias, in most instances, are readily differentiated from carcinoma. In some focal microscopic fields of atypical epithelial hyperplasia, considerable morphologic changes are observed which could cause a misdiagnosis of carcinoma of the prostate (Figure 17–12). In most high-power microscopic fields, the epithelium still consists of a double layer of cells with small basal cells and tall, large surface cells (Figures 17–13; 17–14). If there is a double layer of cells, a diagnosis of cancer is not made. The nucleus in many of the surface cells is large with a very prominent eosinophilic nucleolus (Figure 17–122). The nuclei of the cells have all the cytologic details, similar to those of the neoplastic nuclei of most carcinomas of the prostate, which are properly preserved by formalin or other aldehyde fixing agents (Figure 17–78). Sometimes on microscopic examination one can discern carcinoma arising in atypical epithelial hyperplastic glands. Here they are devoid of basal myoepithelial cells. This finding is more common than that of a de nova carcinoma arising in atrophic glands.[6] Some carcinomatous glands, as they infiltrate the surrounding stroma, may still retain an atrophic pattern. This pattern is a light microscopic descriptive term, and malignant as well as nonmalignant glandular patterns of this type are commonly seen in many surgically removed prostates. This does not imply a transition of this form from the benign to the malignant state. However, in many of the prostates histologically examined, precancerous as well as cancerous changes occur with relative frequency in areas of atypical hyperplasia, but usually not with atrophic glands.

The dividing line between atypical hyperplasia and carcinoma can, at times, be tenuous. There are, however, morphologic criteria that can eliminate many of these ambiguous pathologic findings.

SEMINAL VESICLE VS PROSTATIC CARCINOMA

Biopsy specimens of the prostate gland, when obtained by needle or transurethral resection or by supra- or retropubic prostatectomy, may present more diagnostic variations and dilemmas than can be imagined. One of the problems in making a diagnosis of prostatic carcinoma is that the seminal vesicle and its ducts may be in the pathway of the biopsy instrument which can create an important diagnostic challenge. Similar histologic patterns also may be seen on transurethral resection, where, on occasion, portions of the ducts

of the seminal vesicles may be present. On low-power light microscopy, the histologic pattern of seminal vesicle may be similar to that of carcinoma of the prostate. This is characterized by many glands back-to-back. However, certain cytoplasmic characteristics of seminal vesicular epithelium are helpful in differentiating it from carcinomatous prostatic epithelium.

Histology

The seminal vesicles are evaginations of the vasa deferentia, which are also similar histologically. Seminal vesicle is known to have the ability to secrete a fluid which is added to the sperm from the testis. This fluid manifests itself in surgical specimens and autopsy material as a yellowish, sticky, and viscous substance. Histologically, the cytoplasmic finding of yellow-brown pigment or lipofuscin is of immense help in differentiating seminal vesicular epithelium from carcinomatous prostatic epithelium.

It is not uncommon to find, in prostatic tissue sections of supra- or retropubic prostatectomy, portions of seminal vesicle epithelium in which the glands are back-to-back (Figures 17–51; 17–54). This can result in a misdiagnosis of carcinoma of the prostate. In this type of seminal vesicular epithelium there can be many pleomorphic nuclei, which cytologically can appear to be from a carcinomatous cell. Seminal vesicle epithelium, like prostate, is also thrown up into slender papillary folds which branch freely into secondary and tertiary branches (Figures 17–52; 17–53). These papillary projections protrude into the lumen and anastomose freely with each other. In the center of these papillary folds is a thin fibrovascular core which enables us to distinguish these patterns from some papillary tumors of the prostate. The latter do not possess fibrovascular cores.

Epithelium of the seminal vesicle or vasa deferentia varies considerably. This depends on the age of the patient and the functional state of the epithelium.[7] Moreover, there may be a single layer or a pseudostratified layer of columnar types of cells. When a deeper layer is found, it is usually a round basal cell and contributes to the impression of pseudostratified or a double layer of cells comprising these seminal vesicular glands. This is very significant in distinguishing these glands from carcinomatous glands of the prostate, where there is usually a single layer of cells around a central lumen.

However, an additional feature encountered is lipofuscin, pathognomonic for seminal vesicular epithelium and vasa deferentia. The epithelial surface cells of the seminal vesicle contain numerous secretory granules and/or pigment granule which can be either very fine or clumped in nature to form yellowish-brown masses within the cytoplasm of the cells (Figures 17–55; 17–56; 17–57). This pigment when examined by electron microscopy is normally fatty in nature and negative for iron. It usually appears at puberty. The secretory granules are seen more frequently in the deeper portions of the crypts and have glandlike structures. However, as they approach the surface, they may form droplets or blebs and are ultimately cast off into the lumen. When seminal vesicular epithelium is examined after a period of castration, atrophy develops.[8] The cells are then noted to have a lower cuboidal appearance rather than a tall columnar shape (Figures 17–56; 17–57). The lipofucsin pigment usually remains.

As we know from animal experimentation, the administration of testicular hormones restores these cells to a normal secretory activity. The submucosa or lamina propria, alluded to before as being the central fibrobvascular core or connective tissue which surrounds clusters of these glands which may be almost back-to-back, is composed of a dense connective tissue containing numerous capillaries, lymphatic glands, and nerves. The

smooth muscle layer, when found, may surround clusters of these seminal vesicular glands. They are usually less thick in the seminal vesicle than in the vas deferens. On occasion, smooth muscle cells at the apical ends of their nuclei have a fine granular brown pigment which, on light histologic examination, is similar to the pigment seen in epithelial cells. No such pigment is apparent in the smooth muscle bundles of prostatic muscle tissue.

Light microscopic histology of seminal vesicle epithelium demonstrates a golden brown pigment pathognomonic for seminal vesicular epithelium rather than for prostate. This type of pigment in the epithelium is helpful in the diagnosis of seminal vesicular epithelium when compared with the epithelium of prostatic carcinoma. Although some authors claim that a lipofuscin-like material may, on rare occasions, be present in prostate cancer cells,[9] we do not believe it is present in sufficient amount or confluent enough in prostate to be detected by light microscopy. Over the last decade the surgical specimens examined at Columbia-Presbyterian have not shown this type of pigment to be evident in cancer of the prostate. Summarily, when the epithelial cells contain a confluent yellow-brown pigment, it is diagnostically seminal vesicle, not prostate carcinoma.

MELANOTIC PROSTATIC LESIONS: BLUE NEVUS AND PROSTATIC EPITHELIAL MELANOSIS

Pigmented melanotic lesions that are benign have been described both in the fibromuscular stroma[10–12] and in the epithelium of the prostate.[13] These lesions are being seen with more frequency today because of the greater tendency to take more step-sections of the prostate for histologic detection of prostatic carcinoma. It is important for the urologist to be cognizant that the appellation of melanotic lesion does not always mean a malignant condition. Two lesions of the prostate, blue nevus and prostatic epithe- lial melanosis, have been placed in this cache for the reasons described later. Both lesions are, in themselves, biologically benign.

Gross Pathology

In surgical pathologic processing of either retro- or suprapubic prostatectomy specimens, it is advisable to bread-loaf the gland with a knife so that there will be proper formalin penetrations and fixation of cells comprising these glands. Often, as these gross specimens are cut, areas are encountered that geographically are of different physical consistency and colora- tion. If these areas are firm and yellow- orange, they can be interpreted grossly with some degree of accuracy as car- cinomatous. If the gross areas are noncys- tic, well-circumscribed, and light brown, they can appear, on further histologic sec- tioning, as a benign adenomatous epithe- lial nodule. If it is a lighter brown, also well-circumscribed, and firmer than the epithelial nodule, it will probably even- tuate histologically as a fibrous nodule with occasional muscle cells interdis- persed between the slit-like vascular channels and fibroblasts. However, on certain occasions dark greyish areas are seen, either in the periurethral areas of the gross specimen or in the margin of enucleation.

There are two possible gross anatomic interpretations. The first, which is the most likely, is that it is an infarct of the prostate (Figure 17–28). The second in- terpretation, which is least likely, but still occurs with significant frequency, is that of a pigmented lesion of the prostate.

In several different documented in- stances there have been reports of similar gross anatomic findings in the prostatic gland. Three of these have been described in association with a benign stromal melanotic lesion of the prostate. This is the blue nevus. One report described this in conjunction with melanosis of the

prostatic epithelium.[13] In the last documented reference, there was entail- ment of the prostatic urethra with malig- nant melanoma.[14] However, this was at- tended with a five-year previously pathologically corroborated malignant melanoma of the deltoid region.

Blue Nevus

The presence of melanin in the prostate stroma has been given the appellation of blue nevus of the prostate.[10] Malignant degeneration of prostatic blue nevus ap- pears to be implausible, since malignant changes have not been reported to accrue from this type of blue nevus in the skin.[15] However, malignant metamorphosis has been reported to have occurred in the cellular blue nevus of the skin.[16] Moreover, Berry and Reese[17] have re- ported a possible primary malignant melanoma of the prostate gland. There also are other reports of primary malig- nant melanomas of other visceral or- gans.[18,19] Furthermore, it must be emphat- ically stated that the blue nevus and prostatic epithelial melanosis have not as yet been consorted with malignant melanoma.

On histologic scrutiny of this lesion, the blue nevus (Figures 17–62; 17–63; 17–64; 17–65) manifests itself as numerous melanin-constipated spindle-shaped cells in a fibromuscular stroma. These cells are ovoid or elongated with one or more polar prolongations that insinuate between the individual stromal cells. Large numbers of these cells are present in the stroma, either in close proximity to, or distant from, the epithelial glands. The melanin pigment contained in these stromal cells almost eclipses the ovoid nucleus and nucleolus. The pigment histochemically does not contain iron. Pigmented granules are also cognated as melanin by a positive Fontana silver impregnation and negative Lillie's ferrous iron stain. The pigment is also bleached further by hydrogen peroxide. Unpropitiously, since the tissue is usually fixed in formalin, a dopa oxidase test cannot be performed, but electron microscopy can be done, since the ultrastructure of the melanin granules are formalin stable.

One such case, including our own, was studied by electron microscopy and the pigmented granules were unconditionally confirmed as being diffusely distributed premelanosomes and melanosomes.[12] Electron microscopy of these pigmented cells discloses numerous electron-dense, coarse granules that are diffusely disseminated in the cytoplasm of these cells. Most of the granules are encompassed by a single limiting membrane. The ultrastructural morphology of these electron opaque granules is pathognomonic for mature melanosomes. They are often mixed with premelanosomes which characteristically manifest as parallel arrays of filaments.[12]

Epithelial Melanosis

The prostatic epithelial melanosis occurs with greater frequency than the previously described blue nevus of the prostate. In the surgically removed prostatic glands that have been pathologically studied at our institution, we have not seen prostatic epithelial melanosis associated with stromal melanosis. Guillan and Zelman[13] by utilizing special histochemical stains for melanin have detected the subsistence of this pigment in 13 (4%) of 330 prostates so examined. Dendritic melanoblasts similar to those discerned in the blue nevus were recognized in the stroma of two of these prostates. These configurations were in areas that were contiguous with prostatic epithelium containing melanin. These authors have consequently concluded that the pigment present in the epithelium of the thirteen prostates was formed by the melanoblasts and sequestered by the prostatic epithelium rather than the epithelium itself being melanogenic. Langley and Weitzner[20]

suggestively support the concept that pigment from stromal melanoblasts may be transported to adjacent epithelial cells.

In numerous different prostatic epithelium specimens that we and Goldman[21] have studied by histochemical procedures, we have not observed this relationship. It must, therefore, be construed that prostatic epithelium is melanogenic and that this is unrelated to stromal melanoblasts in the prostate. This histochemical melanin pigment in the epithelium is not refractile as the lipofuscin pigment present in the epithelium of seminal vesicles (Figure 17–55).[22] This melanin pigment is in 10% of the prostates examined at this institution and is localized mostly in ductal rather than in acinar prostatic epithelium (Figure 17–4). These cells contain a fine golden or reddish-brown pigment that is varied in size and in its cytoplasmic distribution (Figures 17–5; 17–6). In some of the cells the pigment is localized to the basal position, whereas in others it assumes a perinuclear distribution, while in some cells it is localized to the apical region. Here it can be large with a dark bluish circumference when tissue sections are stained with hematoxylin, phyloxine and saffaranine (Figure 17–6).

Histopathologic examination of the remainder of the prostatic surgical specimen, however, has usually demonstrated a histologic pattern of atypical hyperplasia of the prostate where the nuclei are very large with conspicuous eosinophilic nucleoli.[23] These are similar to the cancer nuclei previously described by Totten et al.[24] In about one-third of the prostates which contain the epithelial melanosis, there are more overt patterns of prostatic carcinoma. The epithelial cells containing melanin have not been characterized by electron microscopy. The biologic or clinical significance of these atypical hyperplastic glands with cancer nuclei also awaits further elucidation. Do the cancers of the prostate arise in atrophic glands or in areas of atypical hyperplasia?

DIAGNOSTIC CRITERIA FOR HISTOPATHOLOGIC EVALUATION OF PROSTATIC CANCER TISSUE SECTIONS

It has frequently been stated that carcinomas of the prostate are represented by many different patterns that on occasion can be misdiagnosed.[6] This is not only disastrous for the patient but also will allow many false therapeutic interpretations to be perpetuated.

We are all cognizant that a time-proven method for the recognition of prostatic cancer is the light histologic tissue section taken from the prostate at the time of surgery or autopsy. In many instances, there is difficulty in defining pathologically the potential neoplastic activity of the prostate because of the multiform configurations displayed in one microscopic field of this tumor. These patterns could include such morphoses as small as an in situ carcinoma[25] (Figures 17–66 and 17–68), in addition to small and large gland carcinomas, "Indian file" (Figure 17–93), and cribriform patterns (Figure 17–85); as well as other possible and different forms of endometrial and periurethral cancers of the prostate (Figures 17–111 to 17–131). These illustrations should provide some useful guidelines in recognizing the different prostatic cancer morphoses.

For the surgical pathologist or urologist making a histopathologic evaluation of a biopsy or tissue section taken from surgically removed prostates, the following commonly seen structural changes are indications of prostatic malignancy:

1. Prostatic acini back-to-back (Figure 17–67).
2. Cells lining acini, often in single layer. Basal layer of cells are not present (Figure 17–67).
3. Prominent eosinophilic large nucleoli are present. Tissue must be

fixed quickly and properly in formalin or Bouin's solution in order for this to be detected (Figure 17–88).

4. Prostatic acini may or may not be seen as linear infiltrates into the fibromuscular stroma. These look like boats racing up or down a river.
5. Nuclear hyperchromatism may or may not be indicated, depending on the quality of tissue fixation.
6. Perineural invasion may or may not be discerned. When detected, especially on a frozen section, this is very helpful in placing a well-differentiated glandular pattern into a malignant cache.

Variations on a theme or pattern can vary from one microscopic field to another. The tumor may also be seen as a solid cell mass resembling a granuloma. Fortunately, the "Indian file" pattern, and signet-ring cell or mucin-producing carcinomas are rare (Figures 17–96; 17–106). These two forms of prostatic cancer can also be easily obscured by too much electrical current in the resectoscope causing cautery artifact. Caution must be the word because some of the features already mentioned (1–6) may be present and yet the diagnosis is that of benign disease. Not all of the criteria need to be present to make a diagnosis of malignancy.

Microacini are often present in the posterior lobe of the prostate. They also frequently appear in prostatitis and yet, pathologically, they are benign. Many of the microacini are not back-to-back. When examined microscopically, these glands are seen to be lined by a double layer of cells (Figures 17–18; 17–22).

The periacinar ducts as well as the periurethral glands may be filled with cells that are mitotically active, and bizarre, yet they are not the usual type of prostatic cancer (Figure 17–112). This lesion, which is *transitional cell* in type, is often misdiagnosed and treated as prostatic carcinoma. The periurethral ducts as well as the glands around an area of infarction may show extensive squamous cell metaplasia and nuclei with prominent nucleoli. This is not a malignancy but is often misdiagnosed as such if care is not taken. Diethylstilbestrol may induce squamous metaplasia as well as obscure the carcinoma in the tissue section (Figure 17–38).

A group of bizarre glands with pleomorphic nuclei will most likely be seminal vesicles. Look for the brownish refractile cytoplasmic pigment (Figure 17–56).

Mechanical distortion or compression of the hyperchromatic nuclei will definitely confuse the diagnosis either in the direction of malignancy or benignity. If the answer is in doubt, the surgical pathologist should order additional tissue levels from the biopsy. If confusion about the diagnosis still exists, obtain another biopsy.

PROSTATIC CARCINOMA IN SITU

The terminology "carcinoma in situ" of the prostate gland denotes an incidental or clinically detected carcinoma when the neoplasm is found intraacinar.[25] This author favors the use of the term "carcinoma in situ," even though others do not.[25] Usually there is no apparent light microscopic invasion of the surrounding fibromuscular stroma. However, even these microscopic foci of in situ cancer may also be associated with a prostatic neoplasm elsewhere in the gland, with its extension to the prostatic capsule and nerves. When serial sections are taken,[26,27] the incidence of carcinoma of the prostate, upon histologic diagnosis, is increased from 14 to 44%. An almost identical situation is also discerned when prostatic chips are examined by routine histopathologic procedures. Here, it is important that all of the prostatic tissue be embedded and cut properly, and that each prostatic chip be pathologically examined. If the light microscopic examination is astutely executed, then in at least 20% of the tissues examined, numerous combinations of different patterns of prostatic carcinoma will be revealed. In many instances there is only carcinoma in situ and no other form of prostatic cancer. In these cases the surgical pathlogy diagnosis should indicate this fact that there is only a "carcinoma in situ."

The surgical pathologist who reviews these slides is often impressed by the multifocalness of this type of lesion and by its often seen variegated glandular configurations. Many times these multifocal histologic patterns are similar to those seen in Figures 17–66; 17–68; 17–70. These in situ neoplastic areas represent disturbances in architecture and are discernible only under low-power microscopy (×20) in prostatic chips or sections taken from supra- or retropubic prostatectomy. Before the diagnosis of carcinoma in situ can be ascertained, it is often necessary to examine these foci at high magnifications of about ×80 to ×200. Here the glands are almost back-to-back with a small residual amount of stroma interposed between these carcinomatous glands (Figures 17–76; 17–69; 17–71). The stroma is often exiguous, and can only be perceived ultrastructurally, revealing an intact basement membrane surrounding each of these glands. Many of the glands are usually not in a "streaming" pattern, nor do they infiltrate between normal surrounding prostatic glands or ducts, or both.

Occasionally a prostate will be removed for obstructive uropathy which is clinically benign. On pathologic examination, some of these areas disclose numerous large nodular areas of carcinoma in situ (Figure 17–70). In photomicrographs of the carcinoma in situ focus, there still remains a nodular architecture with no "streaming" of the glands into surrounding stroma. Anatomic axes of these oblong glands are not parallel to each other and basal myoepithelioid cells have disappeared. The cells have an eosinophilic cytoplasm and cancer nuclei.[28] There also may be numerous mitotic figures (Figure 17–74). When other step-sections were taken from this surgically removed prostate gland, no foci were found of an infiltrating or invasive carcinoma of the prostate.

The patterns described and illustrated in Figures 17–66 and 17–70 are different from the histologic configurations seen in association with invasive carcinoma of the prostate (Figure 17–89). Various histologic patterns and cell types which are diagnostic for invasive prostatic neoplasia are illustrated in Figures 17–89 to 17–106. It is important to indicate in the surgical pathology report to the urologist that the carcinoma is in either an "in situ" form or else an "invasive" form with perineural invasion.

MUCIN-SECRETING PROSTATIC CARCINOMA

Mucin-secreting neoplasms can be clearly recognized when examined under low-power light microscopy or upon scrutiny of photomicrographs (Figure 17–105). Utilizing the pathologic standards stated in a previous section,[29] demonstration of invasive carcinoma of the prostate with a multitude of different glandular patterns is noted in Figures 17–81 through 17–105. Some of the glands are cribriform in configuration while the remainder are, in part, glandular. In addition, some of the glands have no secretions in their glandular lumens when observed under light microscopy. Others have secretions in their lumen that are very mucoid and stain positive for mucin (Figure 17–105). These latter epithelial glandular configurations have been given the appellation of "mucin adenocarcinoma of the prostate."[30] This type of lesion in the prostate is not common, and only a few cases of this tumor have been reported.[31–36] They are considered to be rare when the mucin-positive form is the only histologic variant. However, we do not deem this to be that uncommon a histologic manifestation of an invasive carcinoma of the prostate.[30] At our institution at least one-tenth of our prostatic carcinomatous glan-

dular specimens will have at least one microscopic focus of mucin production.

Pathobiology

If multiple sections are taken for pathologic processing of tissue from a radical prostatectomy specimen, this pattern can be seen with some frequency. Prostatic tumors that are purely of this nature are biologically less invasive, but are also markedly less responsive to diethylstilbestrol therapy. In the differential diagnosis of mucin-secreting carcinoma of prostate, other mucinous types of carcinomas should be clinically ruled out, namely, mucinous carcinoma of the bladder, carcinoma of the periurethral or Cowper's glands, and invasive carcinomas from the large intestine.

TRANSITIONAL CELL PROSTATIC CARCINOMA

Periurethral neoplasia or transitional cell carcinoma of the prostate is seldom recognized or categorized in the surgical pathology report to the urologist as a distinct morphologic or clinical variety of prostatic carcinoma.[37] However, from cases cited in the literature, and according to our own findings, justification for separating prostatic carcinoma into different histologic patterns is reasonable and possibly of great clinical import.

Melicow and Hollowell[38] referred to transitional cell prostatic cancer when they described 30 cases of Bowen's disease of the urinary tract, of which three cases involved the prostatic urethra. They did not, however, state whether or not two of these patients were devoid of urothelial neoplasia in other parts of the urinary tract. A third patient, who had undergone total cystectomy, including prostatectomy for infiltrating carcinoma of the bladder, on sectioning, presented an intraurothelial carcinoma of the posterior urethra. This had a distinctly different histologic appearance from that of bladder tumor. There was no notation that the periurethral ducts were involved by this process.

A lesion of similar histologic appearance to Melicow and Hollowell's third case was described by Ortega et al.[39] They also observed Pagetoid cells in the prostatic urethra and urinary bladder although they did not describe the process as spreading up the periurethral prostatic ducts into the various lobes of the prostate. Some of their photomicrographs could also be interpreted as demonstrating that the lesions were in situ as well as invasive into the prostatic fibromuscular stroma.

Franks and Chesterman[40] also described in situ undifferentiated carcinoma of a transitional cell type that involved the periurethral prostatic ducts. Their patients also presented an undifferentiated infiltrating tumor of the urinary bladder. It was suggested by these authors that the prostatic lesions were caused by the same carcinogenic stimulus that affected the urothelium of the bladder.

Pathology

Two hundred consecutive cases of prostatic carcinoma were reviewed by Ende et al.[41] They reported that seven of these cases arose in the periurethral prostatic ducts. Three cases were of a pure transitional cell type, whereas four were a mixture of glands and transitional cells that were neoplastic. They postulated that this type of lesion began in the periurethral and prostatic ducts in the junctional area of the columnar and transitional epithelia. Although the tumors had a propensity for causing ureteral obstruction, they did not seem to be especially aggressive and widespread metastases were not commonly seen. The tumors were not associated with elevated blood acid phosphatase. Although their data were scant, these lesions did not appear to have an innocuous clinical course. They extended into the retroperitoneal lymph nodes with subsequent obstructive uropathy and ensuing uremia, but there was no associated

urothelial neoplasia elsewhere in the urinary tract.

Additional pathologic evidence supporting the concept of pathogenesis of this lesion was given by Ullmann and Ross.[42] They cited nine cases in which the epithelium of the periurethral prostatic ducts ranged from an unremarkable hyperplasia through marked atypicality to a definitive carcinoma in situ. They inferred that the rare invasive transitional cell carcinoma of the prostate gland originates in the periurethral prostatic ducts and secondarily invades the prostatic stroma by breaking through the glandular basement membrane. Four of their nine cases demonstrated a urothelium with well-differentiated transitional cells and uniform-sized nuclei. Mitotic figures were rarely observed. However, with the advent of atypical hyperplasia and carcinoma in situ, the number of mitoses was greatly increased. Most forms of prostatic carcinoma, with the exception of the cribriform pattern, do not have great numbers of mitoses per single high-power field.

Karpas and Moumgis[43] took routine serial sections from the prostate of 400 consecutive autopsies. Four cases revealed pronounced epithelial hyperplasia of the periurethral prostatic ducts. One case demonstrated a Grade I papillary transitional cell carcinoma lying wholly within the confines of the prostatic ducts. They believed that hyperplastic transitional cells arose from the indifferent or reserve cells lying between the luminal epithelium and the basement membrane in the periurethral prostatic ducts. They were unable to demonstrate direct continuity of these proliferating cells with the transitional cells lining the prostatic urethra per se. They inferred that these cells were the same as those described in an electron microscopic study of prostatic ducts by Mao and Angrist.[44]

The conclusions of Karpas and Moumgis will also require an ultrastructural study for confirmation of the reserve cell being the cell of origin of the transitional cell hyperplasia and carcinoma. Such a study may possibly explain the pathogenesis or reason for the prostatic urethral and periurethral involvement in approximately 20% of the patients with transitional cell cancer of the bladder. It is not unreasonable to accept a multifocal alteration of the urothelium by a urinary carcinogen to explain the multiple asynchronous development of these urothelial neoplasms that occur within prostatic periurethral glands. However, for a long time, the majority of these neoplasms have been attributed to direct extension from the malignant primary tumor in the urinary bladder.

Finally, Rubenstein and Rubnitz[45] provided data for a pathobiologic evaluation of transitional cell prostatic cancer. Six hundred and seventy cases of prostatic carcinoma were examined and about 2% of them were found to be of the transitional type. Gross observations showed no difference between adenocarcinoma and transitional cell carcinoma of the prostate. Both types produced an enlarged, hard, fixed, and irregular gland. The most important distinction between the two types is found on histologic examination. Adenocarcinoma of the prostate has a characteristic pattern of infiltration, i.e., small hyperchromatic cells that often produce wellformed or abortive glands, or both. Occasionally there is only an insidious infiltration of the fibromuscular stroma by cords or island of small dark-staining cells with no light histologically demonstrable glandular lumens.

Light Microscopy

Various histologic patterns of proliferating transitional cell lesions of the periurethral ducts are shown in Figures 17–111 to 17–115. Transitional cell hyperplasia almost occluding prostatic ducts is seen in Figures 17–42 to 17–46. Figure 17–46 shows, at a higher magnifica-

tion, that there are surface cells of a columnar type surrounding a lumen, and beneath this are numerous cells that are similar to basal cells that are against the basement membrane. The exact nature of these cells awaits ultrastructural confirmation. In Figure 17–115 there is an invasive undifferentiated form of transitional cell carcinoma arising only in the periurethral prostatic ducts. These cells exhibit numerous mitoses. Glandular carcinomas of the prostate usually do not have the number of mitoses that the periurethral prostatic transitional cell carcinomas have.

A distinct in situ transitional cell carcinoma of the periurethral prostatic ducts can be seen in Figure 17–111, on the left. Most of the lumen is occupied by tumor that does not invade fibromuscular stroma. The right side of Figure 17–111 contains some prostatic acini involved by tumor cells. Figure 17–113 contains basal or reserve cells surrounding these neoplastic transitional cells, and Figure 17–114 demonstrates a comedo pattern, often seen with this type of neoplasm. It is important to recognize the neoplastic patterns because transitional cell carcinoma is hormonally unresponsive and other forms of therapy must be instituted immediately.

Pathobiology

The cytologic criteria of malignancy, such as anaplasia and mitoses, may not be present in all cases of transitional cell carcinoma of the prostate gland. Mitoses are usually present in the cribriform pattern of prostatic cancer. Transitional cell carcinoma is, however, often characterized by clusters of large anaplastic tumor cells arising in and filling the periurethral prostatic ducts which spread into the prostatic alveoli. Cellular variation and mitotic figures are often discerned. A propensity for the perineural spaces is not commonly seen in this form of carcinoma, unlike that of adenocarcinoma of the prostate.

In 10 cases of transitional cell carcinoma of the prostate reported by Rubenstein and Rubnitz,[45] hormonal manipulation was of no benefit and the clinical course was steadily downhill, with no patient surviving more than 23 months after diagnosis. Additional evidence of the insidious potential and consequential rapid death with this type of prostatic cancer was also provided by Johnson et al.[46] Six patients without an antecedent history of vesical malignant lesion or coexisting bladder tumor developed transitional cell cancer of the prostate. Diagnosis was established late in the course of the disease, and treatment with radiotherapy did not appear to improve survival rate. These patients died one to three years after the pathologic diagnosis was established. In 14 other patients, prostatic lesions were noted, at the time of treatment, for a noncontiguous bladder lesion (10 patients) or asynchronously in four patients with previous bladder malignancies.

Conservative treatment was advised when the transitional cell cancer was confined to the periurethral prostatic ducts. Radical treatment, using either radiotherapy or surgical extirpation, or a combination of both, was indicated when the fibromuscular stroma was invaded. They concluded from careful histologic observation of tissues from these 20 patients that, in both groups, the lesions began as carcinoma in situ in the periurethral prostatic ducts without subsequent breakthrough into the prostatic fibromuscular stroma. Interestingly, this second group of patients presented chiefly with symptoms of hematuria and vesical irritability rather than with prostatic obstruction.

When the prostatic fibromuscular stroma is invaded by direct extension of a vesical malignant lesion, the assignment, according to the classification of Jewett and Strong,[47] of clinical stage D_1 is certainly warranted. However, indiscriminate assignment of all patients with transitional cell carcinoma of the prostate into such a category most certainly fails to take into account those patients in whom the malignant process originates in the periurethral prostatic ducts. Prostatic and vesical lesions must be staged independently.

It is very important for urologists and pathologists to be aware of these types of lesions because they are biologically different from most forms of prostatic cancer. They should not be considered rare, and they can vary from 2 to 3% of the prostatic carcinomas reported in the literature and up to 4% at our institution.

ADENOID CYSTIC OR SALIVARY GLAND PROSTATIC CARCINOMAS

A histologic variant of prostatic carcinoma that is rarely seen, and even less understood clinically, is the adenoid cystic or salivary gland carcinoma of the prostate.[48] These malignant invasive tumors have a characteristic cribriform histologic pattern[29] and are composed of two cell types. The first variety of cell comprises the duct lining, whereas the second type is of a myoepithelial nature. Composites of both cell types may be arranged in small duct-like structures or as larger masses of myoepithelial cells which may or may not surround a cystic space (Figures 17–108; 17–109).

This form of prostatic cancer represents less than 0.01% of all the carcinomas of the prostate.

Light Microscopy

The histologic appearance of these adenoid cystic prostate tumors, like their salivary gland counterpart, is varied. In the cases that we have examined, they have been extremely varied, even within the same prostate gland. There can be a cribriform pattern with formation of cystic structures. These glands can produce hyaline or mucoid material which may either be in the lumen of the duct-like structures or may likewise surround the myoepithelial cells (Figure 17–110). The mucoid material is PAS positive.

These tumors, as rare as they are, can be histologically confused with transitional cell carcinoma of the prostate.[49] Clinically, the latter tumors are highly malignant and resistant to radiotherapy and hormone therapy.

Pathobiology

The two cases of this type of prostatic cancer seen here were highly invasive and spread to and beyond the prostatic capsule. There is said to be virtually no knowledge of the clinical behavior of these tumors other than the fact that they are probably not amenable to antiandrogen therapy.[48]

ENDOMETRIAL TUMORS AND ASSOCIATED PROSTATIC CARCINOMAS

Malignant neoplasms of the prostate gland may arise not only in the posterior lobe of the prostate gland, but also in the periurethral glands of the prostatic urethra. Transitional cell carcinomas are highly malignant and may arise from the urothelium lining the urethral ends of the prostatic ducts or from the urothelium of the prostatic urethra proper. Periurethral lesions may be of the adenocarcinomatous variety and, as such, may be papillary in form and spread intraductally, as do many carcinomas of the breast. These tumors have their cell of origin in the columnar epithelium lining the numerous varieties of ducts in the prostate. This would include periurethral large prostatic ducts, the ends of the ejaculatory ducts, periurethral glands of Littré, and prostatic utricle which is in the colliculus seminalis and is derived from the müllerian duct.

All of these tumors are markedly different from the various histologic patterns usually demonstrated by the more common microacinar cancer that originates, for the most part, in the posterior lobe of

the prostate gland. The periurethral carcinomas of the prostate not only have a markedly different pathobiologic behavior than those arising in the posterior lobe of the prostate, but they also demonstrate a multiplicity of histologic patterns. They do not respond to radiotherapy and hormonal manipulation.[49] However, in the last several years, the endometrial tumors of the prostatic urethra have assumed a yet to be defined position in regard to their incidence, clinical course, and choice of treatment.[50–52]

Pathology

The majority of cases that have been histologically recognized at this institution have been seen as papillary masses that were present in the region of the verumontanum. One was found lateral to it. They may be exophytic or intraductal. Since 1967 they have been seen at least once a year in fresh surgical specimens of retropubic prostatectomies or transurethral resections. In reviewing the surgical pathology files at this institution, several cases of these tumors were found that had not previously been recognized as endometrial proliferations in the prostate gland. They all appeared in phenotypical normal male patients. In 27 such cases, only three or approximately 10% had elevated serum acid phosphatase levels. Most of these patients (90%) also had an invasive carcinoma of the prostate and/or transitional cell carcinoma of the urothelium.[53]

The majority of cases seen at our institution have been associated with the more conventional microacinar carcinomas of the prostate. This association of conventional prostatic cancers was first recognized by Mostofi and Price[54] and not by previous reports.[50,51] As a consequence, the clinical question then raised is which type of cancer do we treat—the periurethral ductal or endometrial tumor or the more common carcinomas of the prostate? At the present time the only treatment in use is surgery and/or orchiectomy and diethylstilbestrol, and this is performed for the microacinar carcinomas of the prostate. Radiation alone should also be considered.

Histology of Endometrial Tumors

There are several different histologic patterns which this type of endometrial growth can demonstrate. The exophytic masses in the prostatic urethra as well as those that are in situ and spreading up the ducts demonstrate cells having eosinophilic cytoplasm and nuclei with a peripheral clumped chromatin pattern and prominent eosinophilic nucleoli (Figures 17–116; 17–117; 17–118). These cells may have numerous mitotic figures as well as microvilli on their luminal surfaces. More often then not, they do not have fibrovascular stalks. Sparse lymphocytic infiltrates are between the tumor cells which are not detected in other periurethral carcinomas or hyperplasias (Figures 17–119 to 17–122).[55] Another pattern that we believe is an even more benign variant of this type of tumor is shown in Figures 17–123, and 17–125 to 17–131. Here endometrial glands are surrounded by a lamina propria with numerous inflammatory cells. One can see the proximity of endometrial glands to the transitional epithelium of the prostatic urethra as well as a well-differentiated carcinoma of the prostate (Figures 17–123; 17–124). The latter type of tumor is more biologically aggressive and should be treated as such. Cases reviewed by me disclose, both histologically and ultra-structurally, a resemblance to endometrium which is biologically benign. One report stresses the marked biologic aggressiveness of this tumor.[51]

Pathobiology

In most instances the histologic varieties and gross pathology of the endometrial growth are indicative of a non-metastasizing neoplasm. Associated car-cinomas of the prostate, which are contiguous but not continuous to the endometrial tumors, do possess a metastasizing potential. When the surgical specimen contains both these tumors, at the present time it is clinically wiser to treat the more biologically aggressive one, namely, prostatic carcinoma of the microacinar type.

It is imperative that this type of morphologic pattern be differentiated from the other forms of periurethral ductal carcinomas of the prostate. The latter have a much more confirmed malignant course than the endometrial tumors of the prostate (Figures 17–120; 17–121).

CARCINOMA WITH SARCOMATOID CHANGES

Carcinosarcoma of the prostate is rare. However, we frequently discover that either the epithelium or the stroma can be the source of primary malignancy of this gland, rather than both tissue components combined. Even though the epithelial tissue compartment is the source of common prostatic epithelial neoplasm, the stroma as a source of malignancy in this gland constitutes 0.1% of prostatic neoplasms.[56] Sarcomas of the prostate are known to occur in a young age group, whereas epithelial tumors occur in a much older group. Consequently, it is extremely rare for these tumors to coexist in the same individual.[57,58]

Many cases of carcinosarcoma, and especially the three previously reported ones,[57,58] have been discounted as anaplastic variants of epithelial carcinoma.[59] Some epithelial tumors in the genitourinary tract, as well as tumors elsewhere in the body, will occasionally exhibit numerous areas of sarcomatoid change under light microscopy. These sarcomatous findings can predominate in the metastases from these tumors. An exemplary organ of this phenomenon is the kidney. For the prostate to do so is extremely rare, but there have been some well-documented cases examined by light microscopy.

Pathology

Two of the previously cited cases initially had biopsies that were suggestive of carcinosarcoma of the prostate. We have had the same situation occur either on cases studied at this institution or in consultation. One such case is illustrated in Figures 17–132 to 17–135. An epithelial component to the neoplasm (Figures 17–132, left side; 17–133) is observed as is a stroma which is neoplastic (Figure 17–132, right side). It is usually not difficult to recognize that the former epithelial cellular component is cancerous. However, the diagnostic difficulty encountered with this lesion is usually centered around the mesenchymal or nonepithelial part of this type of cancer. It is difficult to determine whether this is a variant of the carcinoma or a separate tumor arising in the mesenchymal elements, although mesenchymal tumors emanating from this portion of the prostate gland are extremely varied.

The histologic patterns examined by us and those reported in the two other documented cases of carcinosarcoma are of the muscular type, namely, neoplasms of the smooth or striated muscle. Neoplasms of the striated or rhabdomyosarcomatous type have many tumor cells with bizarre nuclei (Figures 17–134; 17–135). They may also have a strap-like configuration and on careful scrutiny, cross striations may be indicated.

Difficulty may sometimes be encountered if the tumor is of the small spindle-cell type. Here the diagnosis of leiomyosarcoma or fibrosarcoma must be considered. Special stains, such as trichrome, may be helpful in differentiating between the cell types that compose these two types of malignancies; basically, the cells are fibrocytes or fibroblasts as opposed to smooth muscle cells. Trichrome stain may help since cytoplasm of smooth muscle stains red and that of fibrocytes, blue.

If the tissue is formalin-fixed, the electron microscope can prove of even greater benefit. Numerous filaments of both smooth and striated muscle cells can be seen ultrastructurally. In the smooth muscle cells, there are focal electron-dense condensations that are found with more frequency in the numerous clusters of actomyosin filaments. The striated muscle cell will show cross banding under electron microscopy, whereas the fibrocyte will have none of these ultrastructural findings.

If the stromal malignancy is epithelially derived, then electron microscopy will reveal epithelial stigmata which are not found in smooth, striated, or fibrocytic cells. If it is a sarcomatous epithelial cell, there will be numerous desmosomes and intracytoplasmic lumina which are not demonstrated in any of the stromal tumors.

Mostofi and Price,[60] in their pathologic evaluation of these tumors, state that the lesions designated carcinosarcomas should have tissue stromal components that contain definite neoplastic cartilage or bone formation of sarcomas.

Pathobiology

The metastatic sites for these tumors also include the spine, where they are extensively osteoblastic. Also involved may be the liver, lungs, and abdominal and mediastinal lymph nodes. The cases may behave clinically as a typical carcinoma of the prostate, but the sarcomatous element is believed by Hamlin and Lund[57] to be adversely affected by estrogen therapy. Consequently, it is of great clinical importance to place these tumors in the proper histologic cache. Not all prostatic carcinomas are of the same cell type and all may not respond the same way to estrogen therapy.

PROSTATIC SARCOMAS

The prostate gland not only is an organ in which glandular elements may be involved by a neoplastic process, but it also contains numerous different types of mesenchymal elements that can develop into a primary neoplasm. This process may involve the neurogenic elements and the vascular compartment, as well as the supporting fibromuscular components of the prostate.

We shall primarily discuss the fibromuscular tissue compartment.[29] Even though it is composed mostly of fibrocytes and smooth muscle cells, there is also another type of muscular cell that gives rise to malignant neoplasms that develop primarily in the prostate. This is the skeletal muscle that can be readily seen in normal and benign prostatic tissue obtained after transurethral resection of a suprapubic prostatectomy.[29] This is evidenced by the fact that rhabdomyosarcoma of the prostate is most commonly found in children, whereas leiomyosarcoma and fibrosarcoma occur in a much older age group.

Incidence

These malignant sarcomas constitute approximately 0.1% of all primary neoplasms of the prostate gland.[61] These soft tissue tumors may occur during any decade of life, but at least one-third of them appear in childhood and are usually of the rhabdomyosarcoma type. Stirling and Ash [62] noted that the majority of these sarcomas presented within the first few decades of life, and they coined the phrase "before 50, sarcoma and after 50, carcinoma." Seventy-five percent of the cases occur before the onset age of BPH.

Signs and Symptoms

Clinical findings are as variable as histologic types of sarcomas. Sarcomas of the prostate may produce obstructive uropathy and they may encroach on the rectum and cause constipation, bloody stools, and a sense of fullness, as well as an inability to empty the rectum. These large bowel symptoms, when accompanied by obstructive uropathy, are almost pathognomonic for sarcoma of the prostate gland. Late in the course of the disease, there may be edema of the scrotum, perineum, and lower extremities. On rectal examination, the prostate is enlarged, either symmetrically or asymmetrically. The tumors may be cystic, rubbery, soft, or hard.

Pathobiology

Growth rate of sarcomas of the prostate are explosive when compared to neoplasms of the epithelial tissue compartment. Rhabdomyosarcoma has a greater growth potential than leiomyosarcoma or fibrosarcoma of the prostate. Lymphosarcomas of the prostate have demonstrated a wide spectrum of activity, but this may depend on the specific cell type, namely, a reticulum or lymphoblastic cell. These tumors extend very early in their clinical course into the perivesical and periprostatic connective tissue. There may be early obstruction or compression of the prostatic urethra. Commonly, there is early lymphatic and vascular invasion with eventual progression to the abdominal wall, rectum, regional lymph nodes, and finally to liver, lung, and bone. The bony metastases are mostly osteolytic.

Histologic Types and Differential Diagnosis

It is critical that the tissue obtained for routine light histologic evaluation be free of urologic or crush artifact. If not, there can be numerous different diagnoses, each of which may carry with it a different prognosis and course of treatment. As a consequence, it may be impossible to differentiate malignant lymphoma from severe chronic prostatitis or undifferentiated carcinoma from sarcoma or a sarcomatous variant of bladder cancer that has invaded the prostate.

Lymphosarcoma

Primary lymphosarcoma of the prostate is rare, and there are many who believe that the lesion in the prostate is the initial manifestation of a systemic disease to be seen later in the surrounding lymph nodes.[63] The histopathology of these lesions is described by Cartagena et al.[64] Basically these lesions are of the large cell or reticulum cell type. There is usually a monotonous sea of cells of uniform size. High-power light microscopy reveals numerous cells with pleomorphic nuclei that can compress or completely replace the glandular structure of the prostate gland. A reticulum stain may help in differentiating this type of sarcoma from an undifferentiated carcinoma of the prostate. Individual reticulum fibers will surround each cell in the reticulum cell sarcoma, but in prostate carcinoma it will surround clusters of these cells.

Myosarcomas (Leiomyosarcoma and Rhabdomyosarcoma)

Both varieties of sarcomas are composed of cells that have abundant actomyosin in the cytoplasm. In rhabdomyosarcoma, there will be cross striations in some but not in all cells (Figures 17–136 to 17–140). The phosphotungstic acid stain is of some help in demonstrating these cross striations. Even more helpful in demonstrating cross striations at an ultrastructural level would be electron microscopy. There are many cells that demonstrate this only at submicroscopic levels and not at light microscopic magnification. Properly fixed formalin tissue can also be used if a diagnosis is to be made from light histologic paraffin sections.

Rhabdomyosarcoma usually occurs in the first decade of life and the leiomyosarcoma in a much older age group. However, leiomyosarcoma also contains an actomyosin protein in the cytoplasm which does not have any cross striations, but which will also stain red with a trichrome stain. An even more pathognomonic structure is found when electron microscopy is done. There are numerous fine fibers with focal condensations seen ultrastructurally in the cytoplasm of malignant smooth muscle cells. Many pleomorphic and anaplastic-appearing cells may also be seen that are quite different from the spindle-shaped cells that form a herringbone pattern (Figures 17–141; 17–142).

Fibrosarcoma

This type of tumor also possesses a highly malignant potential and is formed by cells that are spindle- or fusiform-shaped. They are arranged in whorls or bundles. Depending on the way the tissue knife cuts the tissue, there may be histologic patterns of small round cells arranged in a bundle (Figure 17–143). This occurs when the cells are sectioned perpendicular to their axis. A trichrome stain at times can prove helpful. These cells will not have an eosinophilic cytoplasm. Most fibrosarcomas do not have the pleomorphic and anaplastic cells or nuclei that malignant smooth muscle cells have. Electron microscopy of these tumors reveals a type of cytoplasm that ultrastructurally is devoid of myofilaments, but instead is rich in rough-surfaced endoplasmic reticulum. This structure is believed to be of paramount importance by the cell biologist because it is here that amino acid building blocks of collagen are put together.

The most common histopathologic types of sarcomas of the prostate are: (1) rhabdomyosarcoma; (2) leiomyosarcoma; (3) lymphosarcoma, reticulum cell type; (4) fibrosarcoma; (5) angiosarcoma; and (6) fibrous histiocytoma, malignant. Mostofi and Price[65] have observed other histologic type that would include chondrosarcoma, osteogenic sarcoma, neurogenic sarcoma, and neuroblastoma.

Clinical Management

The treatment of choice for malignant lymphomas is radiotherapy, and there have been some favorable results. However, for the other types of sarcomas, if diagnosed when the tumor is still confined to the prostate, a radical vesiculoprostatectomy is believed to be the method of choice. Radiotherapy or chemotherapy, or both, are yet to be validly tested as a method of treatment. In many instances, these tumors have not been properly categorized according to malignant cellular type.

References

1. Tannenbaum, M.: Differential diagnosis in uropathology. II. Urologic artifact and/or pathologist's dilemma. Urology, 4:485, 1974.
2. Tannenbaum, M.: Differential diagnosis in uropathology. III. Melanotic lesions of the prostate. Blue nevus and prostatic epithelial melanosis. Urology, 4:617, 1974.
3. Liavag, L.: Carcinoma of the prostate. Scandinavian University Books, Oslo, Norwegian Monographs on Med. Sci., 1967.
4. Anderson, R.: Carcinoma of the prostate: Clinical observations and treatment. Oslo University Press, Oslo, 1959.
5. Mostofi, F. K., and Price, E. B., Jr.: Malignant tumors of the prostate. In Tumors of the Male Genital System, Atlas of Tumor Pathology, 2nd Series, Fascicle 8, Washington, D.C., Armed Forces Institute of Pathology, 1973, p. 224.
6. Franks, L. M.: Latent carcinoma of the prostate. J. Pathol. Bact., 68:603, 1954.
7. Deane, H. W., and Wurzelmann, S.: Electron microscopic observations on the postnatal differentiation of the seminal vesicle epithelium of the laboratory mouse. Am. J. Anat., 117:91, 1965.
8. Toner, P. G., and Baillie, A. H.: Biochemical, histochemical and ultrastructural changes in the mouse seminal vesicle after castration. J. Anat., 100:173, 1966.
9. Mostofi, F. K., and Price, E. B., Jr.: Tumors of the Male Genital System, Atlas of Tumor Pathology, 2nd Series, Fascicle 8, Washington, D.C., Armed Forces Institute of Pathology, 1973, pp. 258 and 261.
10. Nigogosyan, G., et al.: Blue nevus of the prostate gland. Cancer, 16:1097, 1963.
11. Simard, C., et al.: Le problème du naevus bleu prostatique. Ann. Anat. Pathol., 9:469, 1964.
12. Jao, W., et al.: Blue nevus of the prostate gland. Arch. Pathol., 91:187, 1971.
13. Guillan, R. A., and Zelman, S.: The incidence and probable origin of melanin in the prostate. J. Urol., 104:151, 1970.
14. Lowsley, O. S.: Melanoma of the urinary tract and prostate gland. South Med. J., 44:487, 1951.
15. Upshaw, B. Y., et al.: Extensive blue nevus of Jadassohn-Tièche. Report of a case. Surgery, 22:761, 1947.
16. Dorsey, C. S., and Montgomery, H.: Blue nevus and its distinction from mongolian spot and the nevus of Ota. J. Invest. Dermatol., 22:225, 1954.
17. Berry, N. E., and Reese, L.: Malignant melanoma which had its first clinical manifestations in the prostate gland. J. Urol., 69:286, 1953.
18. Kniseley, R. M., and Baggenstoss, A. H.: Primary melanoma of adrenal gland. Arch. Pathol., 42:345, 1946.
19. Allen, M. S., Jr., and Drash, E. C.: Primary melanoma of the lung. Cancer, 21:154, 1968.
20. Langley, J. W., and Weitzner, S.: Blue nevus and melanosis of prostate. J. Urol., 112:359, 1974.
21. Goldman, R. L.: Melanogenic epithelium in the prostate gland. Am. J. Clin. Pathol., 49:75, 1968.
22. Tannenbaum, M.: Differential diagnosis in uropathology. I. Carcinoma of prostate versus seminal vesicle. Urology, 4:354, 1974.
23. Mostofi, F. K., and Price, E. B., Jr.: Tumors of the Male Genital System. Atlas of Tumor Pathology, 2nd Series, Fascicle 8, Washington, D.C., Armed Forces Institute of Pathology, 1973, p. 225.
24. Totten, R. S., et al.: Microscopic differential diagnosis of latent carcinoma of prostate. Arch. Pathol., 55:131, 1953.
25. Mostofi, F. K., and Price, E. B., Jr.: Malignant tumors of the prostate. In Tumors of the Male Genital System, Atlas of Tumor Pathology, 2nd Series, Fascicle 8, Washington, D.C., Armed Forces Institute of Pathology, 1973, p. 218.
26. Baron, E., and Angrist, A.: Incidence of occult adenocarcinoma of the prostate after fifty years of age. Arch. Pathol., 32:787, 1941.
27. Rich, A. L.: On frequency of occurrence of occult carcinoma of the prostate. J. Urol., 32:215, 1935.
28. Tannenbaum, M.: Atypical epithelial hyperplasia or carcinoma of the prostate gland: The surgical pathologist at an impasse? Urology, 4:758, 1974.
29. Tannenbaum, M.: Diagnostic criteria for histopathologic evaluation of prostatic tissue sections. Urology, 5:407, 1975.
30. Mostofi, F. K., and Price, E. B., Jr.: Malignant tumors of the prostate. In Tumors of the Male Genital System, Atlas of Tumor Pathology, 2nd Series, Fascicle 8, Washington, D.C., Armed Forces Institute of Pathology, 1973, pp. 206–208.
31. Sika, J. V., and Buckley, J. J.: Mucus-forming adenocarcinoma of prostate. Cancer, 17:949, 1964.
32. Joshi, D. P., et al.: Mucogenic adenocarcinoma of the prostate. J. Urol., 98:241, 1967.
33. Balogh, F., and Szendrói, Z.: Cancer of the prostate. Budapest, Akadémiai Kiadó, 1968.
34. Klissoruw, A.: Ein fall von carcinoma gelatinosum prostate. Virchows Arch. Pathol. Anat., 268:512, 1928.

35. Thompson, G. J., et al.: Unusual carcinoma involving the prostate. J. Urol., 69:416, 1953.

36. Edgar, W. M.: Mucin-secreting carcinoma of the prostate. Br. J. Urol., 30:213, 1958.

37. Mostofi, F. K., and Price, E. B., Jr.: Malignant tumors of the prostate. In Tumors of the Male Genital System, Atlas of Tumor Pathology, 2nd Series, Fascicle 8, Washington, D.C., Armed Forces Institute of Pathology, 1973, pp. 269–73.

38. Melicow, M. M., and Hollowell, J. W.: Intraurothelial cancer: Carcinoma in situ, Bowen's disease of the urinary systems. Discussion of thirty cases. J. Urol., 68:763, 1952.

39. Ortega, L. G., Whitmore, W. F., Jr., and Murphy, A. J.: In situ carcinoma of the prostate with intraepithelial extension into the urethra and bladder. Cancer, 6:892, 1953.

40. Franks, L. M., and Chesterman, F. C.: Intraepithelial carcinoma of prostatic urethra, periurethral glands and prostatic ducts (Bowen's disease of urinary epithelium). Br. J. Cancer, 10:223, 1956.

41. Ende, N., et al.: Carcinoma originating in ducts surrounding the prostatic urethra. Am. J. Clin. Pathol., 40:183, 1963.

42. Ullmann, A. S., and Ross, O. A.: Hyperplasia, atypism, and carcinoma in situ in prostatic periurethral glands. Am. J. Clin. Pathol., 47:497, 1967.

43. Karpas, C. M., and Moumgis, B.: Primary transitional cell carcinoma of prostate gland: Possible pathogenesis and relationship to reserve cell hyperplasia of prostatic periurethral ducts. J. Urol., 101:201, 1969.

44. Mao, P., and Angrist, A.: The fine structure of the basal cell of human prostate. Lab. Invest., 15:1768, 1966.

45. Rubenstein, A. B., and Rubnitz, M. E.: Transitional cell carcinoma of the prostate. Cancer, 24:543, 1969.

46. Johnson, D. E., Hogan, J. M., and Ayala, A. G.: Transitional cell carcinoma of the prostate. A clinical morphological study. Cancer, 29:287, 1972.

47. Jewett, H. J., and Strong, G. H.: Infiltrating carcinoma of the urinary bladder: Diagnosis and clinical evaluation of curability. South Med. J., 39:203, 1946.

48. Mostofi, F. K., and Price, E. B., Jr.: Malignant tumors of the prostate. In Tumors of the Male Genital System, Atlas of Tumor Pathology, 2nd Series, Fascicle 8, Washington, D.C., Armed Forces Institute of Pathology, 1973, p. 244.

49. Tannenbaum, M.: Transitional cell carcinoma of prostate. Urology, 5:674, 1975.

50. Melicow, M. M., and Pachter, M. R.: Endometrial carcinoma of prostatic utricle (uterus masculinus). Cancer, 20:1715, 1967.

51. Melicow, M. M., and Tannenbaum, M.: Endometrial carcinoma of uterus masculinus (prostatic utricle). Report of six cases. J. Urol., 106:892, 1971.

52. Carney, J. A., and Kelalis, P. P.: Endometrial carcinoma of the prostatic utricle. Am. J. Clin. Pathol., 60:565, 1973.

53. Tannenbaum, M.: Unpublished results.

54. Mostofi, F. K., and Price, E. B., Jr.: Malignant tumors of the prostate. In Tumors of the Male Genital System, Atlas of Tumor Pathology, 2nd Series, Fascicle 8, Washington, D.C., Armed Forces Institute of Pathology, 1973, pp. 241–244.

55. Dube, V. E., et al.: Prostatic adenocarcinoma of ductal origin. Cancer, 32:402, 1973.

56. Tannenbaum, M.: Sarcomas of the prostate gland. Urology, 5:810, 1975.

57. Hamlin, W. B., and Lund, P. K.: Carcinosarcoma of the prostate, a case report. J. Urol., 97:518, 1967.

58. Haddad, J. R., and Reyes, E. C.: Carcinosarcoma of the prostate with metastasis of both elements, case report. J. Urol., 103:80, 1970.

59. Saphir, O., and Vass, A.: Carcinosarcoma. Am J. Cancer, 33:331, 1938.

60. Mostofi, F. K., and Price, E. B., Jr.: Malignant tumors of the prostate. In Tumors of the Male Genital System, Atlas of Tumor Pathology, 2nd Series, Fascicle 8, Washington, D.C., Armed Forces Institute of Pathology, 1973, p. 257.

61. Melicow, M. M., et al.: Sarcoma of the prostate gland; Review of literature; table of classification; report of four cases. J. Urol., 49:675, 1943.

62. Stirling, W. C., and Ash, J. E.: Sarcoma of the prostate. J. Urol., 41:515, 1939.

63. Waller, J. I., and Shullenberger, W. A.: Lymphosarcoma of the prostate. J. Urol., 62:480, 1949.

64. Cartagena, R., et al.: Primary reticulum cell sarcoma of the prostate gland. Urology, 5:815, 1975.

65. Mostofi, F. K., and Price, E. B., Jr.: Malignant tumors of the prostate. In Tumors of the Male Genital System, Atlas of Tumor Pathology, 2nd Series, Fascicle 8, Washington, D.C., Armed Forces Institute of Pathology, 1973, p. 253.

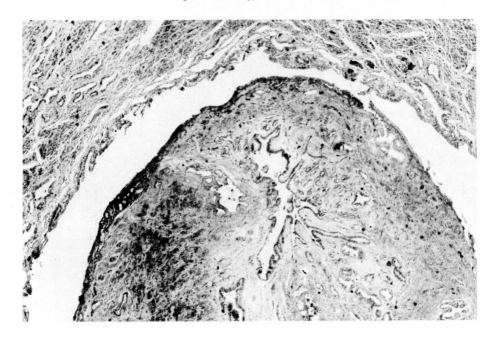

Figure 17–1. Low-power photomicrograph of prostatic urethra region of veru. Note numerous branching ducts. (×38)

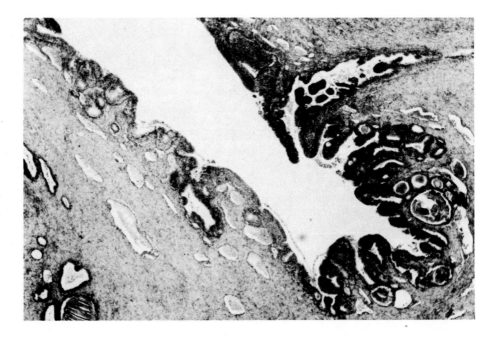

Figure 17–2. Corpora amylacea partially occluding orifice of ducts leading backward to various other lobes of prostate. These ducts are adjacent to fibrovascular proliferations which begin as nodules in periurethral regions of prostate. (×80)

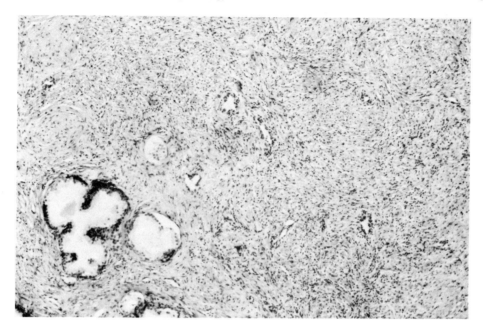

Figure 17–3. Part of nodule with slit-like vascular channels and storiform pattern. Nodules pathologically begin in late twenties. Prostatic tissue in lower left half is often seen to grow into these nodules. (×73)

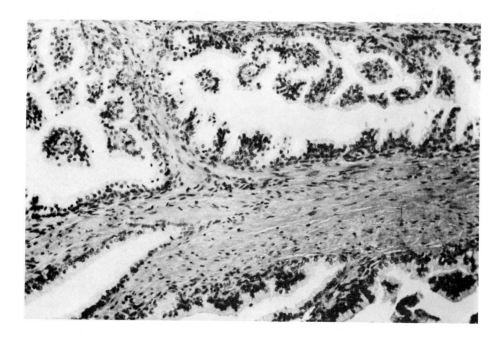

Figure 17–4. Papillary proliferations of periurethral ducts. (×151)

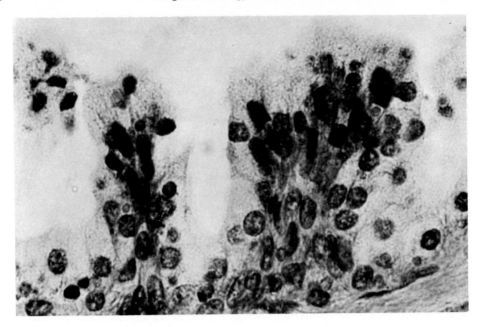

Figure 17–5. Opaque bodies in cytoplasm of periurethral ducts. They vary in size and coloration and are usually reddish-brown on H & E sections. They can be confused with seminal vesicle inclusions. (×911)

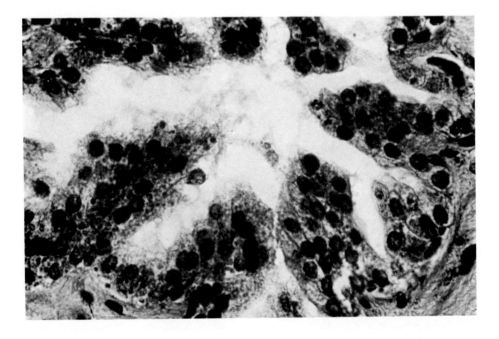

Figure 17–6. Another area of same duct demonstrating different pattern of cytoplasmic granules. The cytoplasmic inclusions found in Figures 17–5 and 17–6 are dopa-positive granules. (×706)

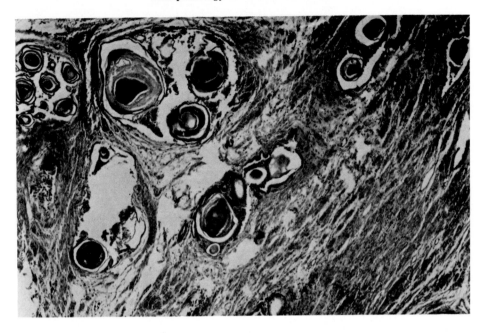

Figure 17–7. Corpora amylacea in periurethral region. (×27)

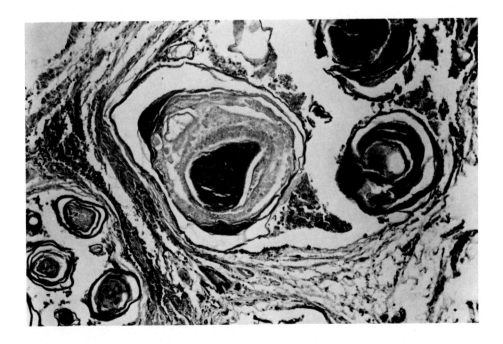

Figure 17–8. Laminated architecture of these structures which can occlude periurethral ducts as well as lie free in benign and malignant acini. (×108)

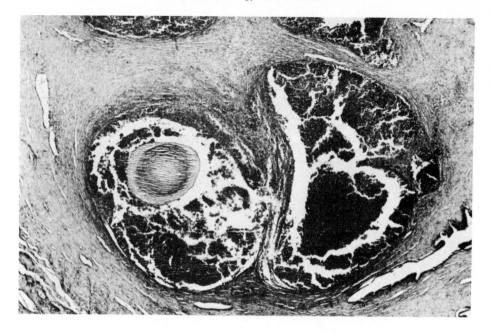

Figure 17–9. Corpora amylacea in occluded acutely inflamed duct in periurethral region of prostate. Bacteria-ridden duct as well as noninflamed periurethral duct in lower right. (×38)

As a consequence of occlusion of periurethral and secondary ducts, numerous atypical hyperplasias are seen throughout prostate that can be misinterpreted as carcinomas of prostate. The next 18 figures represent some patterns that are commonly seen.

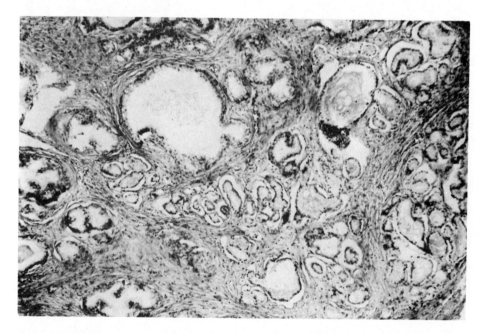

Figure 17–10. Small glands still in arboreal pattern and many glands lined by double layer of cells. (×73)

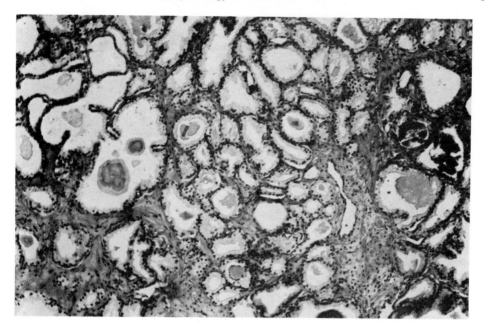

Figure 17–11. Atypical hyperplasia of prostatic epithelium. (×94)

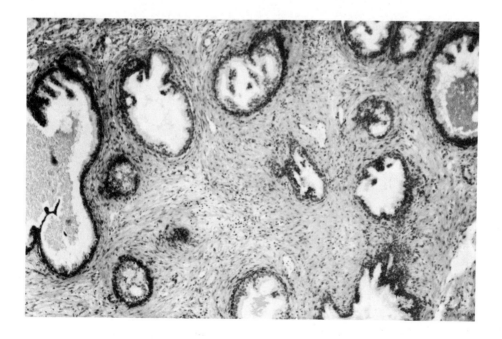

Figure 17–12. Pseudocribriform patterns of epithelia. (×73)

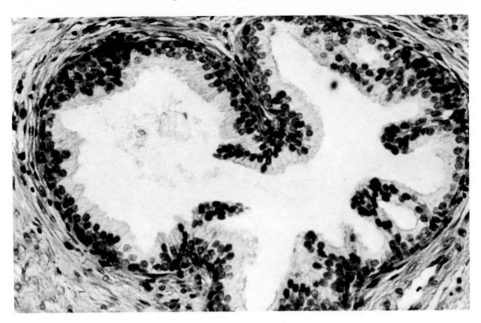

Figure 17–13. Pseudocribriform patterns of epithelia. (×288)

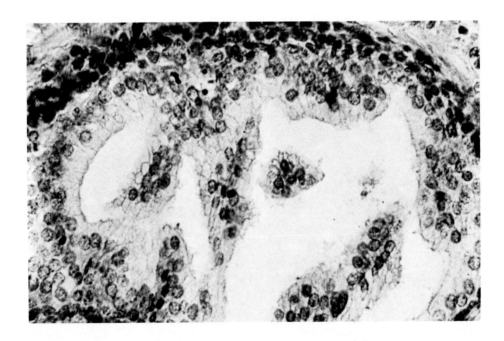

Figure 17–14. Glands exhibit, in part, epithelial proliferations without fibrovascular stalks in which there are glandular lumens. These can be easily confused with cribriform patterns of carcinoma of prostate which are not composed of double layer of cells. (×459)

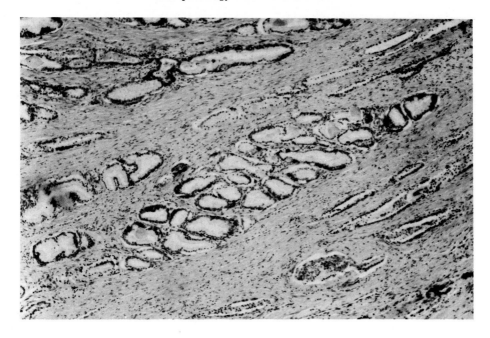

Figure 17–15. Both basal and surface cells should always be looked for in atypical foci that look like carcinoma. (×76)

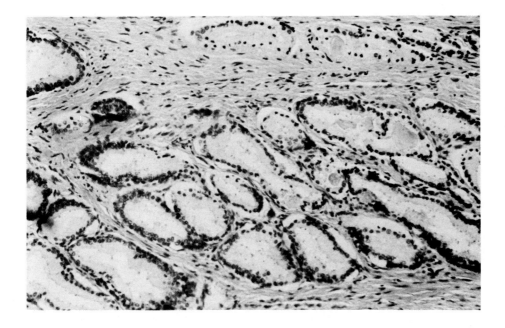

Figure 17–16. Higher magnification of Figure 17–15. (×189)

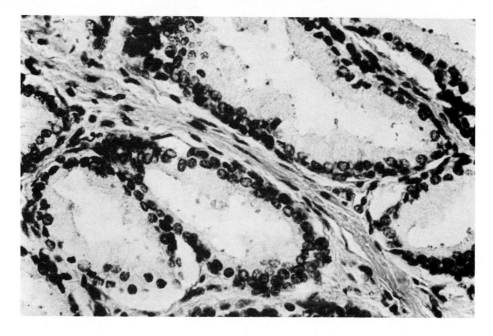

Figure 17–17. Double layer of cells should be present for diagnosis of benign atypical areas of prostate. Basal cells are not present in carcinomatous glands. (×460)

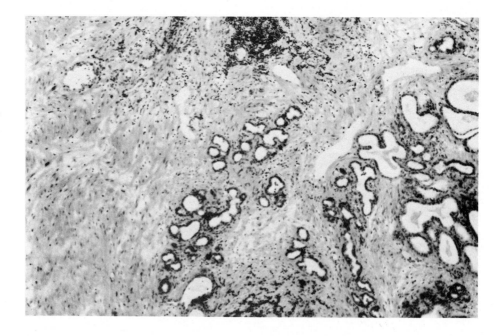

Figure 17–18. Quite often in atypical glands, basal layer may be missing. (×73)

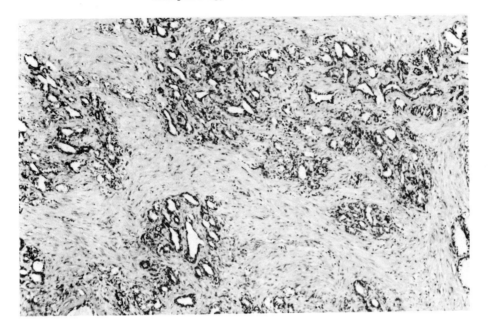

Figure 17–19. Atypical glands. (×76)

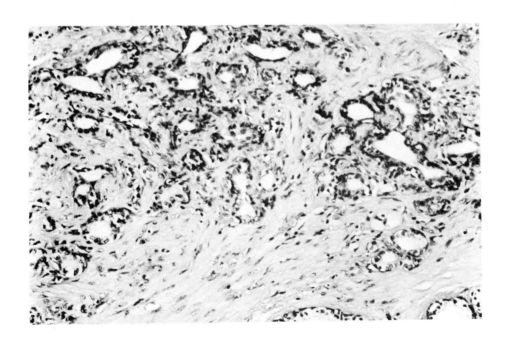

Figure 17–20. Atypical glands. (×189)

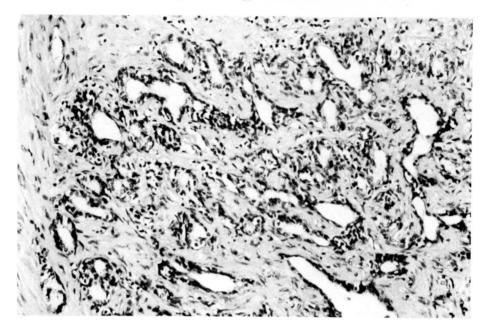

Figure 17–21. Atypical glands. (×189)

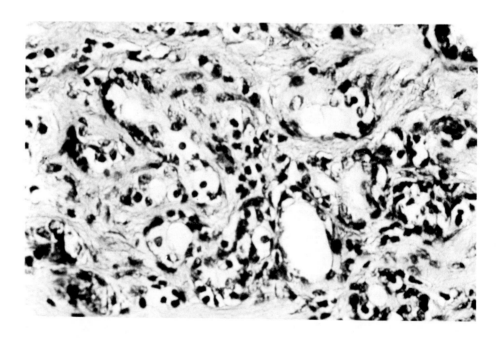

Figure 17–22. Numerous atrophic glands are still in arboreal pattern and not back-to-back. They still have considerable amount of fibromuscular stroma between them with branching of glands and occasional mitosis. Some glands have vacuolated cells simulating carcinomatous glands that have responded to estrogen therapy. A history should always be elicited if there is question of whether specimen is from a patient who has received diethylstilbestrol (DES). (×459)

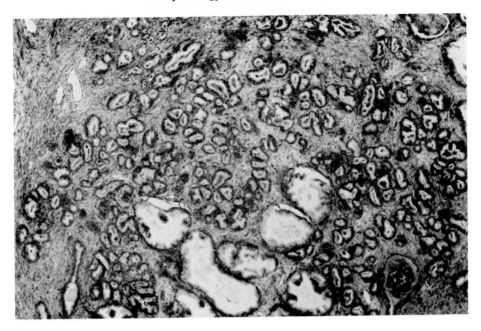

Figure 17–23. Another pattern often seen in prostate removed for obstructive uropathy or else near areas of prostatic infarction are regenerating epithelial nodules. (×45)

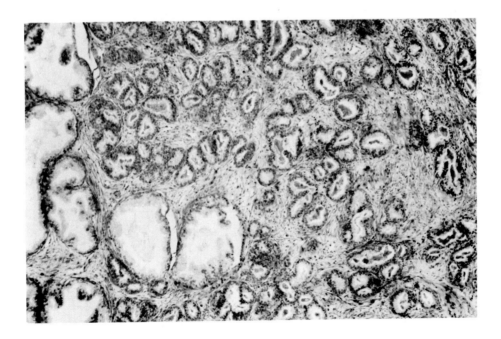

Figure 17–24. Regenerating epithelial nodules. (×73)

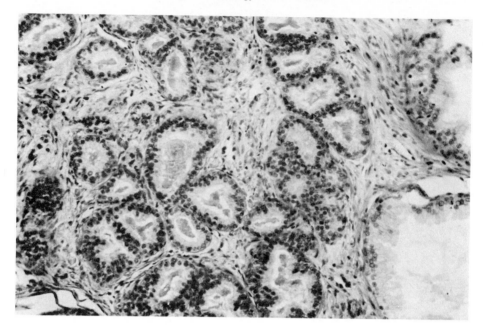

Figure 17–25. Regenerating epithelial nodules. (×189)

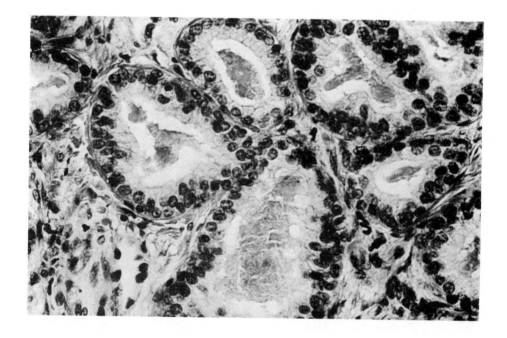

Figure 17–26. Glands are hyperplastic, in arboreal pattern, and lined by double layer of plump prostatic cells. (×459)

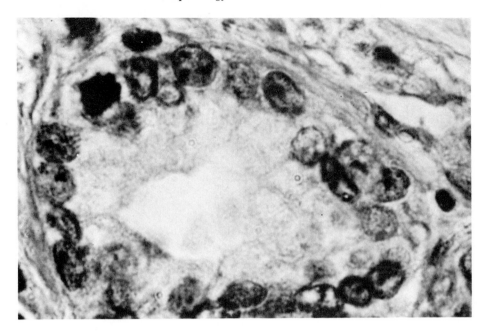

Figure 17–27. Cells have very eosinophilic cytoplasms and very basophilic nuclei, many of which may be in various phases of mitoses. (×1837)

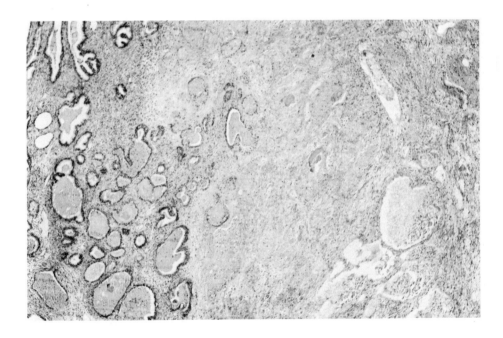

Figure 17–28. Hyperplastic glands often found near infarction area. On left are histologically-intact glands; on right glands have undergone necrosis. (×38)

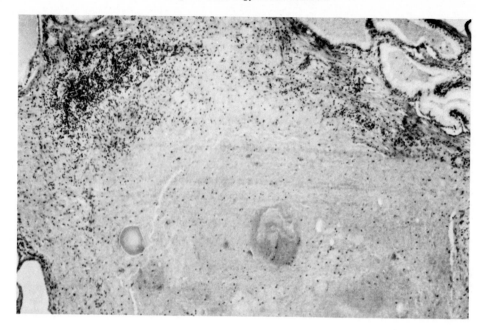

Figure 17–29. Low-power photomicrograph of area of necrosis surrounded by xanthogranulomatous cells. These cells, if taken out of context, can be readily confused with some patterns of carcinoma of prostate (see also Figure 17–103). (×73)

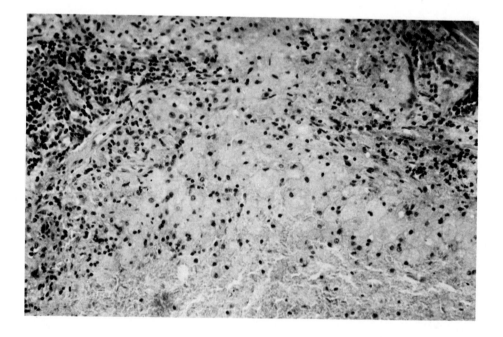

Figure 17–30. Granulomatous cells at edge of infarction and mixed with numerous inflammatory cells. (×189)

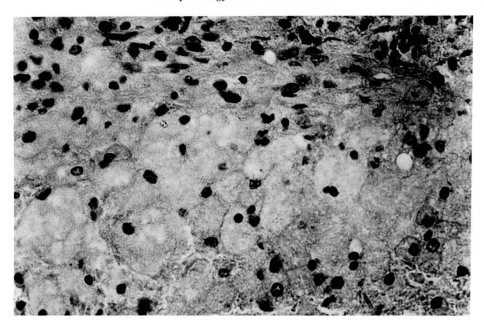

Figure 17–31. Xanthoma cells. (×459)

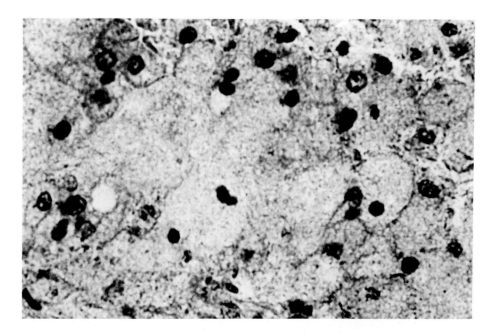

Figure 17–32. Xanthoma cells which reader should compare to confirmed areas of carcinoma (see Figure 17–103). This confusion can readily arise when biopsy has small portions of tissue and clinical diagnosis of carcinoma is suspected. Patterns seen here are typical for granulomatous prostatitis which is benign but which clinically simulates carcinoma of prostate. When reviewing slides, also look for other areas of inflammation and infarction for diagnosis of granulomatous or benign prostatitis. (×706)

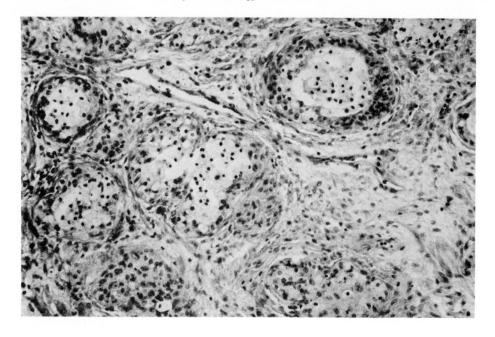

Figure 17–33. Areas often seen when minuscule amounts of tissue are obtained on biopsy. (× 189)

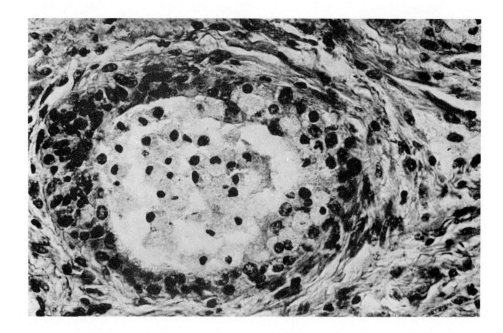

Figure 17–34. Granulomatous cells are found contained within lumen of acini and ducts. (×459)

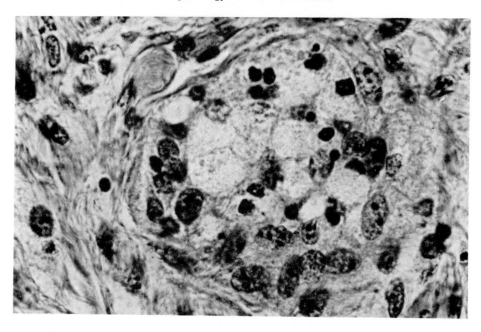

Figure 17–35. Surrounding epithelium of acini may also demonstrate some stigmata of carcinoma with numerous mitoses and nuclei with prominent nucleoli. (×1120)

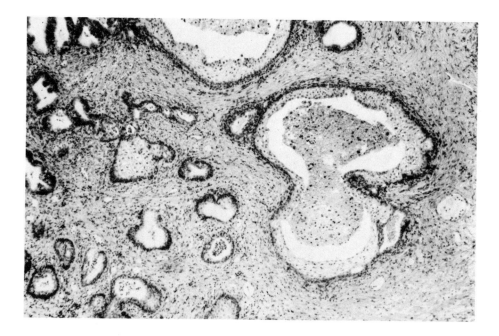

Figure 17–36. Areas of squamous metaplasia of ducts surrounding area of infarct or granulomatous prostatitis. Cytoplasm very eosinophilic and not vacuolated as in squamous metaplasia associated with DES treatment. (×73)

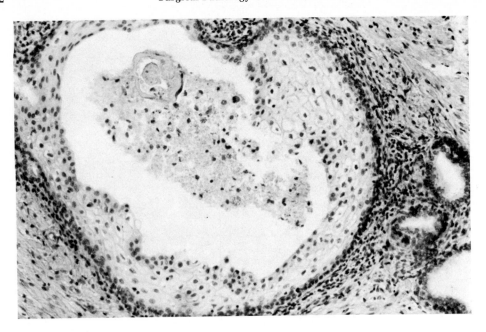

Figure 17–37. Squamous metaplasia. (×189)

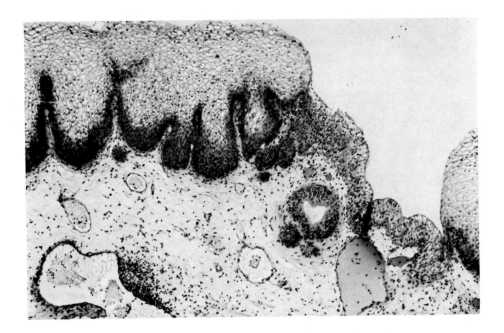

Figure 17–38. Prostatic urethra shows areas of extensive squamous cell metaplasia or transitional cell hyperplasia, or both, which may be accentuated by either infarction, catheterization, or repeated cystoscopies. (×48)

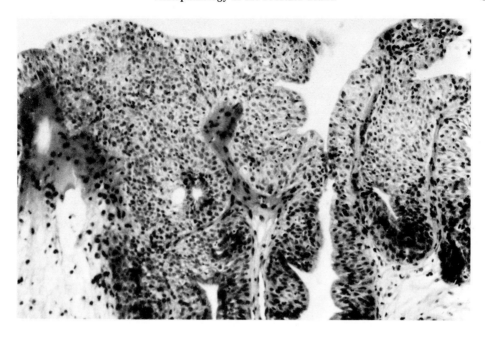

Figure 17–39. Transitional cell hyperplasia may be quite extensive and simulate carcinoma of transitional cell type found in urinary bladder. A history as well as anatomic localization of biopsy site is mandatory. (×189)

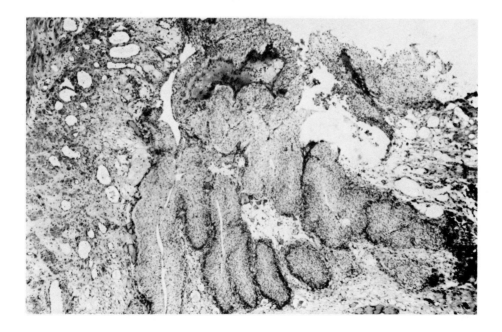

Figure 17–40. Transitional cell hyperplasia. (×48)

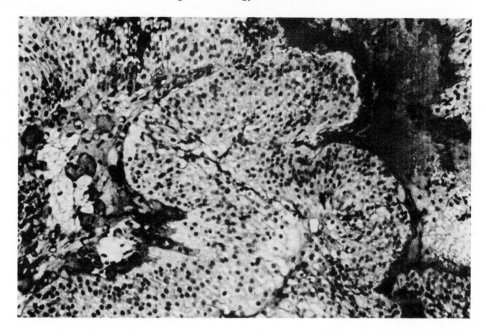

Figure 17–41. Transitional cell hyperplasia that is impossible to distinguish from papillary transitional cell epitheliomas of bladder. It is therefore imperative that surrounding prostatic tissue be critically examined. Transitional cell hyperplasia and metaplasia should extend into periurethral prostatic ducts. (×189)

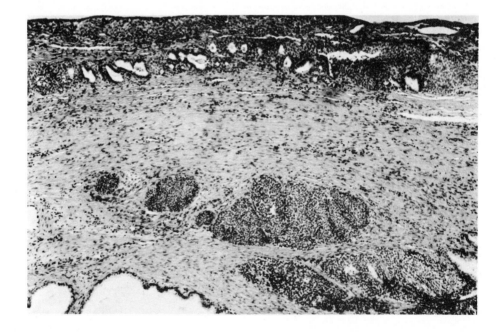

Figure 17–42. Transitional cell epithelium. (×73)

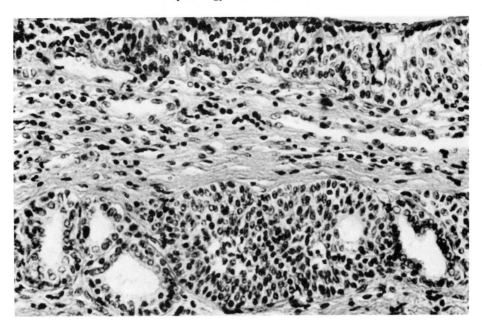

Figure 17–43. Transitional cell epithelium. (×189)

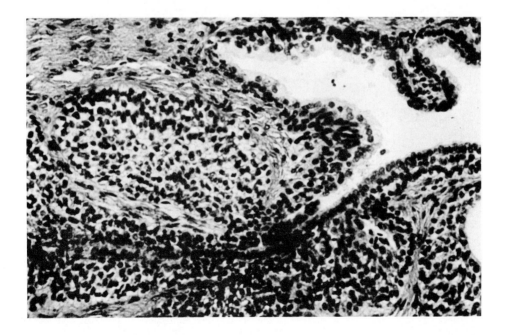

Figure 17–44. Several foci of transitional cell epithelium not only contiguous, but continuous with glandular epithelium of secondary and sometimes tertiary branches of prostatic ducts. (×189)

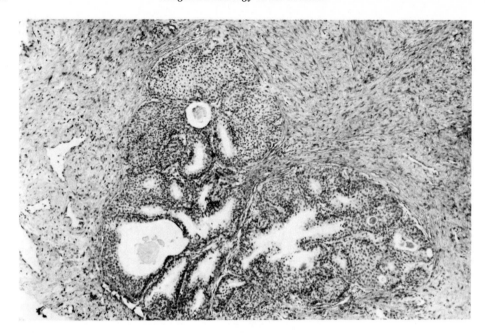

Figure 17–45. Glandular epithelial cells in center of transitional epithelium. (×73)

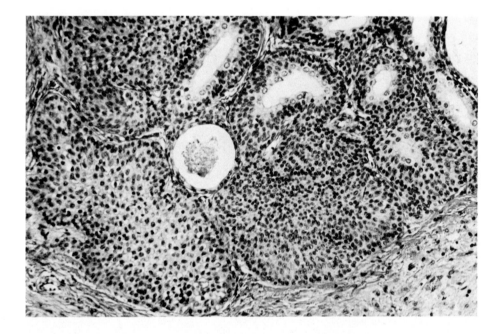

Figure 17–46. Sometimes glandular epithelial cells are not only continuous but may be histologically in center of these foci of transitional epithelium. When there is exuberant amount of transitional epithelium, all cells must be critically examined under high-dry objective (×25–40) to examine cytology of cells. Carcinomas that are either in situ or invasive can be seen to arise in these areas (see Figures 17–111 to 17–115). (×89)

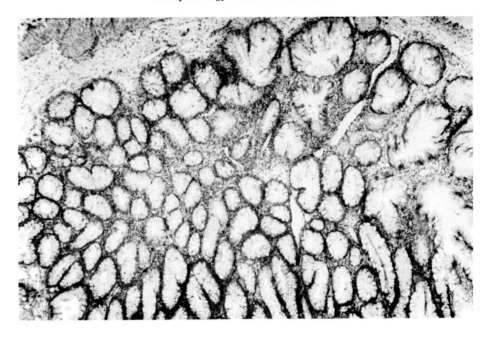

Figure 17–47. Other metaplastic configurations in periurethral area can be seen that simulate colonic epithelium with its surrounding lamina propria. (×76)

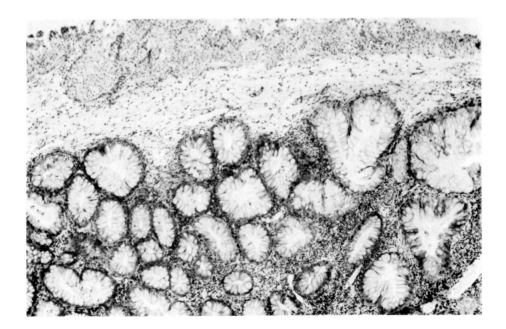

Figure 17–48. In upper half of photomicrograph there is covering urothelial surface above these adenomatous colonic glands. (×76)

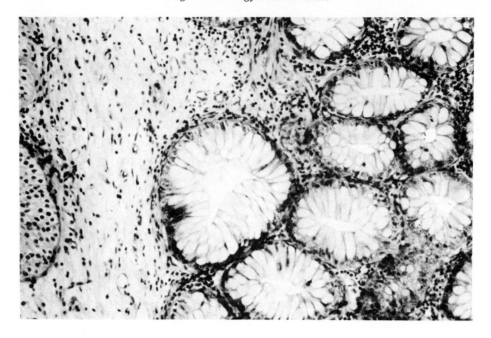

Figure 17–49. Glands and lamina propria. (×189)

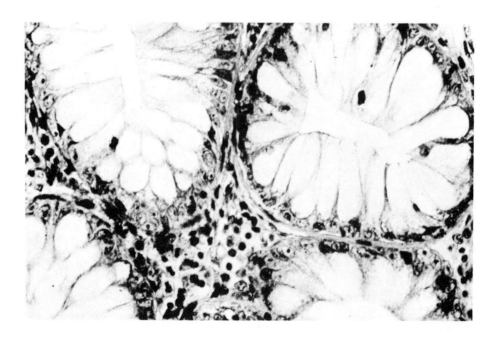

Figure 17–50. There is lamina propria with inflammatory cells surrounding glands containing goblet cells and mitoses. (×459)

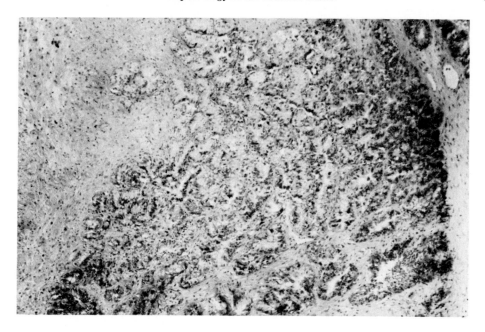

Figure 17–51. Occasionally both transurethral resection and prostatic needle biopsies often have seminal vesicle material or ejaculatory duct structures which can histologically simulate carcinoma of prostate. A glandular, haphazard, almost back-to-back pattern can be seen. Crush artifact or compression artifact from needle biopsy can be noted. (×73)

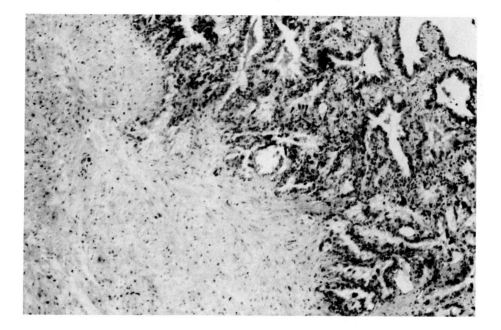

Figure 17–52. Lumens of glands may be occluded but also dilated with secretions. (×94)

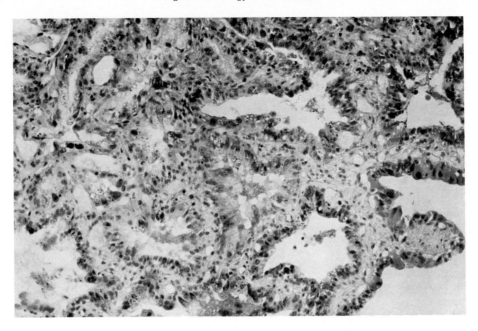

Figure 17–53. When areas like this are seen, microscopist should always turn from low scanning objectives (×2.8–4) to greater magnifying objectives (×10 and above) in order to discern nuclear and cytoplasmic structures that are seen here. (×189)

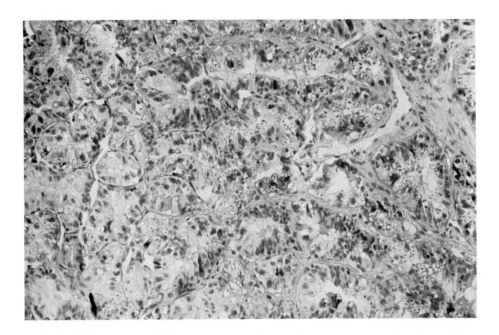

Figure 17–54. Cytoplasm is very eosinophilic and nuclei are almost pyknotic. Glands may or may not be back-to-back, in which case tissue must be examined under higher magnifying objectives in order to discern patterns which are seen in next Figure. (×189)

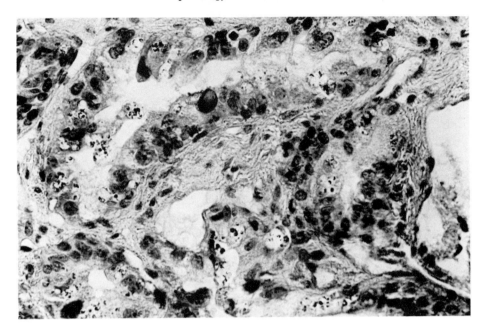

Figure 17–55. Golden-brown refractile pigment. This may be seen in lumen of these glands or in their cytoplasm or extruded into their fibrovascular stroma. (×459)

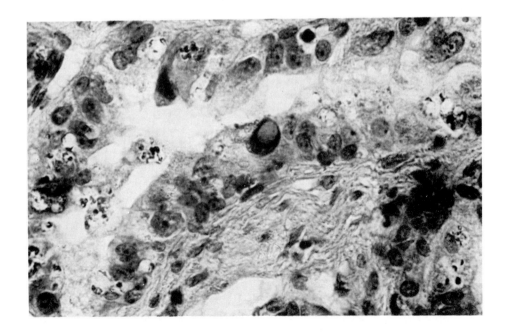

Figure 17–56. Lipofuscin granules or golden-brown refractile pigment. (×706)

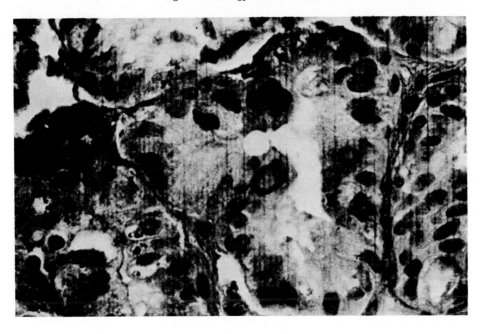

Figure 17–57. Seminal vesicle glands that are back-to-back and contain golden-brown refractile pigment lipofuscin. It is important to see this pigment in order to rule out carcinoma of prostate. (×706)

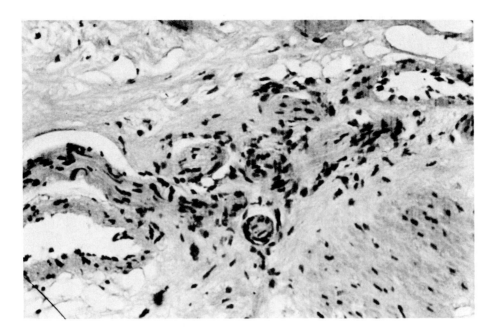

Figure 17–58. Prostatic capsule nerve and blood vessels. (×288)

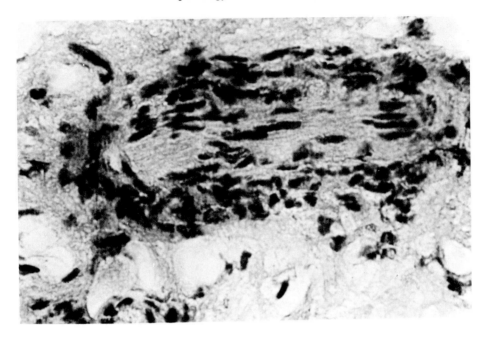

Figure 17–59. Numerous squashed inflammatory cells surrounding nerve. It is difficult at times to be certain that these are indeed inflammatory cells. Further additional levels of histologic blocks are mandatory if there are no other areas indicative of carcinoma. (×706)

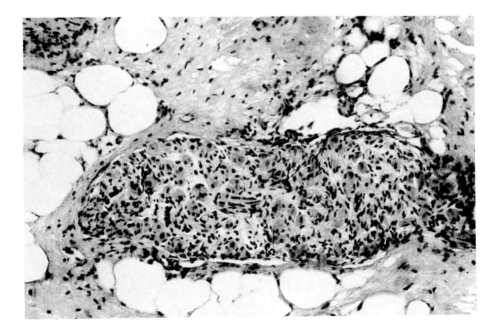

Figure 17–60. Conglomeration of ganglionic cells in area of prostatic capsule. (×189)

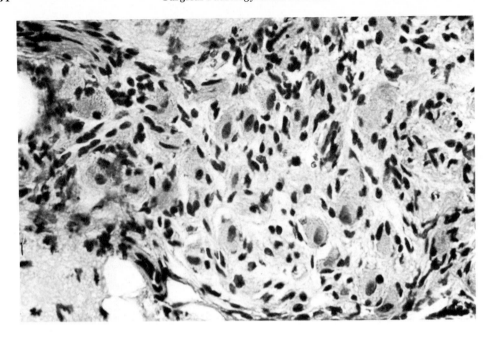

Figure 17–61. Higher magnification of this area with associated crush artifact on left. It is of importance for clinical evaluation of extent of prostatic carcinoma if there is any perineural or prostatic capsular involvement (see also Figure 17–82). (×459)

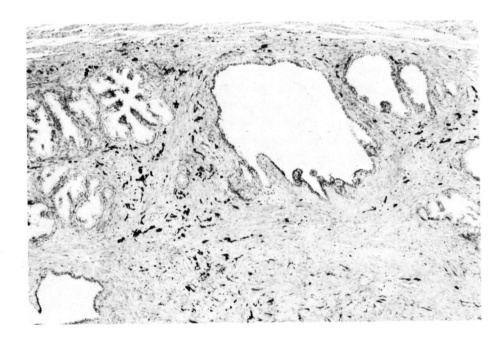

Figure 17–62. Blue nevus demonstrating numerous stellate cells scattered throughout fibromuscular stroma of prostate. (×48)

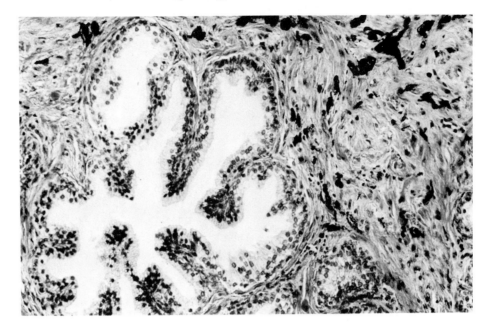

Figure 17–63. Blue nevus demonstrating numerous stellate cells scattered throughout fibromuscular stroma of prostate. (×189)

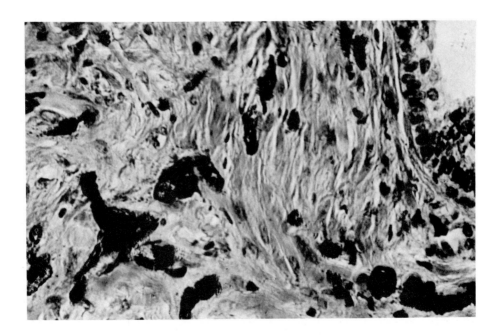

Figure 17–64. Stellate cells engorged with numerous black granules almost occluding their nuclei in blue nevus. (×459)

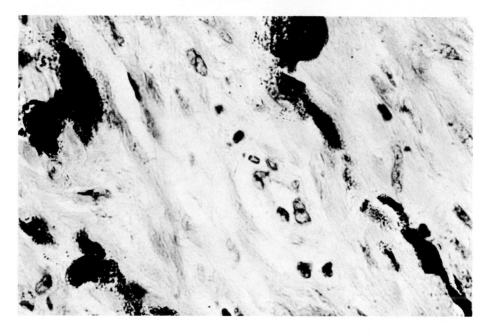

Figure 17–65. Stellate cells engorged with numerous black granules almost occluding their nuclei in blue nevus. (×706)

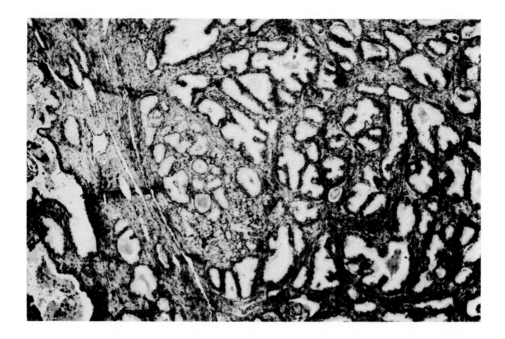

Figure 17–66. Microscopic foci of carcinoma in middle of normal benign glands. (×48)

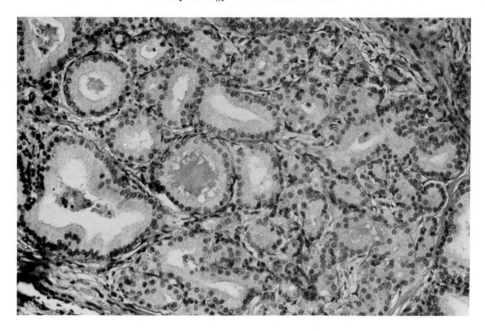

Figure 17–67. Higher magnification revealing many glands back-to-back. (×189)

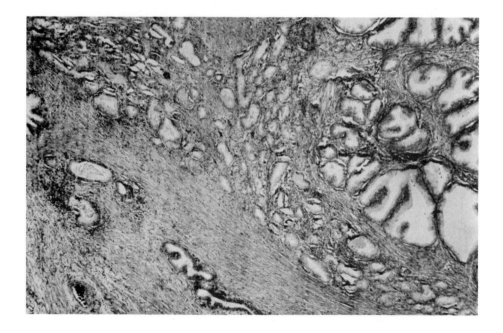

Figure 17–68. Numerous small glands in streaming pattern adjacent to normal glands. (×48)

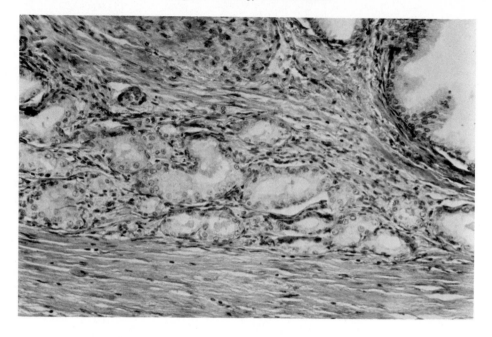

Figure 17–69. Higher magnification of these cancerous streaming back-to-back glands. (×189)

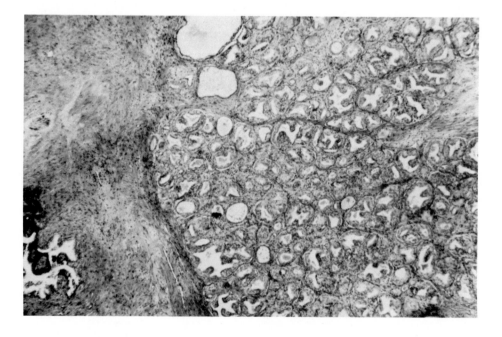

Figure 17–70. Adenomatous focus of carcinoma. (×48)

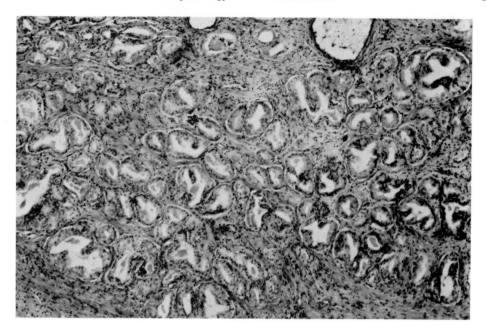

Figure 17–71. Glands are well-differentiated and back-to-back. (×73)

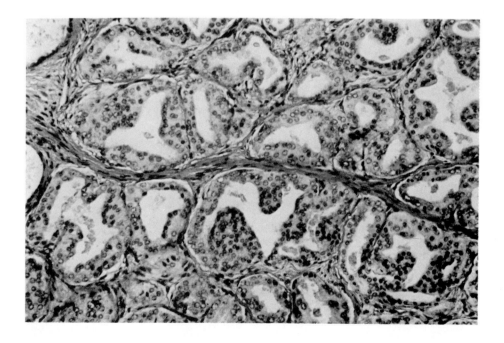

Figure 17–72. Glands composed of papillary projections and numerous cells in thickness without basal cell. (×189)

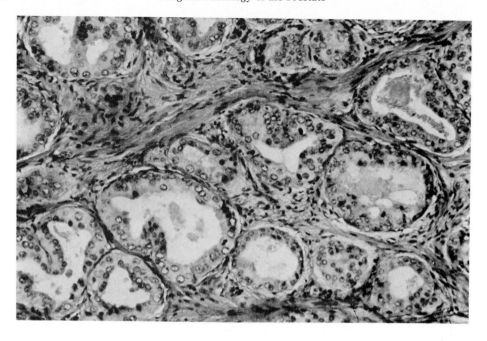

Figure 17–73. Glands composed of papillary projections and numerous cells in thickness without basal cell. (×189)

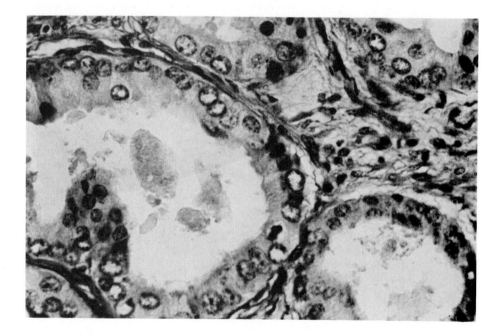

Figure 17–74. Cells may have very prominent nucleolus and mitoses. (×459)

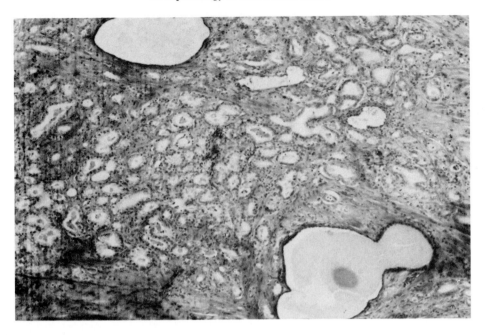

Figure 17–75. Sometimes glands are almost uniform type; small, well-differentiated and diffusely scattered throughout. (×76)

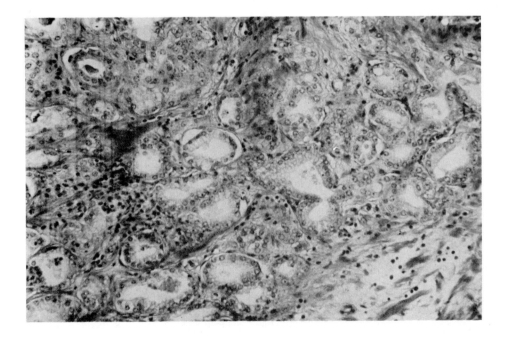

Figure 17–76. Higher magnification shows these glands to be well-differentiated and back-to-back, with sparse infiltration of lymphocytes in stroma. (×189)

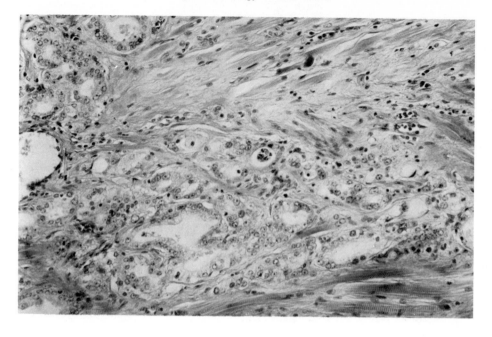

Figure 17–77. Carcinomatous glands adjacent to skeletal muscle. (× 189)

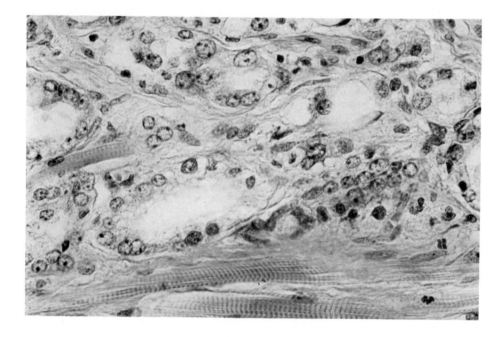

Figure 17–78. Carcinomatous glands adjacent to skeletal muscle. (× 459)

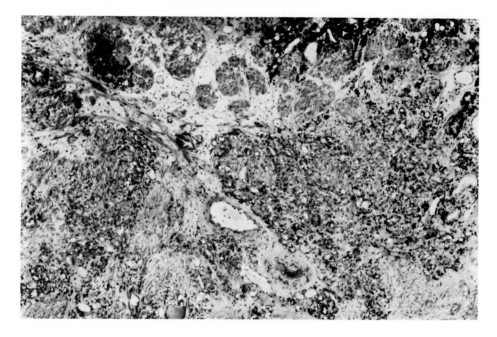

Figure 17–79. Other foci of carcinoma from transurethral resection with cautery artifact in upper part of picture. (×38)

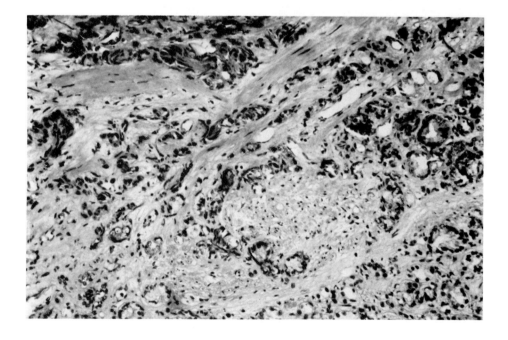

Figure 17–80. Cautery artifact in association with carcinomatous glands. (×189)

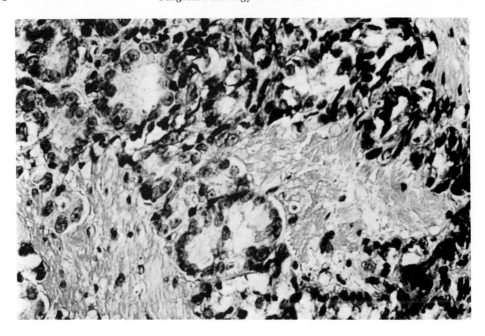

Figure 17–81. Sometimes cautery artifact is so severe that it completely obliterates carcinomatous architecture, giving false impression that no cancer is present. (×459)

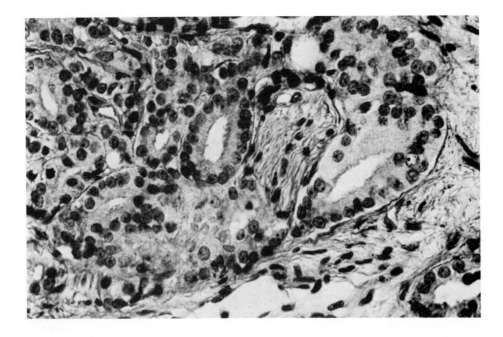

Figure 17–82. A helpful clue, when present, is perineural invasion of well-differentiated carcinomatous glands. (×459)

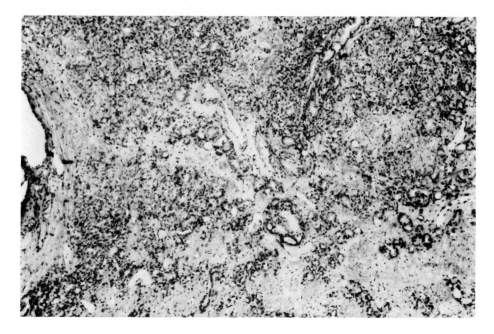

Figure 17–83. Other foci of varying patterns but with cribriform pattern in one focus. (×73)

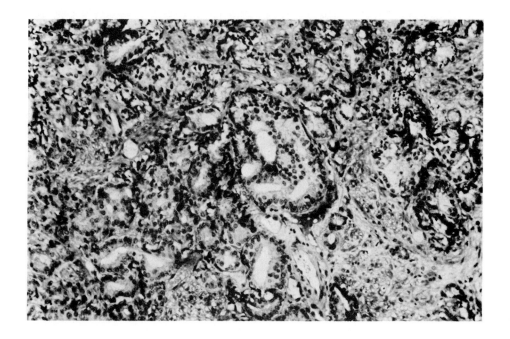

Figure 17–84. Cribriform pattern. (×189)

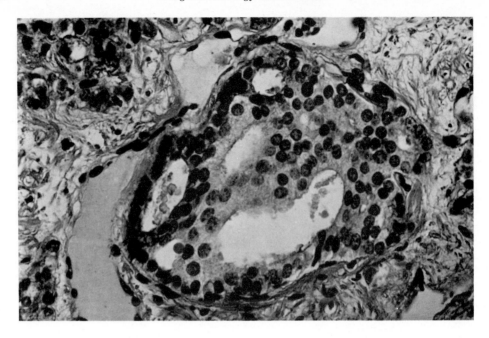

Figure 17–85. Cribriform pattern. (×459)

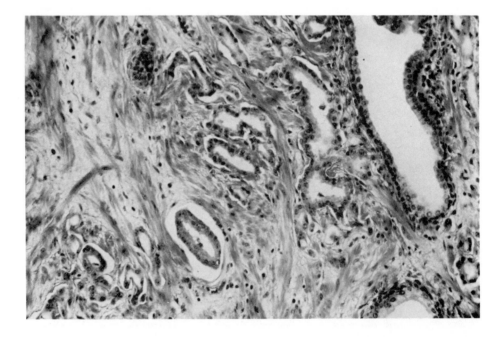

Figure 17–86. At edge of carcinomatous area there are carcinomatous glands of varying size infiltrating fibromuscular stroma. (×189)

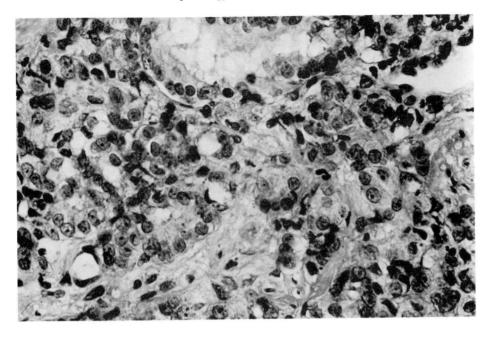

Figure 17–87. Numerous cells having very prominent nucleoli. (×459)

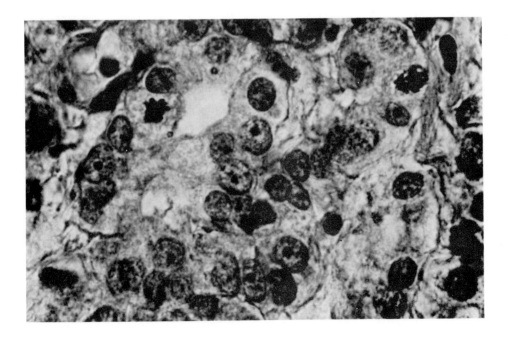

Figure 17–88. Numerous cells undergoing mitoses. (×1126)

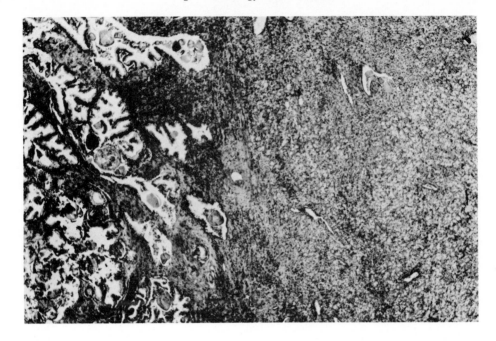

Figure 17–89.   Other foci of various patterns seen in association with benign glands. (×38)

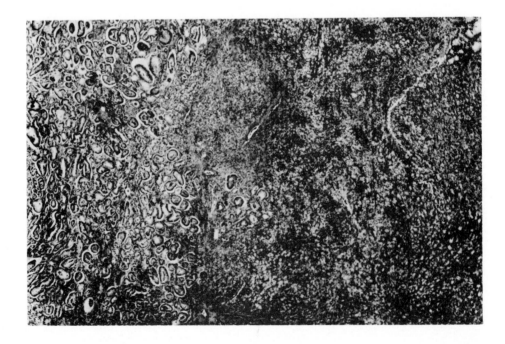

Figure 17–90.   Carcinomatous glands of various sizes; large ones are on left, small ones on right (×38)

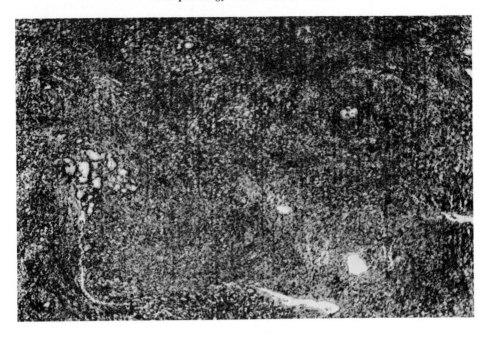

Figure 17–91. Numerous sheets of small gland carcinomas. (×38)

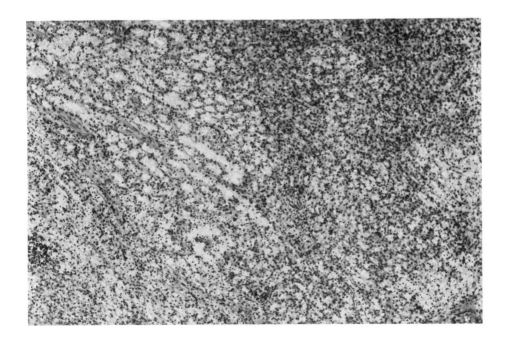

Figure 17–92. Numerous sheets of small gland carcinomas showing even more variability. (×90)

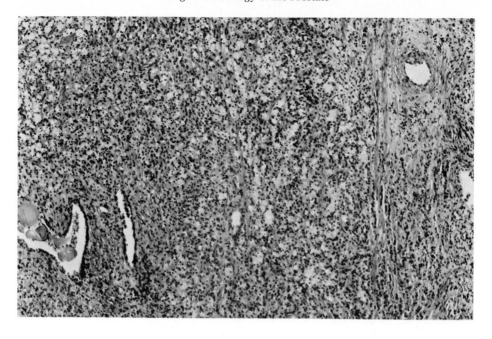

Figure 17–93. Mixture of small gland carcinoma mixed with "Indian-file" pattern of carcinoma of prostate. (×190)

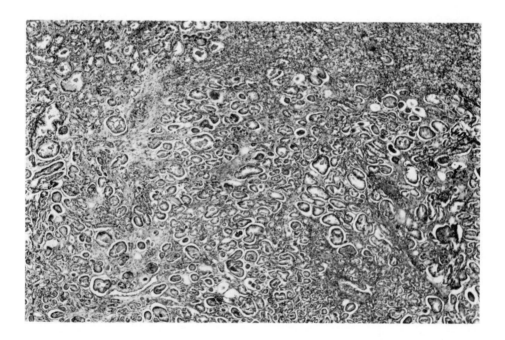

Figure 17–94. Numerous large glands mixed with small glands. (×38)

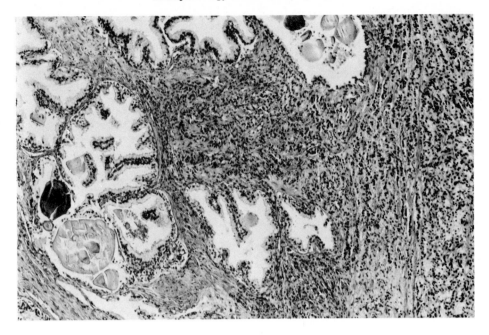

Figure 17–95. "Indian-file" pattern of carcinoma adjacent to normal glands on left. (×90)

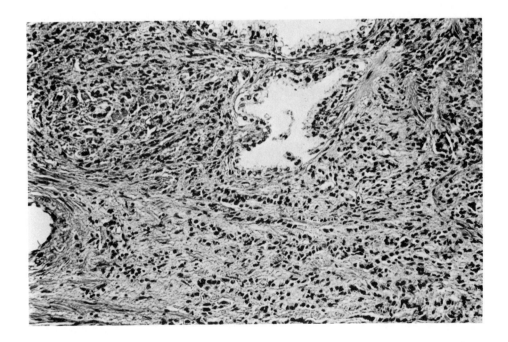

Figure 17–96. Higher magnification of "Indian-file" pattern adjacent to some normal glands. (×189)

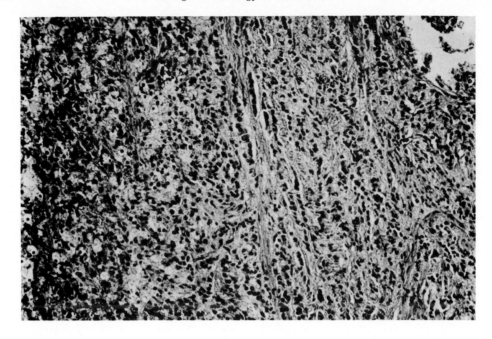

Figure 17–97. Mixture of small carcinomatous glands on left and "Indian-file" pattern on right. (×189)

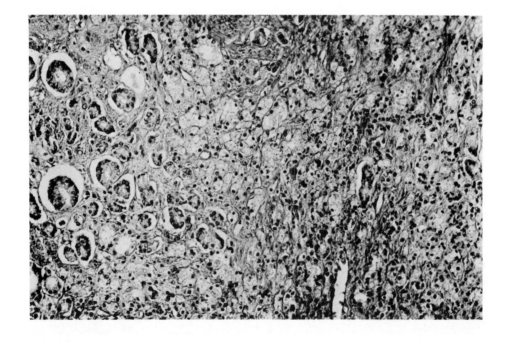

Figure 17–98. Mixture of numerous types of carcinomatous glands in center of which is pattern that looks almost like granulomatous prostatitis. (×189)

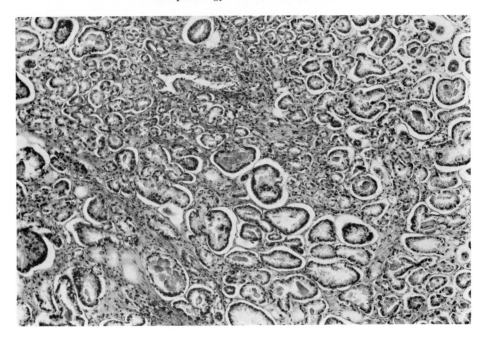

Figure 17–99. Mixture of well-differentiated glands of carcinoma of prostate of slightly different sizes. (×90)

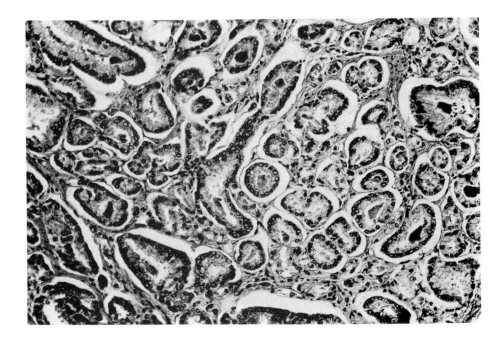

Figure 17–100. Well-differentiated glands at higher magnification. (×189)

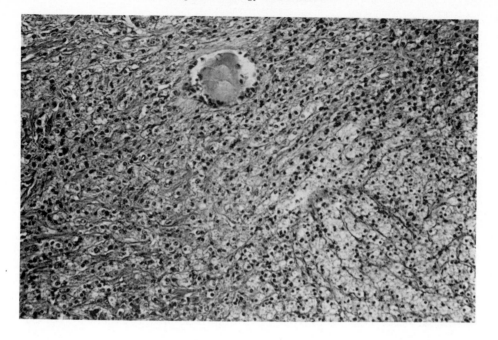

Figure 17–101. Another variation of numerous small carcinomatous glands without lumens. (×189)

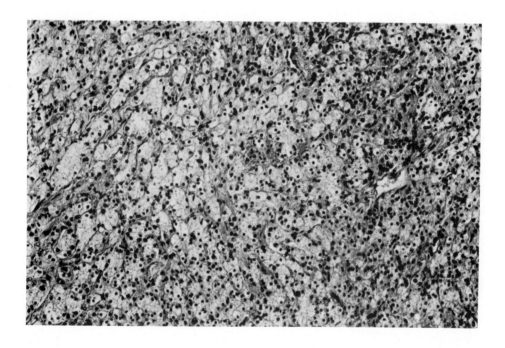

Figure 17–102. Similar glands but of different patterns than those shown in Figure 17–101. (×189.)

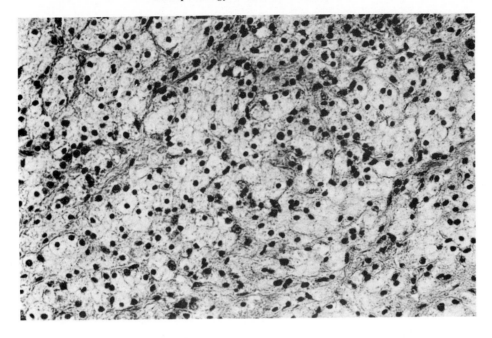

Figure 17–103. Carcinomatous glands that bear resemblance to xanthoma cells found in granulomatous prostatitis (see Figure 17–31). (×364)

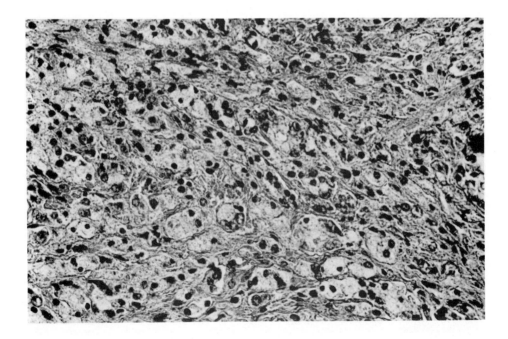

Figure 17–104. Further variation of these small glands with sparse amount of stroma surrounding individual glands. (×364)

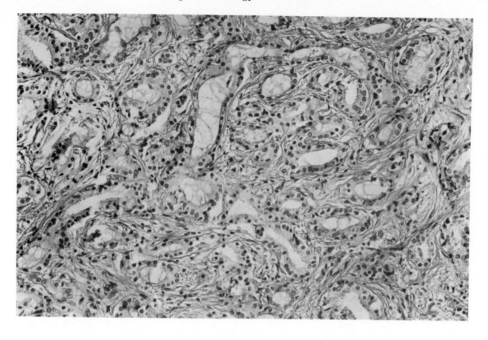

Figure 17–105. Low magnification of mucin-producing carcinoma. (×189)

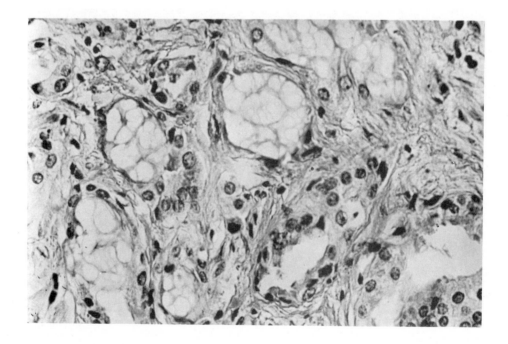

Figure 17–106. Higher magnification of some of these mucin-producing glands. (×459)

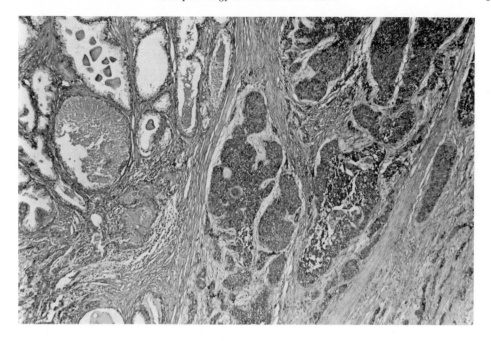

Figure 17–107. Low magnification of adenoid cystic type of prostatic carcinoma where carcinomatous epithelium is composed of two cell types and surrounded by mucoid stroma. (×48)

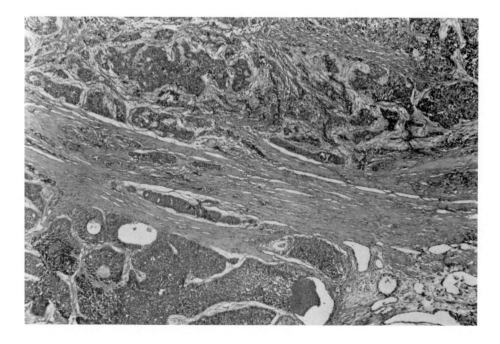

Figure 17–108. Normal prostatic epithelium is seen on left and stroma is almost completely replaced by this adenoid cystic type of carcinoma of prostate. (×48)

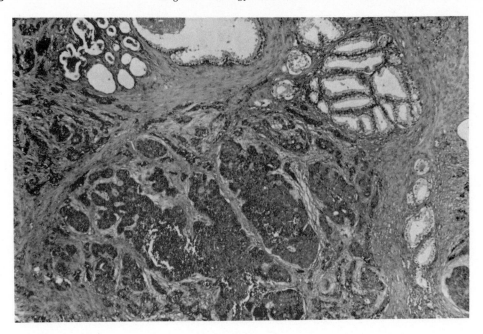

Figure 17–109.   Both forms of this tumor in which on extreme left there is no mucoid matrix surrounding cords of tumor. (×60)

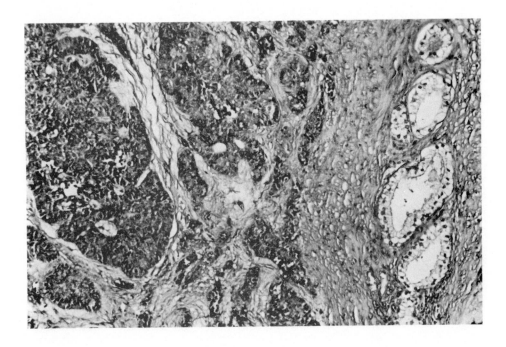

Figure 17–110.   Mucoid matrix surrounding islands of tumor composed of two different cell types. On right are normal prostatic glands. (×189)

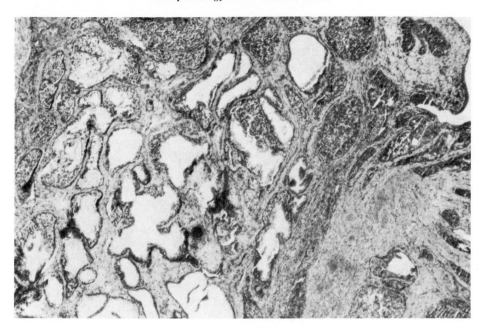

Figure 17–111. Periurethral prostatic ducts may reveal in situ transitional cell tumor spreading from prostatic urethra inward. (×48)

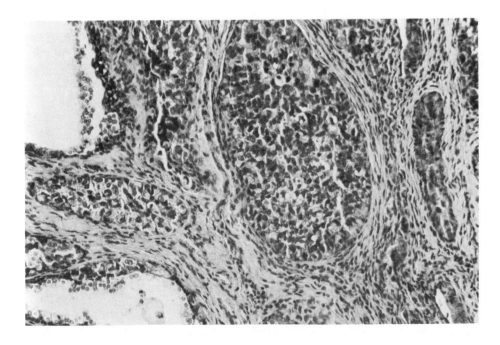

Figure 17–112. Shown at higher magnification is transitional cell epithelial carcinoma plugging ducts and spreading inward toward normal acini and into it. (×189)

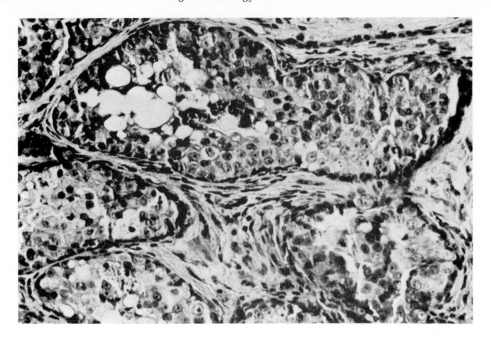

Figure 17–113.   Reveals further spread of tumor up ducts with basaloid cells still intact. (×288)

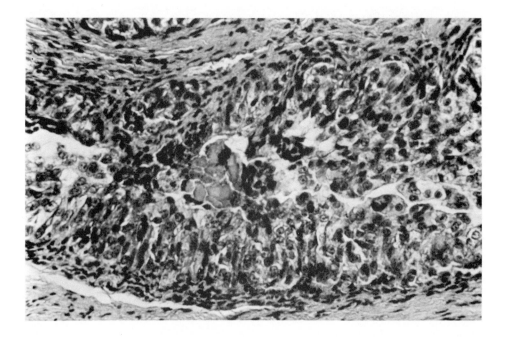

Figure 17–114.   Transitional cell carcinoma of periurethral ducts in comedocarcinoma pattern. (×288)

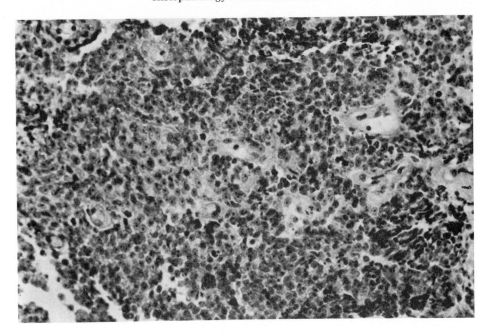

Figure 17–115. Portion of anaplastic infiltrating carcinoma of periurethral prostatic ducts. (×288)

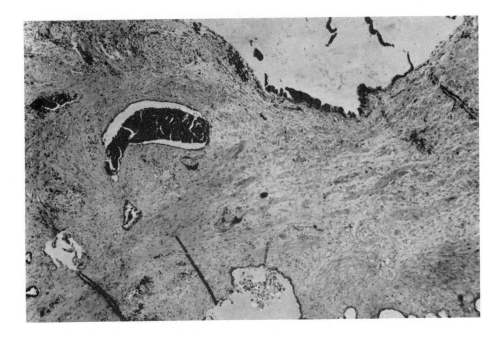

Figure 17–116. Endometrial tumor spreading intraductally through prostate. (×48)

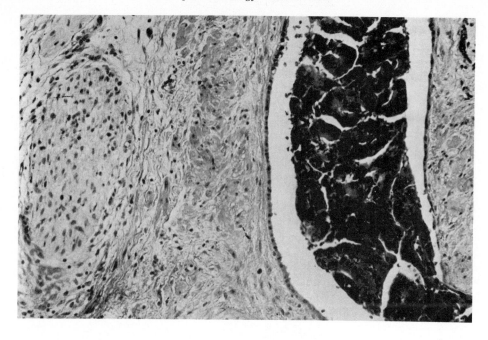

Figure 17–117. Higher magnification of tumor in duct. Note nerve on left. (×189)

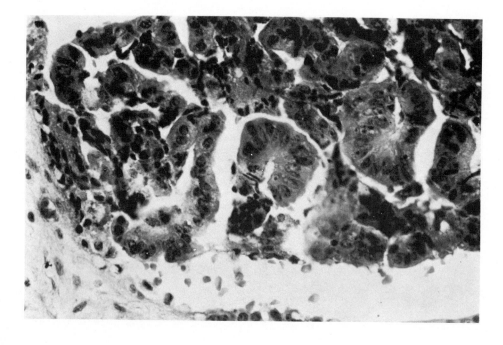

Figure 17–118. Higher magnification of tumor demonstrating palisading tumor cells in glandular pattern. Note eosinophilic cytoplasm. (×459)

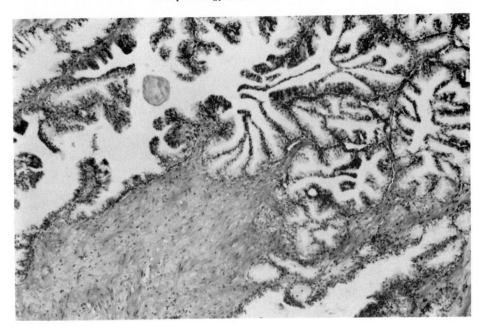

Figure 17–119. Atypical hyperplasia and carcinoma of prostate of other periurethral prostatic ducts found in association with these endometrial tumors. (×76)

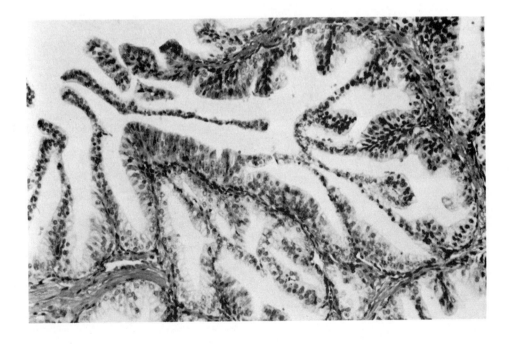

Figure 17–120. Higher magnification of these carcinomatous papillary proliferations. (×189)

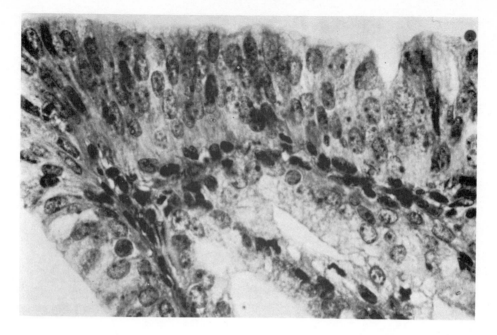

Figure 17–121. Fibrovascular core and cellular nature of these proliferations. (×706)

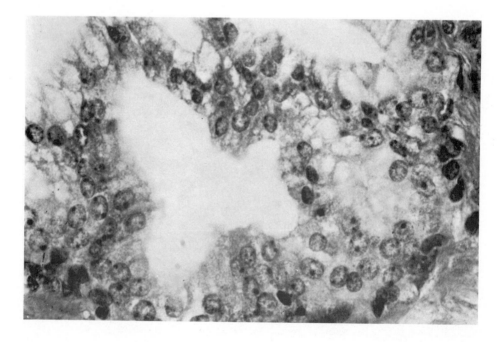

Figure 17–122. "Cancer nuclei" of these cells where there are one or more distinctly prominent nucleoli. These types of ductal carcinomas must also be distinguished from the endometrial tumors. (×706)

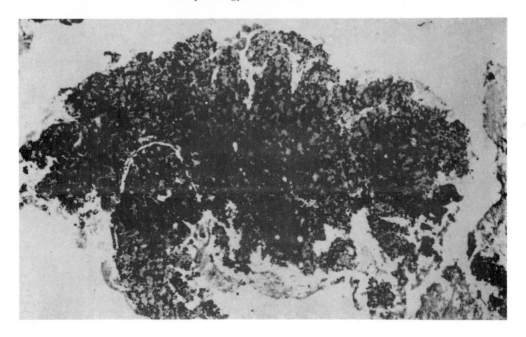

Figure 17–122A. Ductal carcinoma extending into urethra as papillary mass. Microacinar type. (×73)

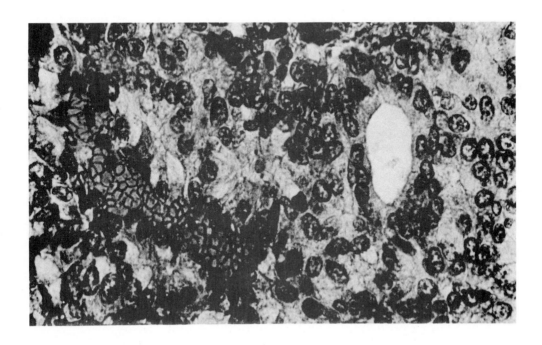

Figure 17–122B. Cancer nuclei, microacinar, and fibrovascular stalks. Here the tumor is primary ductal with a glandular pattern and not transitional. (×706)

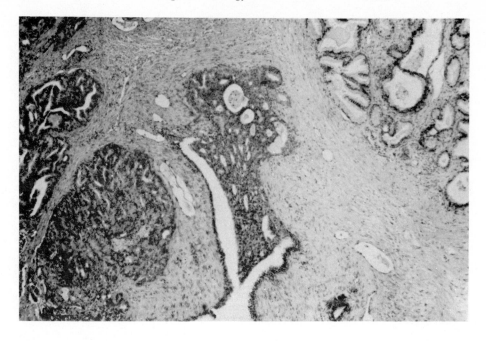

Figure 17–122C. Carcinoma in major ducts. Papillary form with transitional and glandular elements mixed together. (×73)

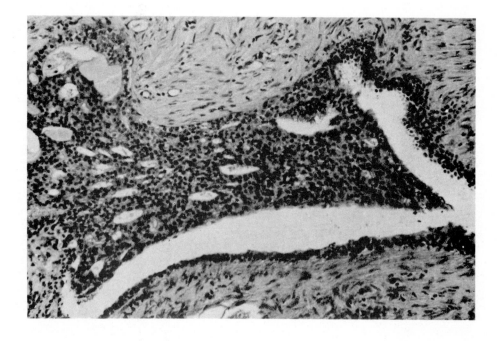

Figure 17–122D. Prostate tumor of periurethral type in duct. Mixed glandular and transitional type. (×189)

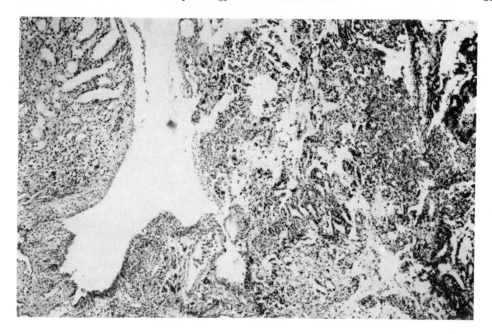

Figure 17–123. Two tumors present in periurethral prostatic duct area. On left is carcinoma of prostate and on right is tumor of endometrial configuration. (×73)

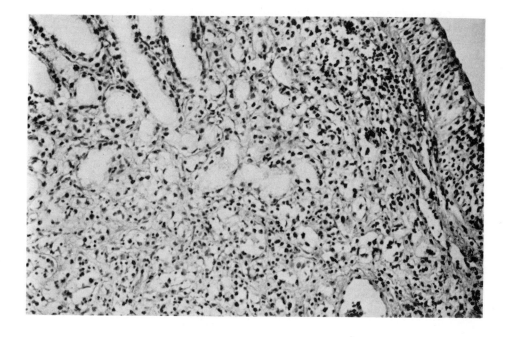

Figure 17–124. Microaciniform carcinoma of prostate beneath urothelial surface on right. (×189)

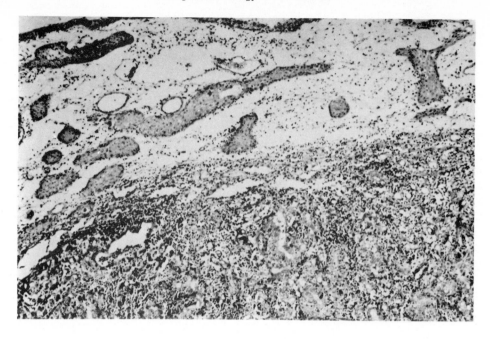

Figure 17–125. Endometrial tumor from same case beneath urethral urothelial surface, which is in upper portion of picture. (×73)

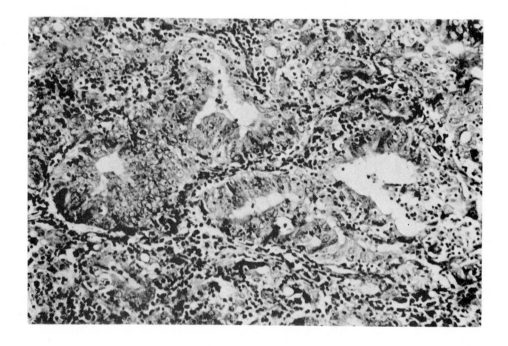

Figure 17–126. Endometrial tumor with surrounding lymphoid stromal infiltrate. (×189)

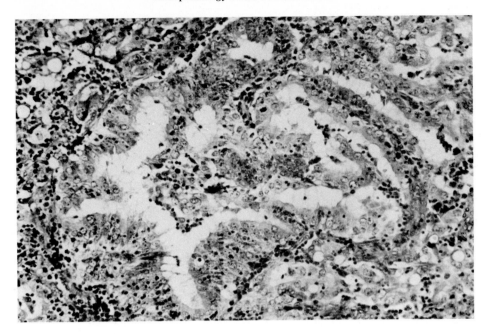

Figure 17–127. Another configuration found in same tumor as shown in Figure 17–126. (×189)

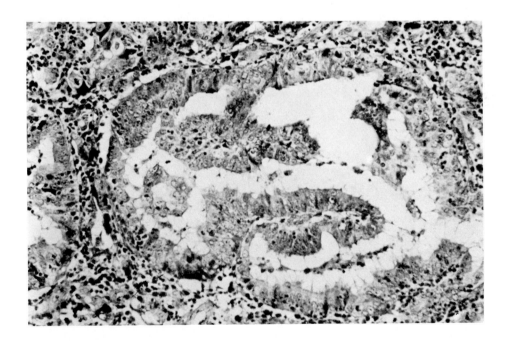

Figure 17–128. Polypoid projection into lumen of gland in this tumor. (×189)

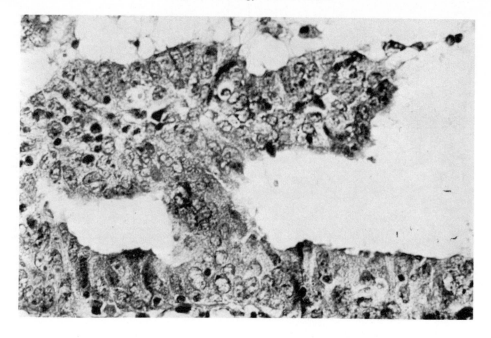

Figure 17–129.   Higher magnification of that polypoid projection into lumen. (×459)

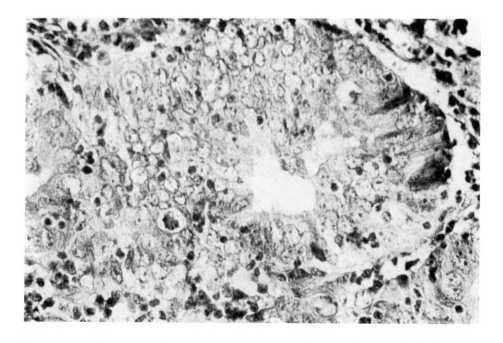

Figure 17–130.   Another area of tumor showing various cell types and lymphoid infiltrate similar to that seen in benign endometrium. (×459)

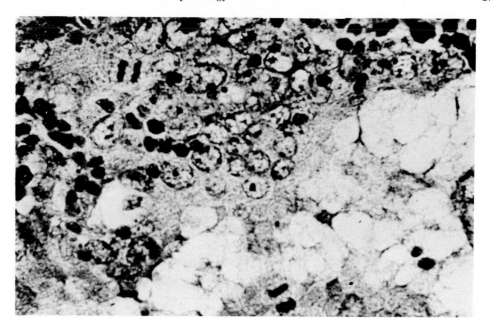

Figure 17–131. At higher magnification, numerous mitoses, lymphoid cell infiltrate, and endometrial epithelium. (×706)

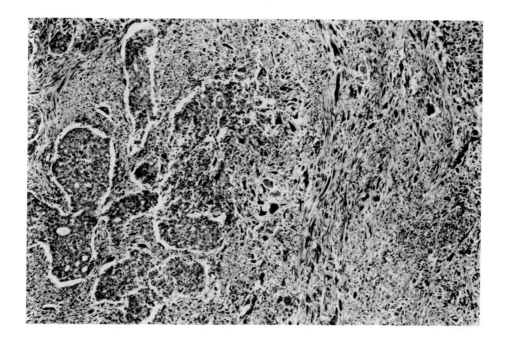

Figure 17–132. Carcinosarcoma of prostate with epithelial component on left and malignant stromal component on right. (×52)

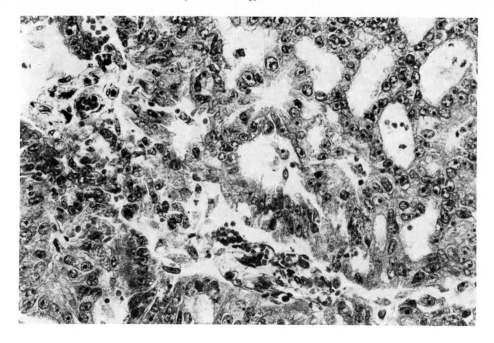

Figure 17–133. Adenocarcinomatous component at higher magnification. (×328)

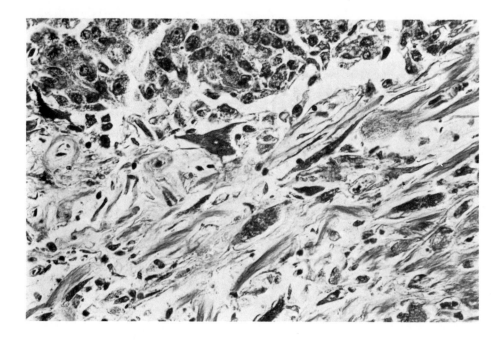

Figure 17–134. Malignant stromal component with bizarre strap-like cells. (×328)

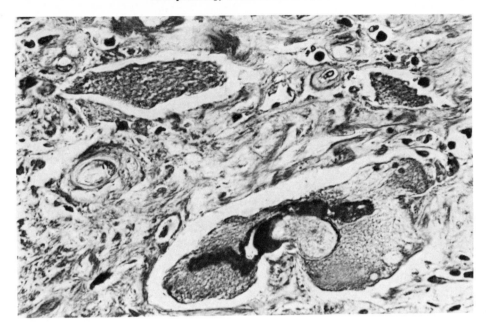

Figure 17-135. Bizarre strap-like cells which are similar to those found in rhabdomyosarcoma. (×504)

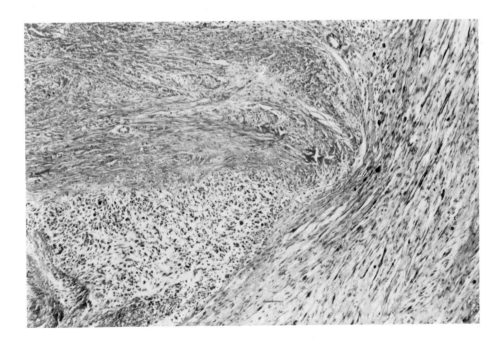

Figure 17-136. Malignant stromal cell tumor of skeletal muscle type in prostate. (×76)

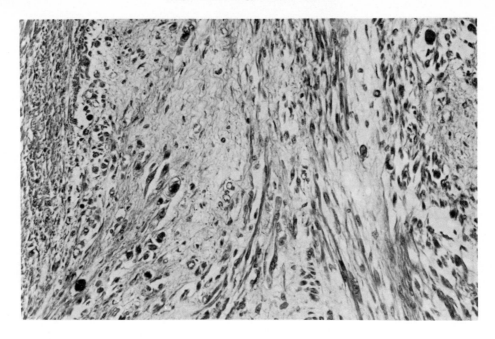

Figure 17–137. At higher magnification, some of the malignant skeletal muscle cells shown in Figure 17–136. (×189)

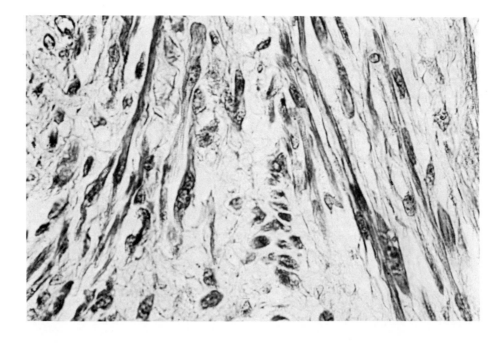

Figure 17–138. At higher magnification with faint cross striations, some of the malignant cells shown in Figure 17–137. (×459)

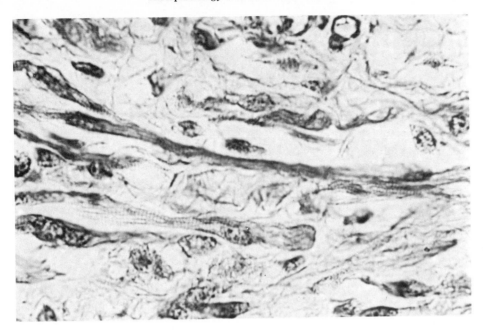

Figure 17–139. At still higher magnification, faint cross striations in these malignant skeletal muscle cells. (×706)

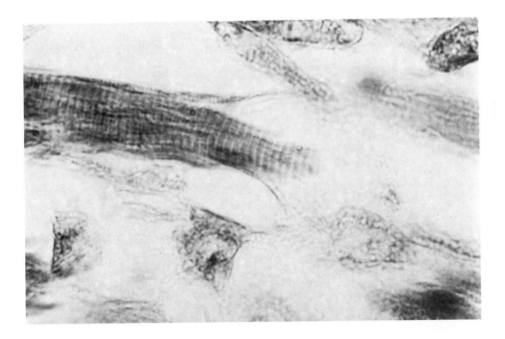

Figure 17–140. Well-differentiated skeletal muscle cell of malignant nature in rhabdomyosarcoma of prostate. (×1820)

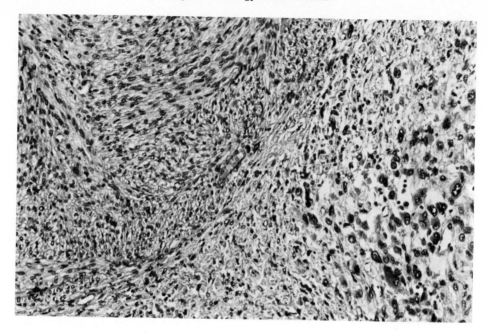

Figure 17–141.   Pattern found in well-differentiated malignant smooth muscle cell tumor or leiomyosarcoma of prostate. (×264)

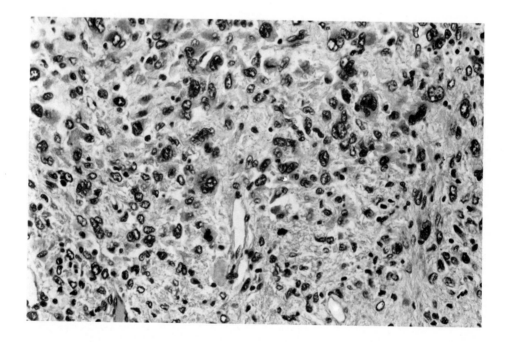

Figure 17–142.   Higher magnification of some multinucleated and bizarre leiomyosarcoma cells. (×260)

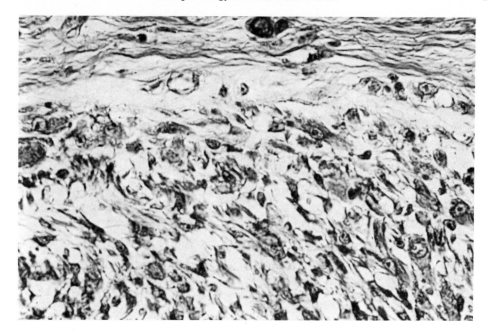

Figure 17–143. Cross-section of numerous closely packed fibrosarcomatous cells in prostate. (×459)

INDEX